INSIGHTS AND PERSPECTIVES IN RHEUMATOLOGY

Edited by **Andrew Harrsion**

Insights and Perspectives in Rheumatology
Edited by Andrew Harrsion

Published by InTech

Janeza Trdine 9, 51000 Rijeka, Croatia

Publishing Process Manager Ivana Zec

Technical Editor Teodora Smiljanic

Cover Designer InTech Design Team

Additional hard copies can be obtained from orders@intechopen.com

Insights and Perspectives in Rheumatology, Edited by Andrew Harrsion
p. cm.
ISBN 978-953-307-846-5

For EU product safety concerns:
IN TECH d.o.o., Prolaz Marije Krucifikse Kozulić 3, 51000 Rijeka, Croatia, info@intechopen.com or visit our website at intechopen.com.

Meet the editor

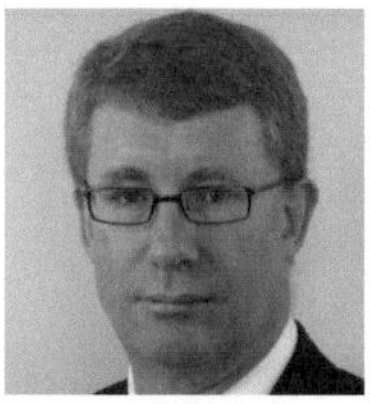

Associate Professor Andrew Harrison is a graduate of the University of Otago Medical School. He undertook a research fellowship at the Royal Postgraduate Medical School at Hammersmith Hospital, London and completed a PhD in the basic biology of inflammation from the University of London in 1995, before returning to Wellington, New Zealand. He is the Clinical Head of the Wellington Regional Rheumatology Unit, Clinical Advisor to Arthritis New Zealand and more recently he held the post of President of the New Zealand Rheumatology Association. He has a clinical interest in musculoskeletal ultrasound, and his research interests include the genetics and pathophysiology of gout, the genetic and environmental causes of spondyloarthropathy, and the economic, geographic and social determinants of access to rheumatology services.

Contents

Preface

Over the past two decades, there has been remarkable progress in the understanding of pathogenesis of rheumatic disease, which has in turn led to dramatic improvements in the ability to control inflammation. In documenting some of the advances that have taken place, this book demonstrates the therapeutic possibilities that fields such as pharmacogenomics might bring, while highlighting the current challenges in rheumatology, such as prevention of treatment-related opportunistic infection and the control of chronic pain.

The first section is concerned with the pathogenesis mechanisms that underlie rheumatic diseases, beginning with a review of autoantibodies and their role in disease pathogenesis. There is a chapter on adipokines; the inflammatory mediators produced by adipose tissue, and the relationship between metabolism and inflammation. The results of microarray studies are outlined within a review on gene expression profiling in rheumatoid arthritis. The role of vitamin D in autoimmune disease is deliberated and there is a chapter that examines the effects of rheumatoid arthritis on bone metabolism. The first section concludes with a review of great clinical relevance – the contribution of TNF inhibitors to the risk of infection in rheumatoid arthritis.

The second section narrows the focus to discuss various aspects of one particular rheumatic disease; Sjögren's syndrome. This section is not intended to be a monograph on this disease, but more of a collection of reviews that put the spotlight on specific interesting facet of Sjögren's syndrome: diagnosis and prognosis, mechanisms of decreased glandular secretion, oral manifestations and salivary proteomics.

The final section of the book moves away from somatic physiology and pathology and examines the impact of the rheumatic diseases on higher functions. The role of psychological stress in the presentation of rheumatic disease is reviewed, and there is a chapter on assessment and management of pain. The transition of JIA patients, from childhood to adulthood, is reviewed in the final chapter of this section.

The hope is, that this book will serve as a resource for those seeking comprehensive reviews of these topics. In its entirety, this book demonstrates the breadth and depth of knowledge that has been accumulated in rheumatology from the molecular level to the highest level of human function.

Dr. Andrew Harrsion
University of Otago,
New Zealand

Part 1

Pathogenic Mechanisms in Rheumatic Disease

1

Natural and Pathologic Autoantibodies

Péter Németh and Diána Simon
University of Pécs, Department of Immunology and Biotechnology
Hungary

1. Introduction

Detection and characterization of autoantibodies reacting with self-antigens is generally used in laboratory diagnostics. However, the presence of different autoantibodies in the blood serum doesn't mean automatically a pathologic condition. Autoantibodies are present both in different diseases as autoimmune diseases, chronic inflammation or infections, and in healthy individuals without any symptoms. The present paper discusses the detailed analysis of recognition pattern and fine epitope specificity of these autoantibodies to better understand of their occurrence and evolution, and their role in physiologic and pathologic conditions.

1.1 Evolution of the immunological recognition

Microorganisms present in the environment continuously come into contact with the human body through external or internal surfaces. Most microorganisms are neutral or useful, but others - so called pathogens - are dangerous for the other living beings including human individuals. During evolution all multicellular organisms have developed defence mechanisms capable of eliminating these invading pathogens without causing damage to self structures. All vertebrates and invertebrates manage self and non-self discrimination. Consequently, discriminating self from non-self is of key importance for directing immune functions effectively, operating on the basis of distinct recognition systems. Any attempt to answer questions concerning recognition must consider the universality of receptor-mediated responses. These may be designated to two forms: pattern recognition receptors and rearranging clonally distributed antigen-specific receptors that distinguish between self and non-self.

1.1.1 Pattern recognition as a basic immune function

Innate immunity serves as first line of defence against pathogens. Its early evolutionary appearance is indicated by its presence in all multicellular organisms including plants, invertebrates and vertebrates. Since invertebrate species rely on innate defence mechanisms only, survival of the species in the presence of environmental pathogens is achieved at the level of the population, which means that individual members, up until a fraction of total population, are dispensable (Kvell et al., 2007). Innate immunity uses receptors that are ancient in their evolutionary origin. These non-clonally distributed receptors have to be able to recognize a wide variety of molecular structures associated with pathogens without damaging self-structures. The problem lies in the discrepancy between the vast heterogeneity of pathogens and the limited number of possible recognizing receptors in the genome. This implies that the relatively few available specific receptors must recognize structures shared by large groups of pathogens, and that the recognized structures have to be pathogen-specific molecular patterns rather than particular molecules specific for pathogens. These pathogen associated molecular patterns (PAMPs) are conserved products of microbial metabolism, they are highly glycosylated, and are essential for microbial survival. The receptors recognizing these PAMPs are termed pattern recognition receptors (PRRs). We distinguish three functional classes of PRRs: endocytic receptors such as cellular C-type lectins, scavenger receptors and Mac-1 (CD11b:Cd18), which facilitate opsonisation and phagocytosis. This type of recognition is predominantly based on sugar-sugar interactions. The second set of PRRs are secreted proteins including mannose binding lectin, C1q, pulmonary surfactant proteins A and D, C-reactive protein and lipopolysaccharide binding proteins, respectively. These molecules facilitate opsonisation for phagocytosis and aid the complement system in destroying pathogens that have been bound by these secreted proteins (Medzhitov 2001). The third functional group is constituted by signalling receptors such as the Toll-like receptors (TLRs), which activate several intracellular signalling cascades, eventually leading to the activation of many immune response genes. PAMPs are targets for many PRRs in innate immunity. PRRs are expressed on cells positioned strategically in the first line of pathogen encounter such as surface epithelia, marginal zone of spleen, and on antigen presenting cells (APCs) such as macrophages and dendritic cells. It is important to note that the relatively broad spectrum of ligands recognized by TLR family members also includes glycoproteins, which points toward the adaptive recognition system (Klein & Nikolaidis 2005). Thus, the TLR family possibly represents an important milestone on the way to a recognition system characteristic for adaptive immunity (Cooper et al., 2006).

Recognition of PAMPs can activate direct effector mechanisms of innate immunity such as phagocytosis, secretion of antimicrobial peptides and induction of nitric oxide synthase in macrophages. Activation of innate immunity results in the secretion of several inflammatory cytokines such as interleukin-1, interleukin-6, tumor necrosis factor-α, type I interferon and many chemokines. One of the most important events caused by PAMPs recognition is the surface expression of CD80 (B7.1) and CD86 (B7.2) co-stimulatory molecules on APCs, which is necessary for the priming of T-dependent adaptive immune responses. Therefore in addition to activate direct first line defence mechanisms, innate immunity substantially contributes to the adaptive response as well. It is important to note that while PRRs recognize molecular patterns instead of specific molecules, and significant redundancy and promiscuity exists in the molecular nature of the recognized ligands, PRRs discriminate infectious non-self from self perfectly. One plausible explanation for this is that PRRs were selected and genetically stabilized over an evolutionary time scale creating an advantage for survival, and organisms possessing self reactive PRRs were eventually eliminated. This process prevents autoimmunity in those organisms which have only the innate recognition system (Cooper et al., 2006; Kvell et al., 2007).

1.1.2 Antigen specific recognition

The adaptive immune system containing specialized organs (bone marrow, thymus, spleen, lymph nodes, highly structured lymphatic tissues associated with the wet and dry body surfaces), that provide appropriate microenvironment for cells which are committed to antigen specific immune defence (T and B cells), appeared later during the evolution. It can be generally found in jawed vertebrates, however the earliest species with a variable antigen receptor based adaptive-like recognition system are jawless fish (lamprey, hagfish). These fish have non-immunoglobulin like clonally distributed receptors with leucine-rich repeats (similar to TLRs) generated with a gene rearrangement mechanism other than the recombination activating genes (RAG-1:RAG-2) characteristic for jawed vertebrates (Pancer et al., 2004). The appearance of adaptive immune system in jawed vertebrates gives the impression of a "sudden" change between jawless and jawed fish. This "big bang" hypothesis concerning gene duplication events, acquisition of a retrotransposon and the appearance of molecules such as major histocompatibilty complex, T- and B-cell receptors (Abi Rached et al., 1999) has been challenged by showing that integration of minor changes accumulated over an extended evolutionary time lead to the appearance of adaptive immune system (Klein & Nikolaidis 2005). Taking into consideration the major immunological recognition and activation theories from Janeway's self/non-self recognition to Polly Matzinger's danger hypothesis and from Burnet's clonal selection to Smith's quantal theory recently, there is a trend to synthesize the self/non-self vs. danger models, particularly proving that receptors distinguish pathogen and danger signals simultaneously (Liu et al. 2009).

In vertebrates the adaptive immunity generates a virtually indefinite pool of recognizing molecules: the T and B cell receptors (TCR, BCR), which repertoire makes the adaptation of each individual to pathogenic challenges possible. According to the clonal selection hypothesis these receptors are clonally distributed, each of them represented by single cell clone. The benefit of the high number of available antigen receptors in adaptive immunity comes with the cost of potentially dangerous recognition of self-structures, leading to autoimmunity. Therefore carefully organized selection mechanisms exist to select the potentially useful clones, and to eliminate or inactivate the autoreactive ones. Germline genes encoding T and B cell receptors are rearranged by the site specific recombinases RAG-1, RAG-2. Once these antigen receptors appear on the cell surface, the cell carrying them has to survive two types of selection. The first of these is probing the utility of the expressed receptor by testing whether it is capable to recognize its ligand in the microenvironment. This selection step is termed positive selection, since in the case of the appropriate engagement of antigen receptor the cell survives. Although the process was described first and in more detail for T cells maturing in the thymus, it was also clearly demonstrated for B cell maturing in the bone marrow and spleen (Cancro & Kearney, 2004). The ligand that activates the antigen receptor is self-peptide-MHC complex and possibly soluble immunoglobulin for T and B cells, respectively. Positive selection operates on a thin margin, the strength of the signal generated by antigen receptor engagement must be lower than in full activation, thus it provides a partial activation signal. The second selection step eliminates clones that possess antigen receptors, which recognize self too strongly, and termed negative selection. This mechanism is based on the full activation of antigen receptor mediated signalling pathways by self antigens and eventually leads either to the deletion of the cell clone, or to long term unresponsiveness of the cell to subsequent stimuli (anergy). Alternatively, in the case of B cells, the recombination machinery could be re-activated and the other immunoglobulin gene harbouring allele could be rearranged (receptor editing), giving the cell a second chance to produce an antigen receptor not reacting with self structures above threshold. Thus, the selection of antigen receptor bearing cells, irrespective of whether they belong to the T or B cell pool, is governed by interaction with self ligands instead of non-self ligands. The generation of the adaptive immune repertoire is therefore strongly self-referential (Janeway 2001).

2. Natural immunity

Since the innate recognition system discriminates self from non-self perfectly, the contribution of innate immunity to the activation of adaptive responses seems to be of vital importance for maintaining tolerance at the periphery. The appearance of co-stimulatory molecules on APC surface is critical for the activation of both T and B cells. In the absence of appropriate co-stimulation the activation signal remains below threshold level and the adaptive immune response will not be activated. The innate and adaptive arms of the immune system differ from each other in several important features and their cooperation is essential for the correct function of immune defence. As a connection bridging the evolutionarily oldest innate and the newly evolved adaptive systems a third compartment of immune machineries, the natural immune system has recently been described. A distinct set of lymphocytes - both T and B cells - with characteristic phenotypes and specialized functions participates in this system. These subsets of cells exhibit common phenotypic characteristics and posses both innate and adaptive features, suggesting a transitional stage in the immune system's evolution. The most important cellular components of the natural immune system according to recent knowledge are the invariant natural killer T (iNKT) cells, mucosa associated invariant T (MAIT) cells, γδ T cells and B1 B cells. The functional character of antigen recognition by these cells (and the immunoglobulins produced by B1 B cells) are closer to the pattern recognition features than to the classical adaptive type immunological recognition, however, the recognizing molecules are genuine T and B cell surface receptors.

2.1 Cellular elements of natural immune system

Among unconventional T cells, only two subsets display both a TCR and selecting MHC class Ib molecules highly conserved between species, the iNKT cells and the mucosal associated invariant T (MAIT) cells. These two populations express highly restricted TCR repertoires consisting of an invariant TCRα chain. Both subsets are selected by hematopoietic cells expressing evolutionarily conserved non-polymorphic MHC class Ib molecules, CD1d for iNKT cells and MHC-related molecule 1 (MR1) for MAIT cells. CD1d-restricted iNKT cells and MR1-restricted MAIT cells constitute two subsets of unconventional T cells that are phylogenetically conserved. Therefore, they are thought to play an essential role within the immune system of mammals (Treiner et al., 2005).

MAIT cells are selected by MR1 in the thymus on a non-B non-T hematopoietic cell, and acquire a memory phenotype and expand in the lamina propria of the gastrointestinal tract and in mesenterial lymph nodes in a process dependent both upon B cells and the bacterial flora. Thus, their development follows a unique pattern at the crossroad of iNKT and γδ T cells. These features suggest that MAIT cells could be involved in tolerance or immunity to infections in the gut. The function of MAIT cells is unknown, but intuitively we can argue that it is related to their localization in the gut mucosa. MAIT cells could somehow be involved in the defense against orally acquired pathogens or in non-immune function important for gut mucosa homeostasis. MAIT cells might also control the type of the gut immune response and/or be involved in oral tolerance. Controlling the balance between tolerance and immune response in the gastrointestinal tract is highly important, and could explain the striking conservation of the MAIT cells across species. The functional relevance of MAIT cells is also underlined by the fact that they represent 1-4% of peripheral T cells in human blood (Treiner et al., 2005).

iNKT cells are selected, expand, and acquire their innate-like phenotype and functions in the thymus. They accumulate in the liver and the spleen, independently of the presence of any exogenous stimuli such as the normal bacterial flora. INKT cells play an important role in both protective and regulatory responses. The nature of the response is determined by the initial cytokine environment: interaction with IL-10-producing cells induces regulatory T cell type iNKT cells and that with IL-12 producing cells results in Th1 type responses, while their production of IFNγ activates both innate and adaptive immune systems. Upon activation of iNKT cells tumor cells can be efficiently eliminated and they also play a role in the development of obesity (Lynch et al., 2009).

The γδ TCR repertoire similarly to the repertoire of innate immune receptors could have been selected through evolution. Thymic selection does little to constrain γδ T cell antigen specificities, but instead determines their effector fate. In general, it is believed that γδ T cells recognize host antigens and play a role in epithelial cell maintenance. Intraepithelial lymphocytes (IEL) ontogeny can show minimal dependency upon the thymus, as they can escape the thymus at a very early stage and migrate into the gut mucosa where they achieve maturation. They may even develop directly from bone marrow derived precursors in specific intestinal lymphoid aggregates called cryptopatches. The absence of positive selection, and the lack of antigen specific priming, seems ideal for γδ T cells to function in the first line of defence. When activated through the T cell receptor, antigen-experienced cells make IFNγ, whereas antigen-unexperienced γδ T cells produce IL-17, a major initiator of inflammation. One of the main functions of IL-17 is to promote the expansion and maturation of neutrophils in the bone marrow. Therefore the rapid IL-17 response mounted by antigen-inexperienced γδ T cells would play a critical role at the onset of an acute inflammatory response to pathogens that the host encounters for the first time, or to host antigens that are only revealed by injury. Furthermore, by acting early in the inflammatory response, γδ T cells may affect the development of antigen specific αβ T cell and B cell responses. Thus γδ T cells may play a much larger role in the adaptive immune response than previously recognized. Since γδ T cells contribute to host immune competence in several ways it is understandable why these cells have been maintained throughout vertebrate evolution, even when αβ T cells and B cells are also present (Konigshofer & Chien 2006).

B1 B cells were originally distinguished from B2 cells on the basis of their expression of CD5, a glycoprotein marker previously considered to be T cell specific. CD5 is a type I transmembrane glycoprotein with three scavenger receptor cysteine rich domains and a highly conserved intracellular domain. Its role in signalling was extensively studied both in T and B cells. As it is associated with antigen receptor signalling complexes, the CD5 molecule considered to be a negative regulator of TCR and BCR signalling. Later on a CD5- B1 B cell population was also identified and termed B1b B cells. Differences in the function and developmental requirements of the two B1 B cell subgroups are poorly characterized; however, it seems that the BCR/CD19 complex is of crucial importance in developmental decisions between B1a and B1b B cells (Haas et al., 2005).

In addition to surface phenotype, B1 B cells have several unique properties distinguishing them from conventional B2 cells. B1 B cells represent a self-renewing population found in high number in the peritoneal and pleural cavities, while they are virtually absent from peripheral lymph nodes and can be found in low number among splenic B cells. They are long lived in vitro, can be forced with phorbol esters to proliferate, and they could not be activated through BCR crosslinking. The immunoglobulin repertoire of B1 B cells is restricted in the number of immunoglobulin genes used; it is dominated by rearrangement of J-proximal V genes and has significantly fever N insertions than the repertoire of B2 cells (Kantor et al. 1997).

There is a long-standing dispute over the developmental origin of B1 B cells in literature (Haas et al., 2005). According to the lineage model, B1 B cells are generated from fetal precursors present in the fetal liver, omentum and splanchnopleura. This view is substantiated by the ability of fetal precursors to reconstitute both the B1 and B2 compartments in irradiated mice, while adult bone marrow-derived cells reconstitute B2 cells only. The induced differentiation model of B1 B cell development proposes that the B1 phenotype is a consequence of T-independent-2 like activation event, thus the specificity of BCR is the key factor which determines the B1 phenotype. The differential ability of fetal vs. adult precursors to generate B1 B cells is due to the different antigen receptor repertoire of these precursors. This argument is supported by several transgenic models in which the origin and specificity of the immunoglobulin transgene determined the B1 phenotype (Chumley et al., 2000).

Functions of B1a cells include the participation in the early phases of immune responses and most importantly the production of natural antibodies with dominantly IgM isotype, which is substantiated by the ability of B1 cells transferred adoptively into irradiated mice to restore normal IgM level. These lines of evidence and the properties of B1 B cell produced natural antibodies indicate that B1 B cells represent an intermediate stage of evolution between innate and adaptive immunity.

2.2 Natural (auto)antibodies

Natural antibodies are immunoglobulins mostly of IgM isotype, and are secreted by B1 cells without immunization with antigen. These antibodies can recognize genetically conserved sequences of pathogens and may serve in the first line of immune defence during an infection. In contrast, natural autoantibodies present in the serum of both healthy humans and patients with chronic inflammatory or systemic autoimmune diseases recognize a set of self-structures that have been conserved during evolution. Most of natural autoantibodies belong to the IgM or IgG isotype, and show polyreactivity with a broad range of affinities for the recognized epitopes (Lacroix-Desmazes et al., 1998).

Several functions have been suggested for natural autoantibodies: they may participate in the selection of immune repertoires, play a role in the acceleration of primary immune responses, and the clearance of apoptotic cells, possess anti-inflammatory effects and contribute to the maintenance of immune homeostasis (Lacroix-Desmazes et al., 1998).

Discrimination of natural antibodies from natural autoantibodies is somewhat artificial since given the limited B1 immunoglobulin gene repertoire driving natural antibody production and the numerous distinct antigens recognized it is probable that specificities with self non-self cross reactivity exist. Based on the above properties of natural antibodies, these molecules could be considered as the "innate like arm" of humoral immune system (Czömpöly et al., 2008).

3. Physiologic and pathologic autoantibodies

The phenomena that natural autoantibodies could recognize self antigens which are also targeted by antibodies in autoimmune diseases are not unprecedented. Several lines of evidence indicate that antibodies recognizing factor VIII, thyreoglobulin, DNA, endothelial cell membrane components etc., are present in sera of both healthy individuals and patients with autoimmune diseases. These findings raise the question whether these detected antibodies are pathologic autoantibodies or belong to the pool of natural antibodies. It is possible that the fine epitope pattern recognized by natural antibodies and disease associated autoantibodies within the targeted antigen is different.

3.1 Characterization of fine epitope structure of the antibodies

There is a need for epitope mapping on circulating autoantibodies both in the basic and clinical immunology and in the immuno-biotechnological research and development. A mixture of different natural and pathologic autoantibodies is present in human blood samples with various antigen specificity. All the classical physico-chemical and immunochemical methods used in antibody characterization are technically difficult in the case of autoantigens.

3.1.1 Methods for determination of epitope specificity

Several techniques are available for the chemical determination of fine specificity of recognition molecules; however, a large scale analysis on serum samples from healthy individuals and patients with autoimmune and other diseases is both theoretically and technically difficult. Epitope mapping with overlapping synthetic peptides is a useful technique, but its constraints include the uncertainties linked to in silico B cell epitope prediction used for selection of antigenic regions, the partial coverage of primary sequence by synthetic peptides and the possible loss of all unpredicted or conformational epitopes. Synthetic overlapping peptides are suitable in the case of well characterized autoantigens. Limited proteolysis and the following mass spectroscopic analysis are generally used techniques in monoclonal antibody characterizations. Random peptide libraries were developed for characterization of epitope specificity on circulating autoantibodies by M13 filamentous phage system. The method was optimized on monoclonal antibodies and applied for serum samples. During our further development lambda phages were used to display fragments of previously determined antigens. Bacteriophage surface display of peptides is a recently used technique for a variety of applications. This technique resembles most the physiological antigen conformation and does not require prior epitope prediction. The technology is based on the expression of recombinant peptides or proteins fused to a phage coat protein. Its key advantage is in the physical coupling of the displayed protein to the nucleic acid coding for it, making the repeated affinity selection and amplification possible. The most commonly used systems are based on fusion to a filamentous phage coat protein. However, the life cycle of these phages limits the size of the displayed peptide, therefore we have chosen phage lambda for the epitope mapping of naturally occurring and pathologic autoantibodies in our different studies. The library contains fragments of the antigen with random starting point and length, consequently it overcomes the theoretical and technical limitations associated with pre-designed fragments or overlapping synthetic peptides (Czömpöly et al., 2008).

3.1.2 Epitope mapping of naturally occurring antibody family specific for the mitochondrial citrate synthase protein antigen

The basic structural elements of living cells such as the cytoskeleton, metabolic organelles, transporters, molecular components of transcription and translation etc., are genetically conserved. The maintainence of immunological tolerance against these structures is a basic functional duty of immune machinery in all of the three levels. The mitochondrion is absolutely necessary for eukaryotic cell function. Genetic alterations which affect mitochondrial proteins have serious consequences, if the mutation is compatible with life at all. Because of their endosymbiotic evolutionary origin, proteins compartmentalized into mitochondria represent an interesting transition from prokaryotic foreign to essential self molecules. To date there are only a limited number of epitope mapping analyses performed on human antigens that are recognized by natural autoantibodies. In particular, little is known about the possible overlap between recognized epitopes of innate and self-reactive natural antibodies. The structural and functional conservation of mitochondrial components makes them candidate antigens for detailed analysis of evolutionary connections between the innate and adaptive immune response. No classical mitochondrion-targeted autoimmune disease - with the exception of the primary biliary cirrhosis is known, suggesting a well established tolerance both at the innate and adaptive level. The inner membrane enzymes, especially the citric acid cycle enzymes offer appropriate models for testing their immunoreactivity, because they are in continuous connection with both innate and adaptive components of the immune system during physiologic turnover of cells. The immunological recognition and the immunoreactivity with these molecules are less studied, and the possible changes in physiological autoreactivity under pathologic autoimmune conditions remain largely unclear (Czömpöly et al., 2006). To address these issues we have chosen a mitochondrial inner membrane enzyme, citrate synthase (CS) as model antigen for epitope mapping using sera of healthy individuals and patients having various systemic autoimmune disease (systemic lupus erythematosus (SLE), rheumatoid arthritis, undifferentiated connective tissue disease, polymyositis/dermatomyosits, systemic sclerosis (SSc), Raynaud's syndrome and Sjögren's syndrome). The CS enzyme is not only a theoretically appropriate model - this is one of the first living protein during the evolution - but has also been studied at gene, protein structure and functional levels.

We demonstrated the presence of antibodies recognizing CS in the sera of both healthy individuals and systemic autoimmune patients. The enzyme specific antibodies with IgM isotype were more frequently present in all investigated groups than those of IgG or IgA isotypes and the incidence of autoantibodies with IgM isotype was significantly higher in autoimmune patients compared to the healthy controls. We found that the reactivity against

CS of individual sera remained permanently constant over a five year period (Fig.1.), in opposite to the anti-CS antibodies with IgG isotype which showed various titer during the investigated period on the same individuals. Our findings, that the majority of these antibodies have IgM isotype, are already present in infants, and the long term stability of their serum titers in adults indicate that these specificities belong to the natural autoantibody repertoire established early in postnatal life. The occurrence of anti-CS antibodies with IgG isotype we can explain as the physiologic dynamics of normal immune defence against different pathogens.

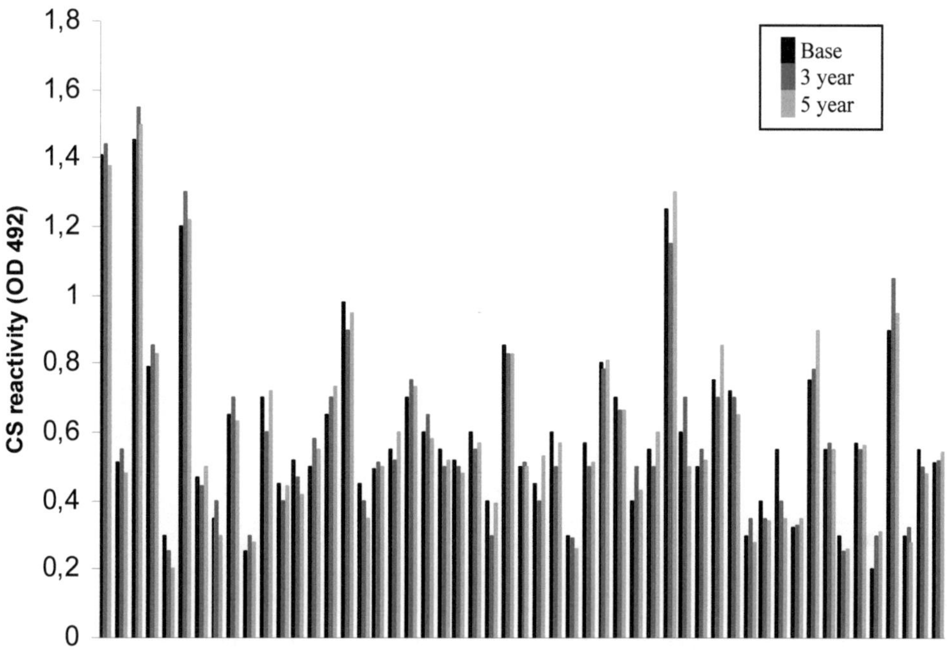

Fig. 1. CS reactivity in healthy individuals - 52 blood donors - followed up during a five year period with IgM isotype specific indirect ELISA.

To compare epitopes recognized by natural autoantibodies in healthy individuals with those recognized in systemic autoimmune patients we performed the epitope mapping of anti-CS antibodies under physiological and pathologic (systemic autoimmune) conditions. Epitope mapping with overlapping synthetic peptides is a widely used technique, but its constraints include the uncertainties linked to in silico B-cell epitope prediction used for selection of antigenic regions, the partial coverage of primary sequence by synthetic peptides and the possible loss of all unpredicted or conformational epitopes. Since these effects could have influenced our results, we sought to perform the epitope mapping using a basically different technique. Bacteriophage surface display of peptides is an extensively used technique for a variety of applications. The most commonly used systems are based on fusion to a filamentous phage coat protein. However, the life cycle of these phages limits the size of the displayed peptide, therefore we have chosen phage lambda for construction of a CS antigen fragment library to analyze the fine epitope structure of anti-CS autoantibodies (Czömpöly et al., 2006). The library contains fragments of CS with random starting point and length; consequently it overcomes the theoretical and technical limitations associated with the overlapping synthetic peptide approach. With this phage display based approach we compared the epitope patterns recognized by anti-CS autoantibodies found in sera of healthy individuals and patients with systemic autoimmune diseases. According to our results there is no favoured region of the CS molecule recognized exclusively either by healthy individuals or patients with systemic autoimmune diseases, but the fine epitope pattern is different in the two groups examined (Fig. 2.).

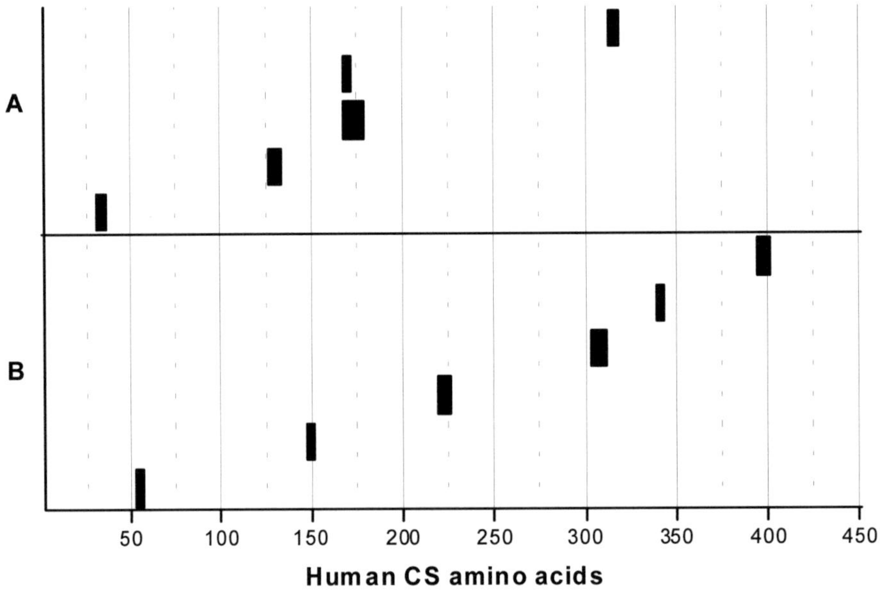

Fig. 2. Amino acid sequences of CS recognized by healthy individuals (A) and patients with systemic autoimmune diseases (B)

3.1.3 Epitope mapping of pathologic autoantibodies specific for a well conserved nuclear antigen, DNA topoisomerase I

Previously described experiments underlined the necessity for the epitope mapping of an autoantibody which is specific for a well defined pathologic condition and has a high diagnostic value. Our aim was to decide whether the target antigen of the disease associated autoantibody is also recognized by naturally occurring autoantibodies. We assumed that comparison of the epitope patterns recognized by natural and disease-associated autoantibodies would contribute to the better understanding of the differences between natural and pathologic autoantibodies. To address these issues we chose DNA topoisomerase I as a model antigen, since anti-topoisomerase I antibodies are important in the diagnosis of SSc.

Using the phage display technique previously developed in our department and optimized by analyzing epitopes of anti-CS antibodies, we performed the epitope mapping of anti-topoisomerase I autoantibodies and examined whether the target antigen of the disease associated autoantibody is also recognized by naturally occurring autoantibodies (Simon et al., 2009).

With the help of the bacteriophage lambda library containing fragments of topoisomerase I with random starting point and length we compared the epitope patterns recognized by anti-topoisomerase I autoantibodies found in sera of patients with diffuse cutaneous SSc (dcSSc), limited cutaneous SSc (lcSSc), and SLE. The results showed that the pattern of recognized epitopes is different between dcSSc, lcSSc and SLE patients (Fig. 3.).

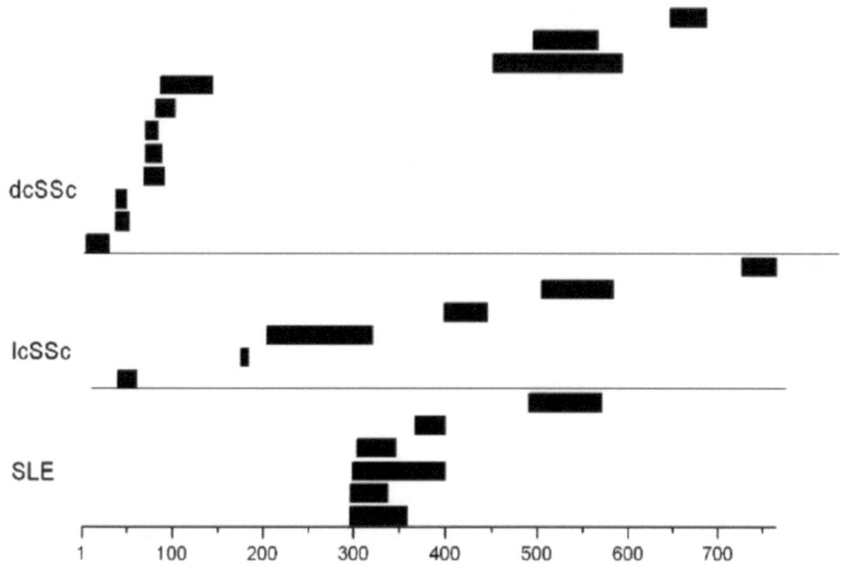

Fig. 3. The pattern of recognized topoisomerase I epitopes is different between dcSSc, lcSSc and SLE patients

A common fragment recognized by all patients' sera was located in the region of amino acid sequence (AA) 450-600, which is in agreement with previously published results. In addition to this, sera of dcSSc patients recognized several short fragments at the N-terminal part of the molecule. Previous studies performed with fusion proteins covering the N-terminal domain starting from AA 70 reported that this part of the molecule is recognized by anti-topoisomerase I antibodies. However, the opposite has also been reported by using a fusion protein covering the entire length of the N-terminal domain and showing that this part of the molecule is not targeted by anti-topoisomerase I antibodies. These seemingly contradictory results may be explained by the different methods and antigen constructs used, and most importantly by possible conformational factors, which could influence the accessibility of short epitopes buried in the tertiary structure. It is important to note that the majority of new epitope containing fragments we identified at the N-terminal part spans only 20-30 AA. The 5-25 AA fragment of the N-terminal part of the molecule contains an experimentally proven granzyme B cleavage site, thus it is possible that in vivo cleavage of topoisomerase I by granzyme B released during T cell mediated cytotoxic responses results in the formation of a neo-antigenic determinant represented by this fragment. In vitro assays using the full length antigen or the full length N-terminal domain may fail to detect antibodies recognizing these short epitopes suggesting strong conformational sensitivity.

On the basis of fragments identified by library selection nine maltose binding protein-topoisomerase I fusion proteins were constructed and expressed (Fig. 4.).

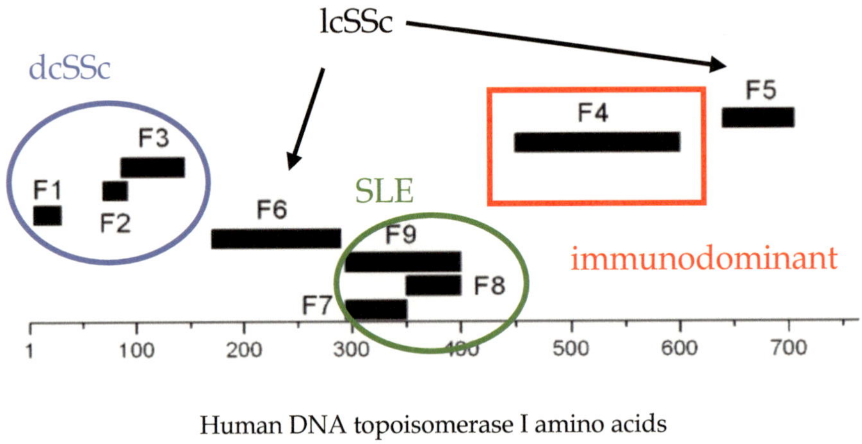

Fig. 4. The constructed and expressed maltose binding protein-topoisomerase I fragment fusion proteins

First we tested recognition of these fusion proteins with sera of healthy individuals and found that a significant portion of healthy individuals posses antibodies with IgM and IgG isotype against fragment F4. Fragment F4 represent a 150 AA long, genetically conserved sequence of topoisomerase I. Using a large number of sera we showed that the presence of antibodies against fragment F4 is essentially independent of the age and geographical origin of healthy individuals. In addition antibodies against fragment F4 could also be detected in sera of patients with inflammatory rheumatic diseases other than SSc and SLE. Anti-F4 antibodies with IgM isotype are present in the highest titer in sera of anti-topoisomerase I antibody positive SSc or SLE patients. It is important to note that all 67 sera from anti-topoisomerase I antibody positive SSc or SLE patients were found to be positive for anti-F4 antibodies with IgG isotype, and the titer of these antibodies was the highest in this group among all groups tested. The fact that these sera were shown to be negative for anti-topoisomerase I antibody by a conventional ELISA test using the full length antigen could indicate that the sequence represented by fragment F4 could be hidden in the three dimensional structure of the full length molecule. These findings raise the possibility that antibodies against fragment F4 present in sera of healthy individuals and patients with systemic autoimmune diseases could belong to the pool of naturally occurring antibodies. To our knowledge these are the first results demonstrating that natural antibodies against topoisomerase I are present in human sera.

It is not unprecedented that natural autoantibodies recognize self antigens which are also targeted by antibodies in autoimmune diseases. Since anti-topoisomerase I antibodies can also be detected in sera of patients with glomerulonephritis, chronic graft versus host disease, primer biliary cirrhosis and in some cases of chronic hepatitis C virus infection induced liver diseases the question arises whether these detected antibodies are pathologic autoantibodies or belong to the pool of natural antibodies. Fragment F4 represents a 150 amino acids long sequence of topoisomerase I, consequently it is possible that the fine epitope pattern recognized by natural antibodies and disease associated autoantibodies within this part of topoisomerase I is different.

The recognition of the majority of fragments (F2, F3, F5-7, F9) seemed to be characteristic for the individual patient sera used for library screening, instead of being characteristic for the given disease subgroup. This is in agreement with result of Henry et al., who found both individual and longitudinal differences in the recognized topoisomerase I epitopes. However, antibodies recognizing the common F4 fragment were detected in all patients' sera tested. In addition to this immunodominant part of topoisomerase I, we identified two new regions (F1 and F8) which were previously not shown to be targeted by anti-topoisomerase I antibodies. Fragment F1 (an evolutionarily relatively new sequence, specific for vertebrates) was recognized by 26% of dcSSc patients and antibodies against fragment F8 (a highly conserved sequence) could be detected in 50% of SLE patients, indicating that these fragments could represent characteristic epitopes for dcSSc and SLE, respectively. Longitudinal analysis showed that reactivity to fragment F4 was stable, while the reactivity to F1 and F8 fragments varied over time.

3.2 Comparative analysis of fine epitope pattern of natural and pathologic autoantibodies

It is possible that the presence of natural antibodies is essential for the appearance of disease associated autoantibodies, since natural autoantibodies can, under appropriate conditions; provide the templates for the emergence of higher affinity and class-switched pathogenic autoantibodies. IgG isotyped disease associated autoantibodies may recognize genetically determined epitopes (epitope patterns) and can be detected in genetically predisposed individuals, which was also suggested by a study examining monozygotic twins suffering from SLE (Silverman et al., 2008). Thus tolerance against conservative antigens might mostly be genetically determined. The permanent impairment of the development and maintenance of tolerance can lead to autoimmune disorders. Pattern recognition mechanisms were thought to be specific for innate immunity and considered to be the defence mechanisms of evolutionarily ancient species. According to our results natural autoantibodies, in terms of their antigen recognizing characteristics, resemble the pattern recognition receptors and recognize epitope patterns. Pathologic autoantibodies detected in autoimmune diseases however are directed mainly against a well defined, disease associated sequence (epitope).

4. Conclusion

A large number of circulating antibodies directed against functional structures of the cell (nucleic acid, nuclear molecules, receptors, or other functional cell components) can be detected in systemic autoimmune diseases. Their presence plays a central role in the diagnosis and classification of this kind of disorder. Moreover, several longitudinal cohort studies have shown that patients may carry autoantibodies many years before they manifest clinical symptoms and detecting these antibodies in serum has been shown to have strong predictive value. Primary structure homologies between the antigens targeted in some autoimmune diseases and conserved sequences of different pathogens (viruses and bacteria) are well known. Although this so called "molecular mimicry" has been extensively studied, direct causality of infections in the development of autoimmune diseases has only been verified in a few patients. Apart from the homologies in primary structure, the similarities in the physico-chemical molecular shape between the mammalian antigens and the structures of microorganisms could provide a real structural basis for the biological recognition suggesting a pivotal role of three-dimensional shape of conserved antigens in both targeting type immunity and tolerance (Czömpöly et al., 2008).

According to the orthodox view of phylogenetic development, immunity has reached its zenith with the emergence of the adaptive immune system. Consequently, we tend to be influenced by anthropocentric views and overlook how other highly developed organisms manage living in hostile environments. As recently more data have become available regarding non-traditional animal models, it has been suggested that the emergence of adaptive immunity is perhaps not the culmination of the evolution of immunity, but simply a successful alternative to using innate immunity alone. For millions of years, many species could keep-up in the continuous arms-race between pathogen and host called co-evolution without the surveillance of adaptive immunity. The complexity of biology should never be underestimated as it turns out that those animals lacking RAG-dependent adaptive immunity can make up for an equal amount of diversity using highly variable elements of innate immunity finally exhibiting adaptive features. On the other hand, in vertebrates, adaptive immunity often simply serves as a sophisticated targeting device that recognizes and then processes the antigen but finally leaves the messy job of actually clearing up pathogens to the immense capacity of innate immunity. Therefore, once again we see that borders are blurring and the strict distinction between innate and adaptive immunity might need revision (Kvell et al. 2007). Network of natural immunity - including wiled range of different cellular elements and naturally occurring antibodies - could explain as the missing evolutionary chain between the "classic" innate and adaptive immune system.

4.1 Clinical relevance of detection of autoantibodies

Analyzing the recognition of epitopes of natural and pathologic autoantibodies could contribute to diagnosis and better understanding of pathomechanisms of systemic autoimmune diseases. The onset of the disease may correlate with a switch from production of IgM to IgG isotyped antibodies. Nevertheless, the exact role of autoreactive IgM in the autoantibody response and the switch to other isotypes is not known. It has to be mentioned that IgM isotyped natural autoantibodies can have a role in protection from autoimmunity by facilitating the removal of apoptotic cells and increasing the tolerance of B cells to self antigen. Since one of the essential functions of the immune system is the prevention of self antigens to stimulate an inflammatory reaction, the presence of autoantibodies is the consequence of a breakdown or failure of B cell tolerance toward the corresponding autoantigens. The timing of exposure, the level of affinity of the autoreactive IgM autoantibodies and their local concentration may determine which scenario applies, i.e., autoimmunity or tolerance. Detection of autoantibodies reacting with self antigens is generally used in laboratory diagnostics. However, their presence in serum samples doesn't mean automatically a pathologic condition. Natural autoantibodies could recognize self antigens which are also targeted by antibodies in autoimmune diseases. The immune response could be explained by a general recognition of the immunodominant part of the molecule, followed by appearance of antibodies directed against disease associated sequences (Czömpöly et al., 2009). Detection of autoantibodies recognizing different epitopes of these antigens could be a useful tool in laboratory diagnostics (Simon et al., 2009).

4.1.1 Diagnostic issues of natural and pathologic autoantibodies

Early diagnosis and initiation of adequate therapy as soon as possible is crucial in systemic autoimmune diseases such as SSc and SLE, because after insidious onset of the disease the development of internal organ manifestations can lead to death of the patient in a few years. Anti-topoisomerase I autoantibodies are considered to be associated with dcSSc. However, the presence of anti-topoisomerase I autoantibodies is not entirely restricted to this subset, since anti-topoisomerase I antibodies have been demonstrated in lcSSc, SLE and other inflammatory diseases. The fact that anti-F4 antibodies were detected in sera which were tested negative for anti-topoisomerase I antibody by a conventional ELISA kit using the full length antigen indicates that an ELISA test using recombinant F4 fragment might be a more sensitive way to determine anti-topoisomerase I positivity and could contribute to early diagnosis and monitoring the activity of SSc (Simon et al., 2009).

4.1.2 Prognostic value of epitope pattern

In systemic autoimmune diseases the prognosis is mostly determined by the activity of the disease and the extent of the developed irreversible lesions. Since anti-topoisomerase I autoantibody is found to be associated with increased mortality, pulmonary fibrosis, musculoskeletal and cardiac involvement, proteinuria and the level of anti-topoisomerase I autoantibody correlates with the extent of fibrosis of the skin and internal organ involvement in dcSSc, it may serve as an activity marker of disease (Minier et al., 2010).

Statistical analysis of clinical data (extent of skin involvement, hand contractures, azotemia and/or malignant hypertension, cardiac involvement, pulmonary artery hypertension, dysmotility and stricture/dilatation of esophagus, extent of lung fibrosis, forced vital capacity) failed to demonstrate associations between anti-topoisomerase I antibody epitope specificity and clinical presentation of the disease. This is in agreement with results also reporting lack of clear association between changes in the anti–topoisomerase I antibody response and clinical parameters (Henry et al., 2005). However, there was a significant difference between F1 negative and F1 positive groups of dcSSc patients in average age and the duration of the disease. The difference in the duration of disease between anti-F1 antibody positive and negative dcSSc patients, together with findings of our longitudinal analysis, may indicate that the anti-topoisomerase I immune response could be explained by a general recognition of the immunodominant part on the molecule (fragment F4), and the disease associated autoantibodies may target the N-terminal part later during the course of the disease. Thus autoantibodies against fragment F1 may represent a new marker of late stage dcSSc (Simon et al., 2009).

Comparison of clinical data of anti-F8 positive and anti-F8 negative SLE patients suggested that SLE patients with antibody against fragment F8 have Raynaud's phenomenon and a milder presentation of the disease (lack of arthritis, central nervous system and kidney involvement).

Discrimination between naturally occurring and pathologic autoantibodies is available according to their recognition patterns, and this is not only a theoretical question but holds important practical - diagnostic and prognostic - consequences in the daily laboratory routine.

5. Acknowledgement

The anti-topoisomerase I work was supported by the Hungarian Scientific Research Fund (OTKA 75912).

6. References

Abi Rached, L.; McDermott, M. F. & Pontarotti, P. (1999). The MHC big bang. *Immunological Reviews,* Vol.167, (February 1999), pp. 33–44, ISSN 1600-065X

Cancro, M.P. & Kearney, J.F. (2004). B cell positive selection: road map to the primary repertoire? *Journal of Immunology,* Vol.173, No.1, (July 2004), pp. 15-19, ISSN 0022-1767

Chumley, M.J.; Dal Porto, J.M.; Kawaguchi, S.; Cambier, J.C.; Nemazee, D. & Hardy, R.R. (2000). AVH11V kappa 9Bcell antigen receptor drives generation of CD5+ B cells both in vivo and in vitro. *Journal of Immunology,* Vol.164, No.9, (May 2000), pp. 4586–93, ISSN 0022-1767

Cooper, E.L.; Kvell, K.; Engelmann, P. & Nemeth, P. (2006). Still waiting for the toll? *Immunology Letters,* Vol.104, No.1-2, (April 2006), pp. 18-28, ISSN 0165-2478

Czömpöly, T.; Olasz, K.; Simon, D.; Nyárády, Z.; Pálinkás, L.; Czirják, L.; Berki, T. & Németh, P. (2006). A possible new bridge between innate and adaptive immunity: Are the anti-mitochondrial citrate synthase autoantibodies components of the natural antibody network? *Molecular Immunology,* Vol.43, No.11, (April 2006), pp. 1761-8, ISSN 0161-5890

Czömpöly, T.; Olasz, K.; Nyárády, Z.; Simon, D.; Bovári, J. & Németh, P. (2008). Detailed analyses of antibodies recognizing mitochondrial antigens suggest similar or identical mechanism for production of natural antibodies and natural autoantibodies. *Autoimmunity Reviews,* Vol.7, No.6, (June 2008), pp. 463-7, ISSN 1568-9972

Czömpöly, T.; Simon, D.; Czirják, L. & Németh, P. (2009). Anti-topoisomerase I autoantibodies in systemic sclerosis. *Autoimmunity Reviews* Vol.8, No.8, (July 2009), pp. 692-6, ISSN 1568-9972

Haas, K.M.; Poe, J.C.; Steeber, D.A. & Tedder, T.F. (2005). B-1a and B-1b cells exhibit distinct developmental requirements and have unique functional roles in innate and adaptive immunity to S. pneumoniae. *Immunity* Vol.23, No.1, (July 2005), pp. 7-18, ISSN 1365-2567

Henry, P.A.; Atamas, S.P.; Yurovsky, V.V.; Luzina, I.; Wigley, F.M. & White, B. (2005). Diversity and plasticity of the anti-DNA topoisomerase I autoantibody response in scleroderma. *Arthritis and Rheumatism,* Vol.43, No12., (December 2005), pp. 2733-42, ISSN 0004-3591

Janeway, C.A .Jr. (2001). How the immune system works to protect the host from infection: a personal view. *Proceedings of the National Academy of Sciences of the United States of America,* Vol.98, No.13., (June 2001), pp. 7461-8, ISSN 0027-8424

Kantor, A.B.; Merrill, C.E.; Herzenberg, L.A. & Hillson, J.L. (1997). An unbiased analysis of V(H)-D-J(H) sequences from B-1a, B-1b, and conventional B cells. *Journal of immunology,* Vol.158, (February 1997), pp. 1175–86, ISSN 0022-1767

Klein, J. & Nikolaidis, N. (2005). The descent of the antibody-based immune system by gradual evolution. *Proceedings of the National Academy of Sciences of the United States of America,* Vol.102, No.1, (January 2005), pp. 169-174, ISSN 0027-8424

Konigshofer, Y. & Chien, Y.H. (2006.) Gammadelta T cells - innate immune lymphocytes? *Current Opinion in Immunology,* Vol.18, No.5, (October 2006), pp. 527-33, ISSN 0952-7915

Kvell, K.; Cooper, E.L.; Engelmann, P.; Bovari, J. & Nemeth, P. Blurring borders: innate immunity with adaptive features. *Clinical and Developmental Immunology,* Vol.2007, (2007), 83671, ISSN 1740-2522

Lacroix-Desmazes, S.; Kaveri, S.V.; Mouthon, L.; Ayouba, A.; Malanchere, E.; Coutinho, A. & Kazatchkine, M.D. (1998). Self-reactive antibodies (natural autoantibodies) in healthy individuals. *Journal of Immunological Methods,* Vol.216, No.1-2, (July 1998), pp. 117–37, ISSN 0022-1759

Liu, Y.; Chen, G. & Zheng, P. (2009). CD40-Siglec G/10 discriminates danger from pathogen associated molecular patterns. *Trends in Immunology,* Vol.30, No.12, (December 2009), pp.557–61, ISSN 1471-4906

Lynch, L.; O'Shea, D.; Winter, D.C.; Geoghegan, J.; Doherty, D.G. & O'Farrelly, C. (2009). Invariant NKT cells and CD1d(+) cells amass in human omentum and are depleted in patients with cancer and obesity. *European Journal of Immunology,* Vol.39, No.7, (July 2009), pp.1893-901, ISSN 1521-4141

Medzhitov, R. 2001. Toll like receptors and innate immunity. *Nature Reviews Immunology,* Vol.1, No.2, (November 2001), pp. 135-145, ISSN 1474-1733

Minier, T.; Nagy, Z.; Bálint, Zs.; Farkas, H.; Radics, J.; Kumánovics, G., Czömpöly, T.; Simon, D.; Varjú, C.; Németh, P. & Czirják, L. (2010). Construct validity evaluation of the European Scleroderma Study Group activity index, and investigation of possible new disease activity markers in systemic sclerosis. *Rheumatology,* Vol.49, No.6, (June 2010), pp. 1133-45, ISSN 1462-0324

Pancer, Z.; Amemiya, C.T.; Ehrhardt, G.R.; Ceitlin, J.; Gartland, G.L. & Cooper M.D. (2004). Somatic diversification of variable lymphocyte receptors in the agnathan sea lamprey. *Nature,* Vol.430, (July 2004), pp. 174-180, ISSN 0028-0836

Simon, D.; Czömpöly, T.; Berki, T.; Minier, T.; Peti, A.; Tóth, E.; Czirják L. & Németh, P. (2009). Naturally occurring and disease associated autoantibodies against topoisomerase I: a fine epitope mapping study in systemic sclerosis and systemic lupus erythematosus. *International Immunology,* Vol.21, No.4, (April 2009), pp. 415-22, ISSN 0953-8178

Silverman, G.J.; Srikrishnan, R.; Germar, K.; Goodyear, C.S.; Andrews, K.A.; Ginzler, E.M. & Tsao, B.P. (2008). Genetic imprinting of autoantibody repertoires in systemic lupus erythematosus patients. *Clinical and Experimental Immunology,* Vol.153, No.1, (July 2008), pp. 102–116, ISSN 0009-9104

Treiner, E.; Duban, L; Moura, I.C.; Hansen, T.; Gilfillan, S. & Lanz, O. (2005). Mucosal-associated invariant T (MAIT) cells: an evolutionarily conserved T cell subset. *Microbes and Infection,* Vol.7, No.3, (March 2005), pp. 552–559, ISSN 1286-4579

2

Adipokines and Systemic Rheumatic Diseases: Linking Inflammation, Immunity and Metabolism

Morena Scotece[1], Javier Conde[1], Veronica Lopez[1], Rodolfo Gómez[1], Francisca Lago[2], Juan J Gómez Reino[1] and Oreste Gualillo[1]

[1]SERGAS, Santiago University Clinical Hospital, Research laboratory 9 (NEIRID LAB: Neuroendocrine Interactions in Rheumatology and Inflammatory Diseases), Institute of Medical Research (IDIS), Santiago de Compostela,

[2]SERGAS, Santiago University Clinical Hospital, Research Laboratory 7 (Molecular and Cellular Cardiology), Institute of Medical Research (IDIS), Santiago de Compostela, Spain

1. Introduction

The cloning of leptin in 1994 introduced a novel concept about white adipose tissue (WAT) (Zhang et al., 1994). Actually, WAT has been recognized as an active tissue able to produce a wide variety of factors, called adipokines. These molecules participate through endocrine, paracrine, autocrine or juxtacrine cross-talk in a great variety of physiological or physiopathological processes, including food intake, insulin sensitivity, immunity and inflammation (Trayhurn & Wood, 2004, 2005).

Moreover, adipokines represent a new family of compounds that can be currently considered as key players of the complex network of soluble mediators involved in the pathophysiology of rheumatic diseases. Adipokines include classic pro-inflammatory proteins such as TNF-α and IL-6, both secreted by adipocytes, but synthesized also by immune cells infiltrating WAT, such as macrophages (Flower et al., 2003; Hotamisligil et al, 1993; Trayhurn et al., 2006).

These pro-inflammatory adipokines appear to significantly contribute to the so-called "low grade inflammation" of obese subjects, a condition associated with increased risk of cancer, type 2 diabetes, cardiovascular complications, autoimmune and inflammatory diseases including rheumatic diseases such as rheumatoid arthritis (RA), osteoarthritis (OA) and systemic lupus (SLE) (Ahima et al, 1996). For instance, it has been reported that obesity that is characterized by abnormal fat accumulation and dysfunction increases the incidence of osteoarthritis (OA). A prevailing hypothesis is that obesity increases mechanical loading on the articular cartilage that finally leads to its degeneration. However, obesity is also associated with OA in non-weight bearing joints such as hand joints, which suggest that metabolic factors, as adipokines, contribute to the high prevalence of OA in obese subjects

(Felson, 2005; Oliveria et al., 1999). Furthermore, adipokines play a pivotal role in other autoimmune and rheumatic diseases such as rheumatoid arthritis (RA) and systemic lupus erythematosus (SLE).

In this book chapter we review the role of adipokines in inflammation and immune response in the context of rheumatic diseases.

2. Leptin

Leptin is the protein product of the *ob* gene, the murine homologue of the human gene LEP, cloned in 1994 (Zhang et al, 1994). This adipokine is mainly produced by white adipose cells and its plasma concentration is directly correlated with the body-fat stores. It has a central role in fat metabolism; in fact leptin is considered a major regulator of body weight by suppressing appetite and stimulating energy expenditure via hypothalamic receptors. This hormone decreases food intake by inducing anorexigenic factors as cocaine amphetamine related transcript (CART) and increases energy consumption by suppressing orexigenic neuropeptides such as neuropeptide Y (NPY). The biological activity of leptin is mediated by specific receptors (Ob-R) that belong to the class 1 cytokine receptor superfamily, and are encoded by the gene diabetes (*db*). Alternative splicing of the *db* gene produce multiple isoforms, but only the long isoform Ob-Rb, appears to be capable of transducing the leptin signal.

Leptin is a hormone with pleiotropic actions. In fact, in addition to regulation of food intake, it also affects a variety of other physiological functions, including fertility, bone metabolism, inflammation, infection, immune responses and others. Recent evidence demonstrates an involvement of leptin in promoting the pathogenesis of different autoimmune and rheumatic diseases such as rheumatoid arthritis, multiple sclerosis and SLE. Several authors have demonstrated a dependence between the risk of aggressive course of RA and leptin levels (Kadowaki & Yamauchi, 2005; Lee et al., 2007; Targonska-Stepniak et al., 2008; Whitehead et al., 2006). It is widely accepted that leptin levels are elevated in patients with RA and that there is a correlation between serum leptin and synovial fluid/serum leptin ratio and disease duration and parameters of RA activity (Olama et al., 2010). Generally, leptin is considered to be pro-inflammatory, but this hormone has been also reported to reduce radiographic joint damage (Rho et al., 2009). This effect could be related to some leptin anabolic effects, such as the stimulation of the synthesis of insulin-like growth factor-1 (IGF-1) and transforming growth factor-β (TGF- β) at both the messenger RNA (mRNA) and protein levels (Dumond et al., 2003)

The actions of leptin in RA are not only targeted to articular tissues, this adipokine also exerts direct modulatory effects on activation, proliferation, maturation and production of inflammatory mediators in a variety of immune cells, including lymphocytes, NK cells, monocytes/macrophages, dendritic cells, neutrophils and eosinophils (Lam & Lu, 2007). In particular, it is known that leptin is able to modulate T regulatory cells that are potent suppressors of autoimmunity. The group of Matarese et al, has recently demonstrated that leptin secreted by adipocytes sustains Th1 immunity by promoting effector T cell proliferation and by constraining Treg cells expansion. Weight loss, with concomitant reduction in leptin levels, induces a reduction in effector T cell proliferation and an increased expansion of Treg cells leading to a down-regulation of Th1 immunity and cell-mediated autoimmune diseases associated with increased susceptibility to infections. On the other hand, an increase in adipocyte mass leads to high leptin secretion, which results in expansion of effector T cells and reduction of $T\text{-}_{Reg}$ cells. This effect determines an overall enhancement of the pro-inflammatory immunity and of T cell-mediated autoimmune disorders. These data suggests that leptin can be considered as a link between immune tolerance, metabolic function and autoimmunity and that future strategies aimed at interfering with leptin signaling may represent innovative therapeutic tools for autoimmune disorders.

Very recently it has been demonstrated that leptin can activate the mammalian target of rapamycin (mTOR) and regulate the proliferative capacity of regulatory T (T_{Reg}) cells. The study of Procaccini et al describes the leptin–mTOR signalling pathway as an important link between host energy status and T_{Reg} cell activity. The authors conclude that oscillating mTOR activity is necessary for T_{Reg} cell activation and suggest that this may explain why T_{Reg} cells are unresponsive to TCR stimulation in vitro, where high levels of leptin and nutrients may sustain mTOR activation (De Rosa et al., 2007; Procaccini et al., 2010).

Leptin also may acts as a catabolic factor involved in the pathogenesis of osteoarthritis.

In fact, Otero et al have demonstrated that in cultured human and murine chondrocytes type 2 nitric oxide synthase (NOS2) is synergistically activated by the combination of leptin plus interferon-γ, and NOS2 activation by IL-1β is increased by leptin via a mechanism involving JAK2, PI3K, and mitogen activated kinases (MEK1 and p38) (Otero M et al., 2003, 2005). Nitric oxide (NO), which is induced by a wide range of pro-inflammatory cytokines, is a well-known pro-inflammatory mediator on joint cartilage, where it triggers chondrocyte phenotype loss, apoptosis, and metalloproteinases (MMPs) activation.

Recently, it was demonstrated that leptin is able to induce also the expression of MMPs involved in OA cartilage damage, such as MMP-9 and MMP-13 (Toussirot et al., 2007). Leptin alone and in combination with IL-1β up-regulates MMP-1 and MMP-3 production in human OA cartilage through the transcription factor NF-κB, protein kinase C and MAP kinase pathways. This hormone is also correlated positively to MMP-1 and MMP-3 in synovial fluid (SF) from OA patients (Koskinen et al., 2011).

It is noteworthy that leptin was recently shown to increase IL-8 production in human chondrocytes (Lago et al., 2008).

Bao et al have defined that leptin enhanced both gene and protein levels of catabolic factors such as MMP-2 y MMP-9, while down-regulated the anabolic factors such as bFGF in articular cartilage of rats. Additionally, the gene expression of ADAMTS-4 and -5 were markedly increased and was observed a depletion of proteoglycan in articular cartilage after treatment with leptin (Bao et al., 2010)

Leptin also could contribute to abnormal osteoblast function in OA. In fact, the elevated production of leptin in OA abnormal subchondral osteoblast is correlated with the increased levels of ALP (alkaline phosphatase), OC, collagen type I and TGF-β1 inducing a dysregulation of osteoblast function (Mutabaruka et al., 2010).

Leptin's and leptin receptor (Ob-Rb) expression levels were significantly increased in advanced OA cartilage and in SF. The induction by leptin of IL-1β production y MMP-9 and

MMP-13 protein expression in chondrocytes indicates a pro-inflammatory and catabolic role of this hormone on cartilage metabolism (Simopoulou et al., 2007).

Ku et al have demonstrated a relation of SF leptin concentrations with the radiographic severity of OA in OA patients, suggesting a role of leptin as an effective marker for quantitative detection of OA (Ku et al., 2009).

All these data have focused on the pro-inflammatory effect of leptin *in vitro* that seems to have an adverse effect on cartilage homeostasis. Very recently, Griffin et al, showed that the incidence of OA was not higher in *ob/ob* and *db/db* female obese mice than in control background strain (C57BL/6J). Nevertheless, in this study, no standard was set for the incidence of OA in obese control mice without leptin mutation (Griffin et al., 2009).

This recent result suggested that obesity alone is insufficient to induce systemic inflammation and knee OA and that leptin has a necessary role in the pathophysiology of OA associated with obesity.

It is also found a relationship between leptin and lupus disease related factors. In fact, patients with SLE have increased concentrations of leptin and these concentrations are associated with insulin resistance, BMI (Body Mass Index) and CRP (C-reactive protein) in these patients (Chung et al., 2009). Figure 1.

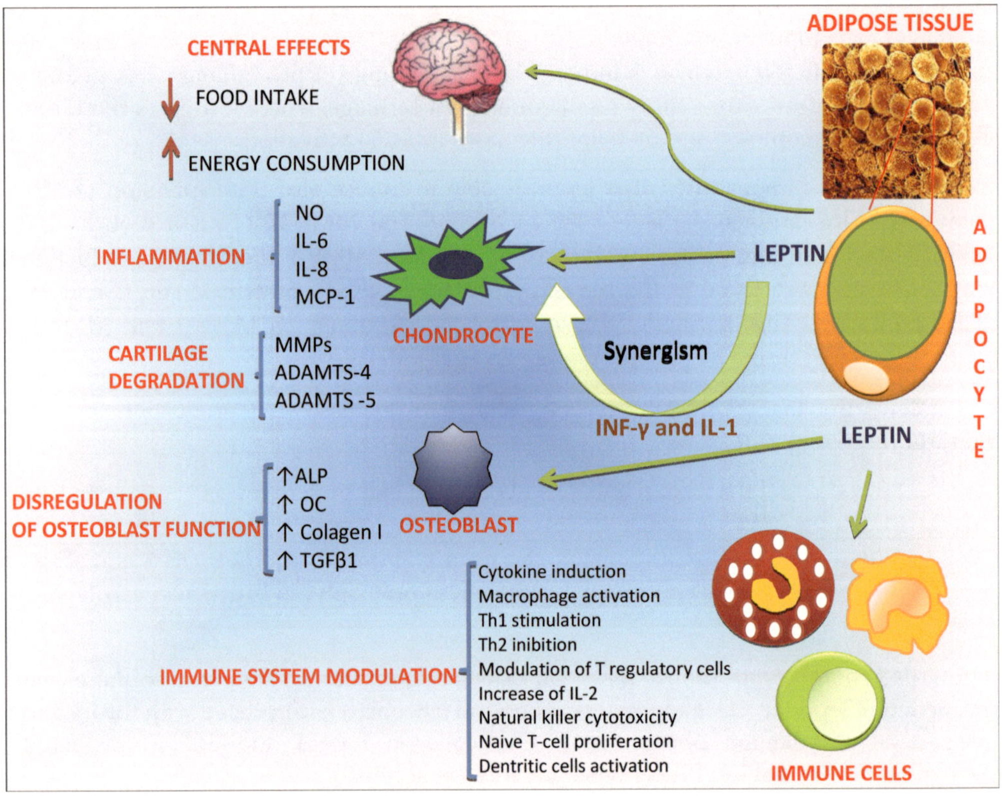

Fig. 1. Schematic representation of the effects of leptin in the brain, immune system, and articular cartilage.

3. Adiponectin

Adiponectin, also known as GBP28, apM1, Acrp30 or AdipoQ, is a 244-residue protein that is produced mainly by WAT. Adiponectin has structural homology with collagens VIII and X and complement factor C1q, and it circulates in the blood in relatively large amounts in different molecular forms (trimers, hexamers and also 12-18-mer forms) (Kadowaki & Yamauchi, 2005; Oh et al., 2007). It increases fatty acid oxidation and reduces the synthesis of glucose in the liver. Ablation of the adiponectin gene has no dramatic effect on-knock-out mice on a normal diet, but when placed on a high fat/sucrose diet they develop severe insulin resistance and exhibit lipid accumulation in muscles (Whitehead et al., 2006). Circulating adiponectin levels tend to be low in morbidly obese patients and increase with weight loss and with the use of thiazolidinediones which enhance sensitivity to insulin (Kadowaki & Yamauchi, 2005; Maeda et al., 2001).

Adiponectin acts via two receptors, one (AdipoR1) found predominantly in skeletal muscle and the other (AdipoR2) in liver. Transduction of the adiponectin signal by AdipoR1 and AdipoR2 involves the activation of AMPK, PPAR-α, PPAR-γ and other signalling molecules (Kadowaki & Yamauchi, 2005). To note, targeted disruption of AdipoR1 and AdipoR2 causes abrogation of adiponectin binding and all its metabolic actions (Yamauchi et al., 2007).

There is evidence that adiponectin has a wide range of effects in pathologies with inflammatory component, such as cardiovascular disease, endothelial dysfunction, type 2 diabetes, metabolic syndrome, OA and RA (Matsuzawa, 2006). Adiponectin acts as a potent modulator of both B and T cells; moreover, it modulates the activity of immune innate response by inducing relevant anti-inflammatory factors such as IL 1 receptor antagonist and IL-10 (Kadowaki & Yamauchi, 2005).

In contrast to its previously described protective role in vascular diseases, there is evidence that adiponectin might act as a pro-inflammatory factor in joints and it could be involved in matrix degradation. Of note, these discrepancies in the functions of adiponectin are linked to the level of oligomerization of the protein and opposite actions have been described for both low molecular weight and high molecular isoforms (Neumeier et al., 2006).

Adiponectin levels in RA patients are higher than in healthy subjects (Otero M et al., 2006) and multiple studies correlated these adiponectin elevated levels with severity of RA (Ebina et al., 2009). Giles and collaborators identified a cross sectional association between serum adiponectin levels and radiographic damage in RA patients (Giles et al., 2009), suggesting that this adipokine may be a mediator of the paradoxical relationship between increasing adiposity and protection from radiographic damage in RA, due to adiponectin circulating levels decreasing as adiposity increases. Therefore, considering that adiponectin may have negative effects on the joint, this adipokine could be a relevant mediator to the inverse relationship between increasing adiposity and radiographic damage observed in RA studies.

In human synovial fibroblasts adiponectin induces IL-6, one of the main mediators of RA, via AMPK, p38, IKKα-β and NF-κB, (Tang et al., 2007). Similarly, IL-8 is induced by adiponectin through an intracellular pathway involving NF-κB (Katano et al., 2009). A recent publication confirms the role of adiponectin in pathogenesis of RA. The authors showed that adiponectin is able to induce the expression of vascular endothelial growth factor, MMP-1 and MMP-13, in synovial cells, at the same levels as IL-1β (Choi et al., 2009). In line with this, it has been reported that adiponectin, in RA synovial fibroblasts (RASFs), increases cyclooxygenase 2 (COX-2), membrane-associated PGE synthase 1 (mPGES-1) and prostaglandin E_2 (PGE_2) mRNA and protein expression in a dose-dependent manner (Kusunoki et al., 2010). This increase was inhibited by siRNA against adiponectin receptors (AdipoR1 and AdipoR2) or using inhibitors of specific proteins involved in adiponectin signal transduction (Kusunoki et al., 2010).

Adiponectin is also implicated in OA pathogenesis. In chondrocytes this hormone is able to induce several pro-inflammatory mediators such as nitric oxide, IL-6, MCP-1, MMP-3 and MMP-9 as well as IL-8 (Gomez et al., 2011; Lago R et al., 2008), generating a pro-inflammatory environment at joint level. However, the implication of adiponectin in OA development is also supported by clinical observations. Laurberg TB et al have reported that plasma adiponectin levels were significantly higher in OA patients than in healthy subjects (Laurberg et al., 2009). Moreover, elevated plasma adiponectin levels were observed in female patients with erosive compared with non-erosive hand OA (Filkova et al., 2009). In addition, adiponectin levels in synovial fluid correlating with osteoarthritis severity (Honsawek & Chayanupatkul, 2010) and aggrecan degradation (Hao et al., 2010). Figure 2.

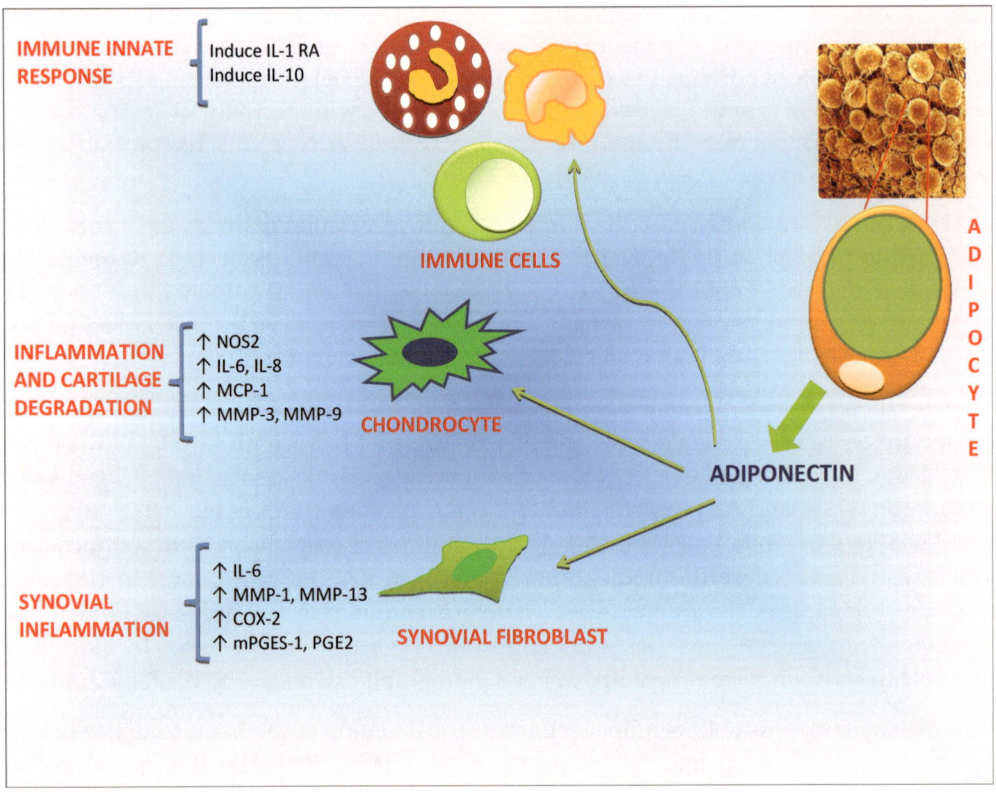

Fig. 2. Schematic representation of the interaction of adiponectin with immune cells, chondrocytes, and synovial fibroblasts.

4. Resistin

Resistin, known as adipocyte-secreted factor (ADSF) or found in inflammatory zone 3 (FIZZ3), was discovered in 2001 and was proposed as potential link between obesity and diabetes (Steppan et al., 2001). It was secreted by adipose tissue, but has been found also in macrophages, neutrophils and other cell types. Serum resistin levels increases with obesity in mice, rats and humans (Degawa-Yamauchi et al., 2003; McTernan et al., 2002). Increasing evidence indicates its important regulatory roles in various biological processes, including several inflammatory diseases.

There are demonstrations that resistin may be involved in the pathogenesis of RA. It has previously been observed increased levels of this adipokine in synovial fluid from patients of rheumatoid arthritis (RA) compared to patients with non-inflammatory rheumatic disorders (Schaffler et al., 2003). Resistin may be a significant mediator in the inflammatory process of RA, in fact the serum resistin levels are associated with disease activity and acute phase reactants, including C-reactive protein and IL-1Ra antagonizing IL-1β (Forsblad d´Elia et al., 2008; Senolt et al., 2007).

Resistin has been found in the plasma and synovial fluid of RA patients, and injection of resistin into joints of mice induces an arthritis-like condition, with leukocyte infiltration of synovial tissues, hypertrophy of the synovial layer, and pannus formation (Bokarewa et al., 2005; Senolt et al., 2007). Bokarewa et al have showed that resistin induces and is induced by several pro-inflammatory cytokines, such as TNF-α or IL-6, in peripheral blood mononuclear cells, via NF-kB pathway, indicating that resistin can increase its own activity by a positive feedback mechanism (Bokarewa et al., 2005).

The pro-inflammatory profile of resistin, together with its association with obesity, suggests that this adipokine might be another potential mediator that links OA with inflammation and obesity. It was demonstrated that this adipokine is elevated in both serum and SF after traumatic joint injuries. Recombinant resistin stimulated proteoglycan degradation in mouse femoral head cultures and the induction of inflammatory cytokines and PGE2 production. Moreover, it inhibited proteoglycan synthesis in human cartilage explants (Lee et al., 2009). However, Berry et al have not identified any association between baseline serum levels of resistin and cartilage volume loss (Berry et al., 2011).

In addition, resistin has a role as a marker of inflammation in other rheumatic diseases, such as systemic lupus erythematous (SLE). In fact, Almehed et al have demonstrated a positive correlation between serum resistin levels, inflammation, bone mineral density and renal functions in patients with SLE (Almehed et al., 2008). Figure 3.

5. Visfatin

Visfatin, also named pre-B-cell colony-enhancing factor (PBEF) and nicotinamide phosphoribosyltransferase (Nampt), was originally discovered in liver, skeletal muscle and bone marrow as a growth factor for B-lymphocyte precursors, however it is also secreted by visceral fat (Fukuhara et al.,2005; Samal et al., 1994). It is supposed that visfatin had insulin mimetic properties, but the role of this adipokine in the modulation of glucose metabolism, as well as its binding to insulin receptors is still debate (Fukurara et al., 2005, 2007).

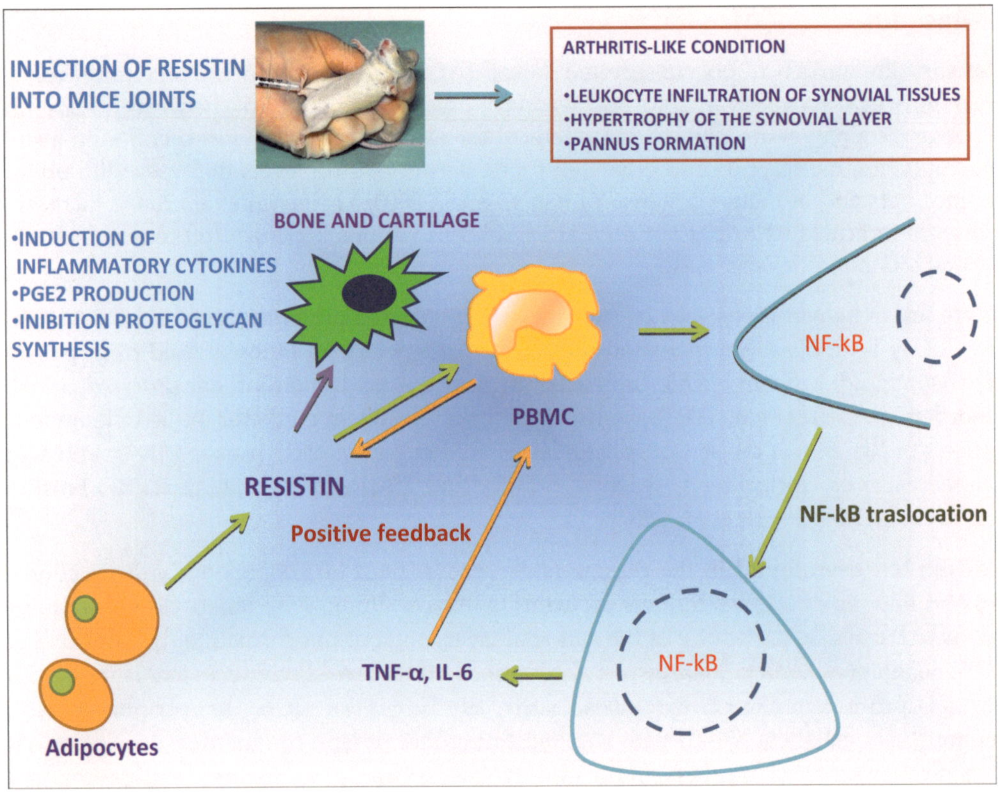

Fig. 3. Schematic representation of resistin interaccion among adipocytes, immune cells and bone and cartilage cells.

It has been reported that visfatin is increased in obesity. Moreover, leucocytes from obese patients produce higher amounts of visfatin compared with lean subjects, and specifically, granulocytes and monocytes are the major visfatin producing cells (Catalan et al., 2011; Friebe et al., 2011). However, leucocytes are not the only non-fat cell-type that synthesizes visfatin. Macrophages have also been described as a source for visfatin production (Curat et al., 2006) and interestingly, this adipokine promoted macrophage survival by reducing apoptosis (Li et al., 2008).

Our group demonstrated that visfatin was increased in RA patients (Otero M et al., 2006), these data were also further confirmed by other authors (Rho et al., 2009). To note, enhanced visfatin levels are associated with augmented joint damage (Rho et al., 2009). Brentano and colleagues reported that visfatin was localized in the site of invasion of synovial tissue in joints of RA patients. Moreover it is able to induce IL-6, MMP-1 and MMP-3 in RA synovial fibroblasts, as well as IL-6 and TNF-α in monocytes (Brentano et al., 2007), concluding that visfatin has relevant pro-inflammatory and catabolic roles in RA pathogenesis and it could be considered a potential therapeutic target.

A recently published study by Busso et al. shows that visfatin is a key mediator in inflammatory arthritis. The administration of a visfatin inhibitor to mice with collagen-induced arthritis reduced arthritis severity with similar effect to that produced by TNF-α inhibitor (Busso et al., 2008). Moreover, pharmacological inhibition of visfatin led to low levels of intracellular NAD in inflammatory cells and decreased the production of TNF-α and IL-6 in affected joints (Busso et al., 2008). However, the mechanism by which visfatin exerts its catabolic effect in arthritic joints is incompletely understood.

At cartilage level, OA chondrocytes are able to produce visfatin and its expression is increased after IL-1β treatment (Gosset et al., 2008). Visfatin administration, like IL-1β, enhances PGE_2 release. In line with this, visfatin also increases MMP-3 and MMP-13 synthesis and release, and ADAMTS-4 and ADAMTS-5 expression in mouse articular chondrocytes (Gosset et al., 2008). Visfatin decreases aggrecan expression, probably due to this increase in the expression of matrix degradative enzymes (Gosset et al., 2008). Taken together, these data suggest that visfatin has a catabolic function in cartilage. Table 1.

6. Chemerin

Chemerin, also known as tazarotene-induced gene 2 and retinoic acid receptor responder 2 (RARRES2), is a novel identified chemoattractant adipokine (Wittamer et al., 2003). It is secreted as an 18 kDa inactive proprotein and activated by post-translational C-terminal cleavage (Zabel et al., 2005). Chemerin acts via the G-coupled receptor chemokine-like receptor 1 (CMKLR1 or ChemR23) (Wittamer et al., 2003). Chemerin and its receptor are mainly expressed, but not exclusively, in adipose tissue (Bozaoglu et al., 2007), for instance, dendritic cells and macrophages express chemerin receptor (Luangsay et al., 2009). Endothelial cells also express ChemR23 and it is up regulated by pro-inflammatory cytokines such as TNF-α, IL-1β and IL-6 (Kaur et al., 2010). Moreover, chemerin exogenous challenge promotes *in vitro* angiogenesis by inducing cell proliferation, endothelial migration and capillary tube formation, critical steps in the development of angiogenesis (Kaur et al., 2010).

Interestingly, chondrocytes express chemerin and its receptor (Berg et al., 2010; Conde et al., 2011) and IL-1β is able to increase chemerin expression (Conde et al., 2011). In the same way, Berg et al. have demonstrated that recombinant chemerin enhances the production of several pro-inflammatory cytokines (TNF-α, IL-1β, IL-6 and IL-8), as well as different MMPs (MMP-1, MMP-2, MMP-3, MMP 8 and MMP-13) in human articular chondrocytes (Berg et al., 2010). These factors play a role in the degradation of the extracellular matrix, by causing a breakdown of the collagen and aggrecan framework, which results in the irreversible destruction of the cartilage in OA and RA. Moreover, these authors reported that the intracellular signalling after ChemR23 activation occurs through p42/44 MAPK and Akt phosphorylation.

Chemerin and ChemR23 expression was found in SLE skin biopsies (Vermi et al., 2005). *In vitro* experiments showed that chemerin acts as a chemotactic factor for plasmacytoid DCs. The tissue distribution of this adipokine, located at the luminal side of inflamed blood vessels suggest that chemerin is involved in the migration of plasmacytoid DCs and the accumulation of this cells in inflamed tissues in SLE patients (Vermi et al., 2005). Moreover, De Palma et al. found chemerin expression in renal tubular epithelial cells from SLE patients with nephritis (De Palma et al., 2011). These authors, using a transendothelial chemotaxis assay, demonstrated that the recruitment of plasmacytoid DCs by TNF-α was mediated by chemerin/ChemR23 interaction, may be due to the induction of the cleavage of pro-chemerin by TNF-α through the local production of serine proteases in proximal tubular epithelial cells (De Palma et al., 2011; Kanalas & Hopfer, 1997; Zabel et al., 2005). Table 1.

7. Lipocalin 2

Lipocalin 2 (LCN2), also termed siderocalin, 24p3, uterocalin and neutrophil gelatinase-associated lipocalin, is a 25 kDa glycoprotein isolated from neutrophil granules, although white adipose tissue (WAT) is thought to be the main source (Triebel et al., 1992). The LCN2 protein has been isolated as a 25 kDa monomer, as a 46 kDa homodimer and in a covalent complex with MMP-9, and its cellular receptor, megalin (GP330), was recently described (Devireddy et al., 2001). LCN2 is involved in apoptosis of haematopoietic cells (Devireddy et al., 2001), transport of fatty acids and iron (Chu et al.,1998), modulation of inflammation (Cowland & Borregaard, 1997) among other processes.

LCN2 has recently been identified in chondrocytes (Owen et al., 2008). In these cells IL-1β, leptin, adiponectin, LPS and dexamethasone act as potent modulators of LCN2 expression (Conde et al., 2011). Lipocalin 2 is likely to be involved in matrix degradation since it forms molecular complexes with MMP-9 (Gupta et al., 2007).

Recently, Katano and colleagues confirmed that the level of NGAL in SF was significantly higher in patients with RA than in those with osteoarthritis. Through proteome analysis Katano et al have showed that GM-CSF may contribute to the pathogenesis of RA by the upregulation of LCN2 in neutrophils, followed by induction of Catepsin D, transitional endoplasmic reticulum ATPase (TERA) and transglutaminase 2 (tg2) in synoviocytes (Katano et al., 2009). These enzymes may contribute to the proliferation of synovial cells and infiltration of inflammatory cells inside the synovia (Katano et al., 2009).

Finally, LCN2 is also a candidate biomarker for the early detection of LN (lupus nephritis) that is an inflammation of the kidney caused by systemic lupus erythematosus (SLE), which is very common in childhood-onset SLE (cSLE). Hinze et al. have demonstrated that urinary and plasma NGAL (U-NGAL and P-NGAL) is an excellent candidate as predictive biomarker for worsening of cSLE renal and global disease activity. (Hinze et al., 2009). Table 1.

Visfatin	LCN2	Chemerin
↑ RA patients	IL-1β, adipokines and dexamethasone increase LCN2 expression	IL-1β increase chemerin expression
↑ IL-6, MMP-1 and MMP-3 in RA synovial fibroblasts	↑ matrix degradation	↑TNF-α, IL-1β, IL-6 and IL-8
↑ IL-6 and TNF-α in monocytes	↑ RA synovial fluid	↑ MMP-1, MMP-2, MMP-3, MMP 8 and MMP-13
↑ PGE2, MMP-3, MMP-13, ADAMTS-4 and ADAMTS-5 in chondrocytes	GM-CSF upregulate LCN2 expression in synovial neuthophils	Chemotactic factor for plasmacytoid DCs
↓ aggrecan expression in chondrocytes	Candidate bionmarker of early detection of lupus nephritis	Involved in the migration and accumulation of plasmacytoid DCs

Table 1. Visfatin, LCN2 and Chemerin: effects relevant to rheumatic diseases.

8. Conclusions

It is now clear that adipokines have multiple relevant roles in the body, and many research efforts are driven to elucidate the intricate network among, metabolic disorders, inflammatory diseases and immune system. Although many aspects are still unclear, this chapter summarizes the present knowledge on the role of adipokines in certain rheumatic diseases.

Several adipokines have catabolic effects in articular cartilage, however some of them showed contradictory results and their involvement in the degeneration of the joint is not well understood.

The data presented here suggest that adipokines could be considered a link between metabolism and rheumatic diseases and their signalling pathways may represent innovative therapeutic strategies for autoimmune and rheumatic disorders.

9. Acknowledgements

Javier Conde is a predoctoral fellow from IDICHUS Foundation. Morena Scotece is a pre doctoral fellow funded by the FPU programme of Spanish Ministry of Education. Rodolfo Gómez is a post-doctoral fellow funded by National Institute of Health "Carlos III", Programme "Sara Borrell". The Instituto de Salud Carlos III and the Xunta de Galicia (SERGAS), through a research-staff stabilization contract, fund the work of O.G. and F.L. OG and FL research is supported by Instituto de Salud Carlos III and Xunta de Galicia. This work was also partially supported by RETICS Program, RD08/0075 (RIER) and REDINSCOR from Instituto de Salud Carlos III (ISCIII), within the VI NP of R+D+I 2008-2011.

10. Abbreviations

Rheumatoid arthritis (RA), osteoarthritis (OA), white adipose tissue (WAT), interleukin (IL), systemic lupus erithematosus (SLE), cocaine amphetamine related transcript (CART), neuropeptide Y (NPY), insulin growth factor-1 (IGF-1), transforming growth factor-β (TGF-β), metalloprotease (MMP), synovial fluid (SF), nitric oxide (NO), alkaline phosphatase (ALP), C-reactive protein (CRP), prostaglandin E2 (PGE2), lipocalin 2 (LCN2).

11. References

Ahima, R.S., Prabakaran, D., Mantzoros, C., Qu, D., Lowell, B., Maratos-Flier, E.,& Flier, J.S. (1996). Role of leptin in the neuroendocrine response to fasting. *Nature* , 382,6588, 250-2, 0028-0836 (Print). 0028-0836 (Linking)

Almehed, K., d'Elia, H.F., Bokarewa, M.,& Carlsten, H. (2008). Role of resistin as a marker of inflammation in systemic lupus erythematosus. *Arthritis Res Ther* , 10,1 , R15, 1478-6362 (Electronic). 1478-6354 (Linking)

Bao, J.P., Chen, W.P., Feng, J., Hu, P.F., Shi, Z.L.,& Wu, L.D. (2010). Leptin plays a catabolic role on articular cartilage. *Mol Biol Rep* , 37,7, 3265-72, 1573-4978 (Electronic). 0301-4851 (Linking)

Berg, V., Sveinbjornsson, B., Bendiksen, S., Brox, J., Meknas, K.,& Figenschau, Y. (2010). Human articular chondrocytes express ChemR23 and chemerin; ChemR23 promotes inflammatory signalling upon binding the ligand chemerin(21-157). *Arthritis Res Ther* , 12,6, R228, 1478-6362 (Electronic). 1478-6354 (Linking)

Berry, P.A., Jones, S.W., Cicuttini, F.M., Wluka, A.E.,& Maciewicz, R.A. (2011). Temporal relationship between serum adipokines, biomarkers of bone and cartilage turnover, and cartilage volume loss in a population with clinical knee osteoarthritis. *Arthritis Rheum* , 63, 3, 700-7, 1529-0131 (Electronic). 0004-3591 (Linking)

Bokarewa, M., Nagaev, I., Dahlberg, L., Smith, U.,& Tarkowski, A. (2005). Resistin, an adipokine with potent proinflammatory properties. *J Immunol* , 174,9, 5789-95, 0022-1767 (Print). 0022-1767 (Linking)

Bozaoglu, K., Bolton, K., McMillan, J., Zimmet, P., Jowett, J., Collier, G., Walder, K.,& Segal, D. (2007). Chemerin is a novel adipokine associated with obesity and metabolic syndrome. *Endocrinology* , 148,10, 4687-94, 0013-7227 (Print). 0013-7227 (Linking)

Brentano, F., Schorr, O., Ospelt, C., Stanczyk, J., Gay, R.E., Gay, S.,& Kyburz, D. (2007). Pre-B cell colony-enhancing factor/visfatin, a new marker of inflammation in rheumatoid arthritis with proinflammatory and matrix-degrading activities. *Arthritis Rheum* , 56,9, 2829-39, 0004-3591 (Print). 0004-3591 (Linking)

Busso, N., Karababa, M., Nobile, M., Rolaz, A., Van Gool, F., Galli, M., Leo, O., So, A.,& De Smedt, T. (2008). Pharmacological inhibition of nicotinamide phosphoribosyltransferase/visfatin enzymatic activity identifies a new inflammatory pathway linked to NAD. *PLoS One* , 3,5, e2267, 1932-6203 (Electronic). 1932-6203 (Linking)

Catalan, V., Gomez-Ambrosi, J., Rodriguez, A., Ramirez, B., Silva, C., Rotellar, F., Cienfuegos, J.A., Salvador, J.,& Fruhbeck, G. (2011). Association of increased Visfatin/PBEF/NAMPT circulating concentrations and gene expression levels in peripheral blood cells with lipid metabolism and fatty liver in human morbid obesity. *Nutr Metab Cardiovasc Dis* , 21,4, 245-53, 1590-3729 (Electronic). 0939-4753 (Linking)

Choi, H.M., Lee, Y.A., Lee, S.H., Hong, S.J., Hahm, D.H., Choi, S.Y., Yang, H.I., Yoo, M.C.,& Kim, K.S. (2009). Adiponectin may contribute to synovitis and joint destruction in rheumatoid arthritis by stimulating vascular endothelial growth factor, matrix metalloproteinase-1, and matrix metalloproteinase-13 expression in fibroblast-like synoviocytes more than proinflammatory mediators. *Arthritis Res Ther* , 11,6, R161, 1478-6362 (Electronic). 1478-6354 (Linking)

Chu, S.T., Lin, H.J., Huang, H.L.,& Chen, Y.H. (1998). The hydrophobic pocket of 24p3 protein from mouse uterine luminal fluid: fatty acid and retinol binding activity and predicted structural similarity to lipocalins. *J Pept Res* , 52,5, 390-7, 1397-002X (Print). 1397-002X (Linking)

Chung, C.P., Long, A.G., Solus, J.F., Rho, Y.H., Oeser, A., Raggi, P.,& Stein, C.M. (2009). Adipocytokines in systemic lupus erythematosus: relationship to inflammation, insulin resistance and coronary atherosclerosis. *Lupus* , 18,9, 799-806, 0961-2033 (Print). 0961-2033 (Linking)

Conde, J., Gomez, R., Bianco, G., Scotece, M., Lear, P., Dieguez, C., Gomez-Reino, J., Lago, F.,& Gualillo, O. (2011). Expanding the adipokine network in cartilage:

identification and regulation of novel factors in human and murine chondrocytes. *Ann Rheum Dis* , 70,3, 551-9, 1468-2060 (Electronic). 0003-4967 (Linking)

Cowland, J.B.&Borregaard, N. (1997). Molecular characterization and pattern of tissue expression of the gene for neutrophil gelatinase-associated lipocalin from humans. *Genomics* , 45,1, 17-23, 0888-7543 (Print). 0888-7543 (Linking)

Curat, C.A., Wegner, V., Sengenes, C., Miranville, A., Tonus, C., Busse, R.,& Bouloumie, A. (2006). Macrophages in human visceral adipose tissue: increased accumulation in obesity and a source of resistin and visfatin. *Diabetologia* , 49,4, 744-7, 0012-186X (Print). 0012-186X (Linking)

De Palma, G., Castellano, G., Del Prete, A., Sozzani, S., Fiore, N., Loverre, A., Parmentier, M., Gesualdo, L., Grandaliano, G.,& Schena, F.P. (2011). The possible role of ChemR23/Chemerin axis in the recruitment of dendritic cells in lupus nephritis. *Kidney Int* , 79,11, 1228-35, 1523-1755 (Electronic). 0085-2538 (Linking)

De Rosa, V., Procaccini, C., Cali, G., Pirozzi, G., Fontana, S., Zappacosta, S., La Cava, A.,& Matarese, G. (2007). A key role of leptin in the control of regulatory T cell proliferation. *Immunity* , 26,2, 241-55, 1074-7613 (Print). 1074-7613 (Linking)

Degawa-Yamauchi, M., Bovenkerk, J.E., Juliar, B.E., Watson, W., Kerr, K., Jones, R., Zhu, Q.,& Considine, R.V. (2003). Serum resistin (FIZZ3) protein is increased in obese humans. *J Clin Endocrinol Metab* , 88,11, 5452-5, 0021-972X (Print). 0021-972X (Linking)

Devireddy, L.R., Teodoro, J.G., Richard, F.A.,& Green, M.R. (2001). Induction of apoptosis by a secreted lipocalin that is transcriptionally regulated by IL-3 deprivation. *Science* , 293, 5531, 829-34, 0036-8075 (Print). 0036-8075 (Linking)

Dumond, H., Presle, N., Terlain, B., Mainard, D., Loeuille, D., Netter, P.,& Pottie, P. (2003). Evidence for a key role of leptin in osteoarthritis. *Arthritis Rheum* , 48,11, 3118-29, 0004-3591 (Print). 0004-3591 (Linking)

Ebina, K., Fukuhara, A., Ando, W., Hirao, M., Koga, T., Oshima, K., Matsuda, M., Maeda, K., Nakamura, T., Ochi, T., Shimomura, I., Yoshikawa, H.,& Hashimoto, J. (2009). Serum adiponectin concentrations correlate with severity of rheumatoid arthritis evaluated by extent of joint destruction. *Clin Rheumatol* , 28,4, 445-51, 1434-9949 (Electronic). 0770-3198 (Linking)

Felson, D.T. (2005). Relation of obesity and of vocational and avocational risk factors to osteoarthritis. *J Rheumatol* , 32,6, 1133-5, 0315-162X (Print). 0315-162X (Linking)

Filkova, M., Liskova, M., Hulejova, H., Haluzik, M., Gatterova, J., Pavelkova, A., Pavelka, K., Gay, S., Muller-Ladner, U.,& Senolt, L. (2009). Increased serum adiponectin levels in female patients with erosive compared with non-erosive osteoarthritis. *Ann Rheum Dis* , 68,2, 295-6, 1468-2060 (Electronic). 0003-4967 (Linking)

Flower, L., Gray, R., Pinkney, J.,& Mohamed-Ali, V. (2003). Stimulation of interleukin-6 release by interleukin-1beta from isolated human adipocytes. *Cytokine* , 21,1, 32-7, 1043-4666 (Print). 1043-4666 (Linking)

Forsblad d'Elia, H., Pullerits, R., Carlsten, H.,& Bokarewa, M. (2008). Resistin in serum is associated with higher levels of IL-1Ra in post-menopausal women with rheumatoid arthritis. *Rheumatology (Oxford)* , 47,7, 1082-7, 1462-0332 (Electronic). 1462-0324 (Linking)

Friebe, D., Neef, M., Kratzsch, J., Erbs, S., Dittrich, K., Garten, A., Petzold-Quinque, S., Bluher, S., Reinehr, T., Stumvoll, M., Bluher, M., Kiess, W.,& Korner, A. (2011).

Leucocytes are a major source of circulating nicotinamide phosphoribosyltransferase (NAMPT)/pre-B cell colony (PBEF)/visfatin linking obesity and inflammation in humans. *Diabetologia* , 54,5, 1200-11, 1432-0428 (Electronic). 0012-186X (Linking)

Fukuhara, A., Matsuda, M., Nishizawa, M., Segawa, K., Tanaka, M., Kishimoto, K., Matsuki, Y., Murakami, M., Ichisaka, T., Murakami, H., Watanabe, E., Takagi, T., Akiyoshi, M., Ohtsubo, T., Kihara, S., Yamashita, S., Makishima, M., Funahashi, T., Yamanaka, S., Hiramatsu, R., Matsuzawa, Y.,& Shimomura, I. (2005). Visfatin: a protein secreted by visceral fat that mimics the effects of insulin. *Science* , 307,5708, 426-30, 1095-9203 (Electronic). 0036-8075 (Linking)

Fukuhara, A., Matsuda, M., Nishizawa, M., Segawa, K., Tanaka, M., Kishimoto, K., Matsuki, Y., Murakami, M., Ichisaka, T., Murakami, H., Watanabe, E., Takagi, T., Akiyoshi, M., Ohtsubo, T., Kihara, S., Yamashita, S., Makishima, M., Funahashi, T., Yamanaka, S., Hiramatsu, R., Matsuzawa, Y.,& Shimomura, I. (2007). Retraction. *Science* , 318,5850, 565, 1095-9203 (Electronic). 0036-8075 (Linking)

Giles, J.T., Allison, M., Bingham, C.O. 3rd, Scott, W.M. Jr,& Bathon, J.M. (2009). Adiponectin is a mediator of the inverse association of adiposity with radiographic damage in rheumatoid arthritis. *Arthritis Rheum* , 61,9, 1248-56, 0004-3591 (Print). 0004-3591 (Linking)

Gomez, R., Scotece, M., Conde, J., Gomez-Reino, J.J., Lago, F.,& Gualillo, O. (2011). Adiponectin and leptin increase IL-8 production in human chondrocytes. *Ann Rheum Dis* , 1468-2060 (Electronic). 0003-4967 (Linking)

Gosset, M., Berenbaum, F., Salvat, C., Sautet, A., Pigenet, A., Tahiri, K.,& Jacques, C. (2008). Crucial role of visfatin/pre-B cell colony-enhancing factor in matrix degradation and prostaglandin E2 synthesis in chondrocytes: possible influence on osteoarthritis. *Arthritis Rheum* , 58 ,5, 1399-409, 0004-3591 (Print). 0004-3591 (Linking)

Griffin, T.M., Huebner, J.L., Kraus, V.B.,& Guilak, F. (2009). Extreme obesity due to impaired leptin signaling in mice does not cause knee osteoarthritis. *Arthritis Rheum* , 60,10, 2935-44, 0004-3591 (Print). 0004-3591 (Linking)

Gupta, K., Shukla, M., Cowland, J.B., Malemud, C.J.,& Haqqi, T.M. (2007). Neutrophil gelatinase-associated lipocalin is expressed in osteoarthritis and forms a complex with matrix metalloproteinase 9. *Arthritis Rheum* , 56,10, 3326-35, 0004-3591 (Print). 0004-3591 (Linking)

Hao, D., Li, M., Wu, Z., Duan, Y., Li, D.,& Qiu, G. (2010). Synovial fluid level of adiponectin correlated with levels of aggrecan degradation markers in osteoarthritis. *Rheumatol Int* , 1437-160X (Electronic). 0172-8172 (Linking)

Hinze, C.H., Suzuki, M., Klein-Gitelman, M., Passo, M.H., Olson, J., Singer, N.G., Haines, K.A., Onel, K., O'Neil, K., Silverman, E.D., Tucker, L., Ying, J., Devarajan, P.,& Brunner, H.I. (2009). Neutrophil gelatinase-associated lipocalin is a predictor of the course of global and renal childhood-onset systemic lupus erythematosus disease activity. *Arthritis Rheum* , 60,9, 2772-81, 0004-3591 (Print). 0004-3591 (Linking)

Honsawek, S.&Chayanupatkul, M. (2010). Correlation of plasma and synovial fluid adiponectin with knee osteoarthritis severity. *Arch Med Res* , 41,8, 593-8, 1873-5487 (Electronic). 0188-4409 (Linking)

Hotamisligil, G.S., Shargill, N.S.,& Spiegelman, B.M. (1993). Adipose expression of tumor necrosis factor-alpha: direct role in obesity-linked insulin resistance. *Science* , 259,5091, 87-91, 0036-8075 (Print). 0036-8075 (Linking)

Kadowaki, T.&Yamauchi, T. (2005). Adiponectin and adiponectin receptors. *Endocr Rev* , 26,3, 439-51, 0163-769X (Print). 0163-769X (Linking)

Kanalas, J.J.&Hopfer, U. (1997). Effect of TGF-beta 1 and TNF-alpha on the plasminogen system of rat proximal tubular epithelial cells. *J Am Soc Nephrol* , 8,2, 184-92, 1046-6673 (Print). 1046-6673 (Linking)

Katano, M., Okamoto, K., Arito, M., Kawakami, Y., Kurokawa, M.S., Suematsu, N., Shimada, S., Nakamura, H., Xiang, Y., Masuko, K., Nishioka, K., Yudoh, K.,& Kato, T. (2009). Implication of granulocyte-macrophage colony-stimulating factor induced neutrophil gelatinase-associated lipocalin in pathogenesis of rheumatoid arthritis revealed by proteome analysis. *Arthritis Res Ther* , 11,1, R3, 1478-6362 (Electronic). 1478-6354 (Linking)

Kaur, J., Adya, R., Tan, B.K., Chen, J.,& Randeva, H.S. (2010). Identification of chemerin receptor (ChemR23) in human endothelial cells: chemerin-induced endothelial angiogenesis. *Biochem Biophys Res Commun* , 391,4, 1762-8, 1090-2104 (Electronic). 0006-291X (Linking)

Kitahara, K., Kusunoki, N., Kakiuchi, T., Suguro, T.,& Kawai, S. (2009). Adiponectin stimulates IL-8 production by rheumatoid synovial fibroblasts. *Biochem Biophys Res Commun* , 378,2, 218-23, 1090-2104 (Electronic). 0006-291X (Linking)

Koskinen, A., Vuolteenaho, K., Nieminen, R., Moilanen, T.,& Moilanen, E. (2011). Leptin enhances MMP-1, MMP-3 and MMP-13 production in human osteoarthritic cartilage and correlates with MMP-1 and MMP-3 in synovial fluid from OA patients. *Clin Exp Rheumatol* , 29,1, 57-64, 0392-856X (Print). 0392-856X (Linking)

Ku, J.H., Lee, C.K., Joo, B.S., An, B.M., Choi, S.H., Wang, T.H.,& Cho, H.L. (2009). Correlation of synovial fluid leptin concentrations with the severity of osteoarthritis. *Clin Rheumatol* , 28,12, 1431-5, 1434-9949 (Electronic). 0770-3198 (Linking)

Kusunoki, N., Kitahara, K., Kojima, F., Tanaka, N., Kaneko, K., Endo, H., Suguro, T.,& Kawai, S. (2010). Adiponectin stimulates prostaglandin E(2) production in rheumatoid arthritis synovial fibroblasts. *Arthritis Rheum* , 62,6, 1641-9, 1529-0131 (Electronic). 0004-3591 (Linking)

Lago, R., Gomez, R., Otero, M., Lago, F., Gallego, R., Dieguez, C., Gomez-Reino, J.J.,& Gualillo, O. (2008). A new player in cartilage homeostasis: adiponectin induces nitric oxide synthase type II and pro-inflammatory cytokines in chondrocytes. *Osteoarthritis Cartilage* , 16,9, 1101-9, 1522-9653 (Electronic). 1063-4584 (Linking)

Lam, Q.L.&Lu, L. (2007). Role of leptin in immunity. *Cell Mol Immunol* , 4,1, 1-13, 1672-7681 (Print). 1672-7681 (Linking)

Laurberg, T.B., Frystyk, J., Ellingsen, T., Hansen, I.T., Jorgensen, A., Tarp, U., Hetland, M.L., Horslev-Petersen, K., Hornung, N., Poulsen, J.H., Flyvbjerg, A.,& Stengaard-Pedersen, K. (2009). Plasma adiponectin in patients with active, early, and chronic rheumatoid arthritis who are steroid- and disease-modifying antirheumatic drug-naive compared with patients with osteoarthritis and controls. *J Rheumatol* , 36,9, 1885-91, 0315-162X (Print). 0315-162X (Linking)

Lee, J.H., Ort, T., Ma, K., Picha, K., Carton, J., Marsters, P.A., Lohmander, L.S., Baribaud, F., Song, X.Y.,& Blake, S. (2009). Resistin is elevated following traumatic joint injury and causes matrix degradation and release of inflammatory cytokines from articular cartilage in vitro. *Osteoarthritis Cartilage* , 17,5, 613-20, 1522-9653 (Electronic). 1063-4584 (Linking)

Lee, S.W., Park, M.C., Park, Y.B.,& Lee, S.K. (2007). Measurement of the serum leptin level could assist disease activity monitoring in rheumatoid arthritis. *Rheumatol Int* , 27,6, 537-40, 0172-8172 (Print). 0172-8172 (Linking)

Li, Y., Zhang, Y., Dorweiler, B., Cui, D., Wang, T., Woo, C.W., Brunkan, C.S., Wolberger, C., Imai, S.,& Tabas, I. (2008). Extracellular Nampt promotes macrophage survival via a nonenzymatic interleukin-6/STAT3 signaling mechanism. *J Biol Chem* , 283,50, 34833-43, 0021-9258 (Print). 0021-9258 (Linking)

Luangsay, S., Wittamer, V., Bondue, B., De Henau, O., Rouger, L., Brait, M., Franssen, J.D., de Nadai, P., Huaux, F.,& Parmentier, M. (2009). Mouse ChemR23 is expressed in dendritic cell subsets and macrophages, and mediates an anti-inflammatory activity of chemerin in a lung disease model. *J Immunol* , 183,10, 6489-99, 1550-6606 (Electronic). 0022-1767 (Linking)

Maeda, N., Takahashi, M., Funahashi, T., Kihara, S., Nishizawa, H., Kishida, K., Nagaretani, H., Matsuda, M., Komuro, R., Ouchi, N., Kuriyama, H., Hotta, K., Nakamura, T., Shimomura, I.,& Matsuzawa, Y. (2001). PPARgamma ligands increase expression and plasma concentrations of adiponectin, an adipose-derived protein. *Diabetes* , 50,9, 2094-9, 0012-1797 (Print). 0012-1797 (Linking)

Matsuzawa, Y. (2006). Therapy Insight: adipocytokines in metabolic syndrome and related cardiovascular disease. *Nat Clin Pract Cardiovasc Med* , 3,1, 35-42, 1743-4297 (Print). 1743-4297 (Linking)

McTernan, P.G., McTernan, C.L., Chetty, R., Jenner, K., Fisher, F.M., Lauer, M.N., Crocker, J., Barnett, A.H.,& Kumar, S. (2002). Increased resistin gene and protein expression in human abdominal adipose tissue. *J Clin Endocrinol Metab* , 87,5, 2407, 0021-972X (Print). 0021-972X (Linking)

Mutabaruka, M.S., Aoulad Aissa, M., Delalandre, A., Lavigne, M.,& Lajeunesse, D. (2010). Local leptin production in osteoarthritis subchondral osteoblasts may be responsible for their abnormal phenotypic expression. *Arthritis Res Ther* , 12,1, R20, 1478-6362 (Electronic). 1478-6354 (Linking)

Neumeier, M., Weigert, J., Schaffler, A., Wehrwein, G., Muller-Ladner, U., Scholmerich, J., Wrede, C.,& Buechler, C. (2006). Different effects of adiponectin isoforms in human monocytic cells. *J Leukoc Biol* , 79,4, 803-8, 0741-5400 (Print). 0741-5400 (Linking)

Oh, D.K., Ciaraldi, T.,& Henry, R.R. (2007). Adiponectin in health and disease. *Diabetes Obes Metab* , 9,3, 282-9, 1462-8902 (Print). 1462-8902 (Linking)

Olama, S.M., Senna, M.K.,& Elarman, M. (2010). Synovial/Serum leptin ratio in rheumatoid arthritis: the association with activity and erosion. *Rheumatol Int* , 1437-160X (Electronic). 0172-8172 (Linking)

Oliveria, S.A., Felson, D.T., Cirillo, P.A., Reed, J.I.,& Walker, A.M. (1999). Body weight, body mass index, and incident symptomatic osteoarthritis of the hand, hip, and knee. *Epidemiology* , 10,2, 161-6, 1044-3983 (Print). 1044-3983 (Linking)

Otero, M., Gomez Reino, J.J.,& Gualillo, O. (2003). Synergistic induction of nitric oxide synthase type II: in vitro effect of leptin and interferon-gamma in human chondrocytes and ATDC5 chondrogenic cells. *Arthritis Rheum* , 48,2, 404-9, 0004-3591 (Print). 0004-3591 (Linking)

Otero, M., Lago, R., Gomez, R., Lago, F., Dieguez, C., Gomez-Reino, J.J.,& Gualillo, O. (2006). Changes in plasma levels of fat-derived hormones adiponectin, leptin, resistin and visfatin in patients with rheumatoid arthritis. *Ann Rheum Dis* , 65,9, 1198-201, 0003-4967 (Print). 0003-4967 (Linking)

Otero, M., Lago, R., Lago, F., Reino, J.J.,& Gualillo, O. (2005). Signalling pathway involved in nitric oxide synthase type II activation in chondrocytes: synergistic effect of leptin with interleukin-1. *Arthritis Res Ther* , 7,3, R581-91, 1478-6362 (Electronic). 1478-6354 (Linking)

Owen, H.C., Roberts, S.J., Ahmed, S.F.,& Farquharson, C. (2008). Dexamethasone-induced expression of the glucocorticoid response gene lipocalin 2 in chondrocytes. *Am J Physiol Endocrinol Metab* , 294,6, E1023-34 , 0193-1849 (Print). 0193-1849 (Linking)

Procaccini, C., De Rosa, V., Galgani, M., Abanni, L., Cali, G., Porcellini, A., Carbone, F., Fontana, S., Horvath, T.L., La Cava, A.,& Matarese, G. (2010). An oscillatory switch in mTOR kinase activity sets regulatory T cell responsiveness. *Immunity* , 33,6, 929-41, 1097-4180 (Electronic). 1074-7613 (Linking)

Rho, Y.H., Solus, J., Sokka, T., Oeser, A., Chung, C.P., Gebretsadik, T., Shintani, A., Pincus, T.,& Stein, C.M. (2009). Adipocytokines are associated with radiographic joint damage in rheumatoid arthritis . *Arthritis Rheum* , 60,7, 1906-14, 0004-3591 (Print). 0004-3591 (Linking)

Samal, B., Sun, Y., Stearns, G., Xie, C., Suggs, S.,& McNiece, I. (1994). Cloning and characterization of the cDNA encoding a novel human pre-B-cell colony-enhancing factor. *Mol Cell Biol* , 14,2, 1431-7, 0270-7306 (Print). 0270-7306 (Linking)

Schaffler, A., Ehling, A., Neumann, E., Herfarth, H., Tarner, I., Scholmerich, J., Muller-Ladner, U.,& Gay, S. (2003). Adipocytokines in synovial fluid. *JAMA* , 290,13, 1709-10, 1538-3598 (Electronic). 0098-7484 (Linking)

Senolt, L., Housa, D., Vernerova, Z., Jirasek, T., Svobodova, R., Veigl, D., Anderlova, K., Muller-Ladner, U., Pavelka, K.,& Haluzik, M. (2007). Resistin in rheumatoid arthritis synovial tissue, synovial fluid and serum. *Ann Rheum Dis* , 66,4, 458-63, 0003-4967 (Print). 0003-4967 (Linking)

Simopoulou, T., Malizos, K.N., Iliopoulos, D., Stefanou, N., Papatheodorou, L., Ioannou, M.,& Tsezou, A. (2007). Differential expression of leptin and leptin's receptor isoform (Ob-Rb) mRNA between advanced and minimally affected osteoarthritic cartilage; effect on cartilage metabolism. *Osteoarthritis Cartilage* , 15,8, 872-83, 1063-4584 (Print). 1063-4584 (Linking)

Steppan, C.M., Bailey, S.T., Bhat, S., Brown, E.J., Banerjee, R.R., Wright, C.M., Patel, H.R., Ahima, R.S.,& Lazar, M.A. (2001). The hormone resistin links obesity to diabetes. *Nature* , 409, 6818, 307-12, 0028-0836 (Print). 0028-0836 (Linking)

Tang, C.H., Chiu, Y.C., Tan, T.W., Yang, R.S.,& Fu, W.M. (2007). Adiponectin enhances IL-6 production in human synovial fibroblast via an AdipoR1 receptor, AMPK, p38, and NF-kappa B pathway. *J Immunol* , 179 ,8, 5483-92, 0022-1767 (Print). 0022-1767 (Linking)

Targonska-Stepniak, B., Majdan, M.,& Dryglewska, M. (2008). Leptin serum levels in rheumatoid arthritis patients: relation to disease duration and activity. *Rheumatol Int* , 28,6, 585-91, 0172-8172 (Print). 0172-8172 (Linking)

Toussirot, E., Streit, G.,& Wendling, D. (2007). The contribution of adipose tissue and adipokines to inflammation in joint diseases. *Curr Med Chem* , 14,10, 1095-100, 0929-8673 (Print). 0929-8673 (Linking)

Trayhurn, P., Bing, C.,& Wood, I.S. (2006). Adipose tissue and adipokines--energy regulation from the human perspective. *J Nutr* , 136,7 Suppl, 1935S-9S, 0022-3166 (Print). 0022-3166 (Linking)

Trayhurn, P.&Wood, I.S. (2004). Adipokines: inflammation and the pleiotropic role of white adipose tissue. *Br J Nutr* , 92,3, 347-55, 0007-1145 (Print). 0007-1145 (Linking)

Trayhurn, P.&Wood, I.S. (2005). Signalling role of adipose tissue: adipokines and inflammation in obesity. *Biochem Soc Trans* , 33,Pt 5, 1078-81, 0300-5127 (Print). 0300-5127 (Linking)

Triebel, S., Blaser, J., Reinke, H.,& Tschesche, H. (1992). A 25 kDa alpha 2-microglobulin-related protein is a component of the 125 kDa form of human gelatinase. *FEBS Lett* , 314,3, 386-8, 0014-5793 (Print). 0014-5793 (Linking)

Vermi, W., Riboldi, E., Wittamer, V., Gentili, F., Luini, W., Marrelli, S., Vecchi, A., Franssen, J.D., Communi, D., Massardi, L., Sironi, M., Mantovani, A., Parmentier, M., Facchetti, F.,& Sozzani, S. (2005). Role of ChemR23 in directing the migration of myeloid and plasmacytoid dendritic cells to lymphoid organs and inflamed skin. *J Exp Med* , 201, 4, 509-15, 0022-1007 (Print). 0022-1007 (Linking)

Whitehead, J.P., Richards, A.A., Hickman, I.J., Macdonald, G.A.,& Prins, J.B. (2006). Adiponectin--a key adipokine in the metabolic syndrome. *Diabetes Obes Metab* , 8,3, 264-80, 1462-8902 (Print). 1462-8902 (Linking)

Wittamer, V., Franssen, J.D., Vulcano, M., Mirjolet, J.F., Le Poul, E., Migeotte, I., Brezillon, S., Tyldesley, R., Blanpain, C., Detheux, M., Mantovani, A., Sozzani, S., Vassart, G., Parmentier, M.,& Communi, D. (2003). Specific recruitment of antigen-presenting cells by chemerin, a novel processed ligand from human inflammatory fluids. *J Exp Med* , 198,7, 977-85, 0022-1007 (Print). 0022-1007 (Linking)

Yamauchi, T., Nio, Y., Maki, T., Kobayashi, M., Takazawa, T., Iwabu, M., Okada-Iwabu, M., Kawamoto, S., Kubota, N., Kubota, T., Ito, Y., Kamon, J., Tsuchida, A., Kumagai, K., Kozono, H., Hada, Y., Ogata, H., Tokuyama, K., Tsunoda, M., Ide, T., Murakami, K., Awazawa, M., Takamoto, I., Froguel, P. , *et al.* (2007). Targeted disruption of AdipoR1 and AdipoR2 causes abrogation of adiponectin binding and metabolic actions. *Nat Med* , 13,3, 332-9, 1078-8956 (Print). 1078-8956 (Linking)

Zabel, B.A., Allen, S.J., Kulig, P., Allen, J.A., Cichy, J., Handel, T.M.,& Butcher, E.C. (2005). Chemerin activation by serine proteases of the coagulation, fibrinolytic, and inflammatory cascades. *J Biol Chem* , 280,41, 34661-6, 0021-9258 (Print). 0021-9258 (Linking)

Zhang, Y., Proenca, R., Maffei, M., Barone, M., Leopold, L.,& Friedman, J.M. (1994). Positional cloning of the mouse obese gene and its human homologue. *Nature* , 372,6505, 425-32, 0028-0836 (Print). 0028-0836 (Linking)

3

Gene Expression Profiling in Rheumatoid Arthritis

Cornelis L. Verweij and Saskia Vosslamber
Department of Pathology and Rheumatology; VU University Medical Center, Amsterdam, The Netherlands

1. Introduction

Rheumatoid arthritis (RA) is a systemic chronic inflammatory disease that primarily affects the joints. Aetiology of RA is unknown. Once symptoms are present RA manifests itself as a heterogeneous disease with a clinical spectrum ranging from mild to severe disease, and variable involvement in secondary organ systems. The heterogeneous nature is reflected by variation in responsiveness to treatment. The heterogeneity most likely has its origin in its multifactorial nature, whereby specific combinations of environmental factor(s) and genetic factors are likely to influence not only susceptibility but also the disease severity and prognosis. Unfortunately, our understanding of the molecular complexity of RA is incomplete, and criteria for subtyping of patients, e.g. for prognosis to select those patients who will benefit from a specific treatment, are currently lacking.

By definition, nearly every aspect of a disease phenotype should be represented in the pattern of active genes and subsequent transcripts and proteins that are expressed. DNA microarray technology is a powerful technique that enables studying of mRNA levels of all the genes in the genome simultaneously. Application of large-scale gene expression profiling using DNA micro arrays (genomics) of blood and tissue samples from patients with RA allows an open-ended survey to identify comprehensively the fraction of active genes that are specific for a clinical condition (figure 1). This information provides insight in biological pathways contributing to disease and to identify classifiers for early diagnosis, prognosis, and response prediction.

Due to the complexity of the microarray technology and sometimes not optimal powered studies, and high costs associated with use of this technology, several important aspects need to be considered when analyzing micro array data. In almost all cases, the number of transcripts that is measured on an array is much higher than the number of samples included in a study and therefore there is a high change of 'false positives' of which one should be aware and account for in the analysis. Thus, good laboratory proficiency for data acquisition needs to be ensured and appropriate and properly used data analyses practices are essential.

Initially several pitfalls were experienced using this multistage technology. Factors that could influence the sensitivity and reproducibility range from differences in sample storage and processing, variation in amount and quality of starting RNA, RNA amplification and labeling strategies, solid-phase DNA sequences and hybridization conditions. In addition the lack of standardized approaches for normalization and usage of data analysis algorithms could influence the outcome. Hence, the application of perfectly standardized conditions is crucial to generate high quality data points. Moreover, verification of results became an essential step in microarray studies. In order to set quality criteria for performing and publishing microarray studies, standards for microarray experiments and data analysis were created (Brazma et al., 2001).

Cluster algorithms are very useful in visualizing huge datasets obtained with microarray experiments. Data can be clustered according a predetermined separation of the patient samples (supervised), or driven by molecular variation (unsupervised). Very often the data set becomes more comprehensive by selecting only genes that are differentially expressed between groups of patients/samples. Filtering of expression data by applying a threshold for a certain fold change compared to the median expression levels in at least a certain number of patients studied results in a condense and informative set of differentially expressed genes. Additional, pathway-level analyses, and classifier and prediction algorithms can provide more insight in the functional pathways or biological processes and markers for stratification, prognosis and response prediction.

Now, after years of technical and analytical improvement, the technology and algorithms for data analysis are robust and reproducible across properly designed and controlled experiments between different research groups. In addition the introduction of PAXgene (PreAnalytix, GmbH, Germany) whole blood aspiration system, whereby cells are directly lysed and the RNA stabilized, excludes *ex vivo* processing artifacts and forms an essential step in the standardization process. However, careful standardization is still required for cell subsets and tissues that are obtained via *ex vivo* manipulation.

This review describes developments in transcriptomics research to identify novel pathways that contribute to disease and to uncover clinically relevant biomarkers. Ultimately this information may help clinicians to improve disease management.

2. Gene expression profiling in affected target tissues and cells

2.1 The rheumatoid synovium

Since synovitis is the hallmark of rheumatoid arthritis, gene expression analysis was initially aimed to provide insight in the molecular features and biological pathways at play in the affected synovium. The first study on gene expression profiling in rheumatoid synovium highlighted the increased expression of genes involved in chronic inflammation such as immunoglobulins and HLA-DR in RA synovium when compared with normal synovium (Zanders et al., 2000) Comparative analysis of synovial tissue specimen from RA and osteoarthritis (OA) patients revealed that these diseases were characterized by distinct synovial gene signatures (van der Pouw Kraan et al., 2003a; van der Pouw Kraan et al., 2003b; Sha et al. 2003; Devauchelle et al., 2004; Kato et al. 2007; Nzeusseu et al. 2007; Huber et al. 2008). The finding that genes involved in the adaptive immunity (B and T cell regulation) were upregulated in RA tissues confirmed histological findings of increased infiltration of T cells and B cells in the rheumatoid synovium compared to OA. In addition, a number of non-immune genes were found to be differentially expressed between the RA and OA synovium, which were involved in diverse biological processes such as extracellular matrix biology (e.g. fibronectin, fibulin-3 and collagen type IIIa1), transcription and cell cycle regulation (CAK, DNA replication licensing factor, CDK7, FOS, CHD2), receptor/signaling (GBP1 IL1R1, CXCL2, PDGFRA), protease biology (Cathepsin L and Cathepsin D, adhesion paxillin, integrina2, D66) and apoptosis (BECN1). Analysis of 3265 genes led to the discovery of a 21 gene discriminator between RA and OA synovial tissue (Kato et al. 2007). Devauchelle found a 48 gene discriminator out of 5670 genes studied (Devauchelle et al. 2004). Using an array with 1050 gene sequences with a combination of a binary probit model with bayesian variable selection, Sha and colleagues found several small gene sets that led to good classification results. A similar study was performed by Huber and colleagues (Huber et al. 2008) who identified three pathways with significantly higher variances in RA (e.g. B-cell receptor signaling and vascular endothelial growth factor signaling) compared to OA. Functionally, the majority of the identified pathways are involved in the regulation of inflammation, proliferation, cell survival and angiogenesis.

Additional comparative analyses of synovial biopsy tissue from patients with RA, OA and systemic lupus erythematosus (SLE) confirmed and extended observations that distinct diseases were characterized by distinct molecular synovial signatures (Nzeusseu et al. 2007). Overall, tissue profiling in RA and other rheumatic diseases has led to an increase in our understanding of disease pathogenesis. These findings highlight the molecular differences between the RA, OA and SLE synovia and demonstrate that transcriptome analysis provide a rich source for the establishment of diagnostic tools and may lead to identification of novel drug targets.

2.1.1 Heterogeneity between rheumatoid synovial tissues

The lack of a consistent comprehensive transcript profile in RA synovium may be due to the small samples sizes, heterogeneity between disease tissues, differences in appropriate control tissues, and/or technical differences such as the variation in the type and the complexity of the arrays used by the different research groups.

A large-scale gene expression profiling study of 30 synovial tissue specimens from patients with erosive RA revealed considerable heterogeneity among patients (van der Pouw Kraan et al., 2003a; van der Pouw Kraan et al., 2003b). Also Huber and colleagues noted the broad intra-group inter-individual expression variances in RA for genes representing different pathways (e.g. Toll-like receptor signaling pathway, T-cell receptor signaling pathway, Fc epsilon receptor I signaling pathway, adherence junction, classical TGF-β sub-pathway and the anti-apoptotic sub-complex (Huber et al., 2008). Accordingly, Lindberg and colleagues showed that synovial biopsies had gene expression signatures that were unique for each patient (Lindberg et al., 2006a). Heterogeneity is not surprising known the variation in clinical presentation, differences in treatment outcome and complex pathogenesis that changes over time.

Systematic characterization of the differentially expressed genes highlighted the existence of at least two molecularly distinct forms of RA tissues (van der Pouw Kraan et al., 2003a; 2003b). One group, referred to as the RA high inflammation group, was characterized by genes involved in inflammation and adaptive immune response. The genes involved in the high inflammation tissues consist of immunoglobulin genes and genes indicative for an activated IFN/STAT-1 pathway. Seven of these (TIMP2, PDGFRA, GBP1, Fos, CTSL, TUBB and BHLHB2) were also described by Devauchelle and colleagues, of which 2 (GBP1 and CTSL) are known to be regulated by type I IFN (Devauchelle et al., 2004). The second group of RA tissues was characterized by a low inflammation gene signature that was reminiscent of that of tissues from patients with OA. While inflammation and immune-related genes were decreased, these tissues showed an increased expression of genes involved in tissue remodeling activity, which is associated with fibroblast dedifferentiation. Remarkably, the high and low inflammation tissues revealed reciprocal expression of specific matrix metalloproteinases (MMP). Whereas levels of MMP11 and 13 were increased in low inflammation tissues, levels of MMP1 and 3 were increased in high inflammation tissues (van der Pouw Kraan et al., 2003a).

Histological analyses already revealed the existence of different tissue types in the rheumatoid synovium that are related to differences in the cell distribution (Takemura et al., 2001). In approximately 10% of synovial tissues T cells, B cells, and follicular dendritic cells (FDCs) are organized into germinal centres (GC) like structures. The other tissue types lack FDCs and show either a diffuse or an aggregated T-cell and B-cell infiltrate.

The tissues with these so called ectopic GCs were selectively present in the high inflammation tissues. These tissues revealed increased Ig transcript expression with the concomitant presence of B cells and/or plasma cells, which may support local production of antibodies. Gene expression revealed concomitant expression of genes encoding the chemokines CXCL12 and CCL19 and the associated receptors CXCR4 and CXCR5, which are important for the attraction of T cells, B cells, and dendritic cells, in GC containing tissues (Timmer et al., 2007). In addition genes involved in T-cell and B-cell specific pathways, and Fc-receptor type I and JAK/STAT signaling. Elevated expression of IL-7 receptor α(IL-7Rα)/IL-2Rγ chains and IL-7) suggest a role for the IL-7 pathway in synovial lymphoid neogenesis in RA. Tissues with a diffuse type of infiltrate exert evidence of repressed angiogenesis and increased extracellular matrix remodeling.

Overall, the gene expression profiling of rheumatoid synovium has provided insight into the molecular basis of the heterogeneous nature of synovial disease pathogenesis in RA and may facilitate subclassification of patients based on a synovial marker profile *(figure 1)*. However, it remains to be determined if a specific molecular profile applies to all affected synovia in a single patient, and if the profile is stable during the course of disease.

2.2 Gene expression in mesenchymal cells derived from affected target tissues

Fibroblast-like synoviocytes (FLS) are major players in joint destruction in RA. FLS have a transformed phenotype and act as sentinel cells that contribute to leucocyte migration and local immune response through the production of various immune modulators (Smith et al., 1997; Hogaboam et al., 1998; Brouty-Bové et al. 2000). Reversibly, the soluble factors, such as cytokines and growth factors released from the immune cells, in combination with cell-cell interactions likely activate FLS and influence their behavior. One of the first gene expression analyses of in-vitro cultured FLS clearly demonstrated over-expression of genes responsible for tumor-like growth (Watanabe et al., 2002). Analysis of the expression of 588 known cancer-related genes revealed increased expression of PDGFRα, PAI-1 and SDF1A by FLS from five patients with RA compared to FLS from five traumatic control patients. Galligan and colleagues performed a comparative gene expression analysis on FLS cultured from RA

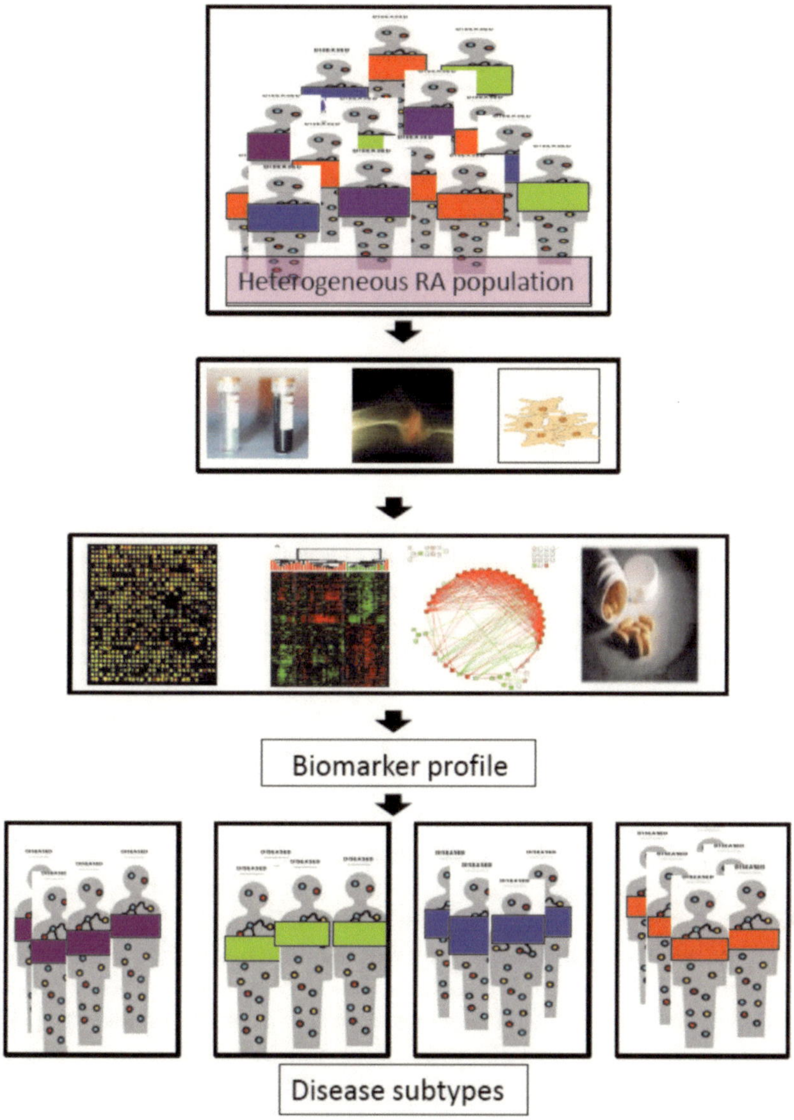

Fig. 1. Schematic outline for disease subclassification in RA

Legend: RA patients reveal a striking heterogeneity based on clinical, biological and molecular criteria. Categorization of patients is crucial for decision making in clinical practice. Recent developments in high-throughput screening technologies makes it possible to characterize patients based on their molecular profile. Application of DNA-microarrays enables the generation of a transcript profile (barcode) of an individual patient. When associated with clinical read-outs clinical useful molecular markers could be selected and applied in day-to-day clinical practice. The procedure starts with collecting biosamples (e.g. peripheral blood cells) from each patient. The biosample can be processed to isolate mRNA and then further analyzed using DNA-microarray technology. Subsequently, computational algorithms will be applied to select biomarkers that allow subtyping of patients. This approach helps to elucidate the distinct pathological mechanisms that can explain the inter-patient variation, disease progression, and treatment response.

(17), OA (20) and trauma (6) joint tissue using affymetrix microarrays (Galligan et al., 2007). A total of 34 genes were significant differentially expressed between RA and OA FLS. Genes highly and exclusively expressed by RA FLS are HOXD10, HOXD11, HOXD13, CCL8 and LIM homeobox 2. Genes encoding CLU, sarcoglycan-y, GPR64, POU3F3, peroxisome proliferative activated receptor-y and tripartite motif-containing 2 were exclusively expressed in OA FLS. Interestingly, only a few of the significant differently expressed in FLS also differed between the total synovial tissue expression profiles, suggesting that the contribution of the synovial lining cells is not dominant in the total tissue profile. Alternatively, the transcriptome of in-vitro cultured FLS may not be representative for the genuine transcriptome of in situ FLS. Evidence that in vitro cultured FLS gene expression changes are beyond the 10% when passaged less than 6 times, as was done by Galligan and colleagues, suggest that this was not the case (Nuemann et al., 2010). However, formal proof by comparison of in-vitro cultured FLS with in-situ FLS (via e.g. Laser Capture Microscopy derived cells) is lacking.

Others investigated the effects of tumour necrosis factor (TNF) and IL-1b on FLS. TNF and IL-1b have been shown to be of primary importance in the effector phase of the disease. Defining TNF-α and IL-1b response signatures in FLS may be instrumental for application in pharmacology studies to monitor the effects of TNF and IL-1b blockade. In an early microarray study 96 inflammatory genes were studied in cytokine-stimulated RA-FLS cells. A number of cytokine-regulated genes such as IL-6, CXCL8, CXCL1, MMP-1, MMP-3, MMP-8 and VCAM-1 were identified (Heller et al., 1997). Additional studies using arrays with higher complexity (12.600 genes) revealed that TNF affected the expression of genes representing cytokines and inflammatory mediators, extracellular matrix and adhesion molecules, cell cycle and proliferation related proteins, transcription related proteins, and apoptotic mediators (Gallagher et al., 2003). One of these TNF-response genes, Nef-associated factor-1 (Naf1, an A20-binding, nuclear factor kappa B (NFkB) inhibitory protein), was identified as indicator for TNF-bioactivity. This analysis revealed higher expression in synovial biopsies from patients with active RA and seronegative arthropathy than in those from patients with OA. Taberner and colleagues showed that there exists a broad overlap between TNF- and IL-1b response genes. Out of 12600 genes tested 126 genes were regulated by both TNF and IL-1b, 65 genes were specifically regulated by IL-1b (e.g. G-CSF, CXCL6, CCL4, PAI-1, OAS 40kD and VEGF) and 21 genes by TNF (e.g. CXCL19, CXCL11, PIAS3, ID1, MAPKKK4) (Taberner et al., 2005). It is likely that these response signatures contain numerous genes that contribute critically to the pathogenesis of RA and provide a framework to unravel IL-1b and TNF driven effector pathways.

Detailed analysis of the gene expression profiles clearly revealed that the profiles are not uniform between RA patients, analogous to the gene expression of the synovial tissues. Transcriptome analysis of FLSs derived from 19 RA patients using microarrays with a complexity of 24,000 cDNA elements, revealed 3 molecular profiles, indicative for the existence of 3 FLS subtypes (Kasperkovitz et al., 2005). Accordingly, others also noted marked heterogeneity in both the gene expression profile (Galligan et al. 2004) as well as the sensitivity to proinflammatory cytokines between FLS derived from different RA patients (Taberner et al. 2007). Correlation studies of paired synovial tissue and FLS clustering revealed that heterogeneity at the synovial tissue level is associated with a specific phenotypic characteristic of the cultured resident FLS (Kaperkovitz et al., 2005). The high inflammation tissues were associated with an FLS subtype that exhibits similarity with so-called myofibroblasts. The myofibroblast is a specialized fibroblast that has acquired the capacity to express α-smooth muscle actin, an actin isoform that is typical of vascular smooth muscle cells. The myofibroblast is a specialized fibroblast that plays a key role in connective tissue remodelling and contributes to cell infiltration. These cells are characterized by a markedly increased expression of genes that represent the transforming growth factor (TGF)-β response programme. Among these response genes were SMA, SERPINE1, COL4A1 (type IV collagen-α chain), IER3 (immediate early response 3), TAGLN (transgelin) and the gene encoding activin A, which is a potential agonist for the induction of the TGF-β response programme. Similar cells were recently identified in the human $TNF^{+/-}$-transgenic mouse model of arthritis (Aidinis et al., 2005). Moreover, Pohlers and colleagues noted constitutive activation of the TGF-β pathway in RA FLS (Pohlers et al., 2007). A significant positive correlation were observed between the constitutive expression of TGF-β1 mRNA (but not protein) and the serum levels of C-reactive protein was observed. Myofibroblasts may play a crucial role in angiogenesis through the production of extracellular matrix proteins, chemokines and growth factors, as has been shown in the field of oncology. Hence, it is proposed that these cells contribute to angiogenesis in the rheumatoid synovium. This finding supports the hypothesis that phenotypic variation between FLS may be causally related to the inflammation status of the target tissue.

2.3 Gene expression in rheumatoid bone marrow

Evidence exists that bone marrow-derived mononuclear cells (BMMC) contribute to the pathogenesis of RA (Ochi et al., 1988; Jongen-Lavrencic et al., 1997; Hirohata et al., 2004). The bone marrow harbors three types of stem cells: the mesenchymal stem cells, the hematopoietic stem cells and the endothelial stem cells. The local cell-cell interactions and soluble factors act in a sophisticated network that regulates the proliferation and differentiation of these cells. Elevated levels of IL-6 and IL-8 in RA bone marrow serum was reported to be associated with synovial hyperplasia (Tanabe et al., 1994). Comparative gene expression profiling between RA and OA BMMC revealed marked variation between the two diseases (Nakamura et al., 2006; Lee et al., 2011). Transcriptome analysis identified 2,674 genes which were differentially expressed between RA and OA BMMC (Lee et al., 2011). Marked upregulated genes were classified as immune response genes, which were highly relevant to the antigen presentation pathway (e.g. HLA-E, HLA-F, HLA-G, tapasin (TAP), TAP binding protein) and interferon (IFN) signaling (e.g. IFITM1, IFITM3, IFI16, MAPK14, MyD88, IL8). In a third network IFNγ played a central role (e.g. PSM8, PSM9, CLEC5A, CLEC4E). A fourth network was centered around HNF4 and involved in lipid metabolism, coagulation and negative regulation of cell growth. The downregulated genes were dominantly related to cell cycle and DNA metabolism. These findings provide important information to abnormal BMMC biology in RA. It remains to be determined why these processes are disturbed and how these abnormalities contribute to the pathogenesis of RA.

2.4 Gene expression in blood cells

Known the systemic nature of RA and the communication between the systemic and organ specific compartments, whole blood and/or peripheral blood mononuclear cells (PBMC) is a useful compartment to study the disease-related gene expression profiles. Because of the low-invasiveness blood aspiration this compartment is extremely suitable for explorative studies in large cohorts of patients to identify clinically relevant biomarkers.

Several investigators studied gene expression levels in peripheral blood cells to address the question, whether disease specific features were present in peripheral blood cells. Bovin and colleagues identified 25 genes immune related genes (e.g. calcium-binding proteins S100A8 and S100A12) that discriminated between PBMC of RA patients (n=14) and healthy controls (n=7) (Bovin et al., 2004). S100A8 and S100A12 (calgranulins C) belong to a class of inflammatory mediators, and function as heterodimers. These proteins are released by e.g. activated monocytes upon interaction with activated endothelial cells under inflammatory conditions and mediate leukocyte migration and adhesion to vascular endothelium. Liao et al. used tandem mass spectrometry (MS/MS), coupled with multidimensional liquid chromatography (LC) to identify biomarkers of disease severity in the synovial fluid and serum of patients with RA (Liao et al., 2004). Levels of CRP, S100A8, S100A9 and S100A12 were elevated in the serum of patients with erosive disease compared with patients with non-erosive RA. No significant differences between RF positive and RF negative RA were observed. In a larger study with 29 RA patients and 21 healthy controls Batliwalla and colleagues identified 81 differentially expressed genes (e.g glutaminyl cyclase, IL1RA, S100A12 and Grb2-associated binding protein (GAB2) as the main discriminators. This profile correlated with an increased monocyte count (Batliwalla et al., 2005). Studies with a preselected set of 96 genes in PBMC from IBD, psoriasis and RA patients, and healthy controls revealed genes (e.g. ADM, AQQ9, CXCL12, IL10, NAMPT) that were specific for the chronic inflammatory diseases in general, and disease specific genes (Mesko et al., 2010). Genes that were specific for RA included mainly downregulated genes e.g CCL4, CCL5, CDNK1C, CYP51A1, FGL2, HMGB1, IL23R, and PTPN22, and only IL-8 as upregulated gene. Additional studies on peripheral blood cells, including analyses on whole blood cell samples (PAXgene) confirmed and further extended the molecular differences between the peripheral blood compartment between healthy controls and RA patients (van der Pouw Kraan et al., 2007; 2008; Teixeira et al., 2009). Additional genes that Teixeira and colleagues identified include Ly96/MD2, NFAT5, thioredoxin, CAP/LL37, ORM1, ORM2, SLC11A1, PGLyRP1 and Factor V.

Van der Pouw Kraan and colleagues observed that a prominent cluster of IFN-response genes was significantly upregulated in patients with RA indicating that this pathway is systemically activated in RA (van der Pouw Kraan et al., 2007). This cluster contains highly correlated genes such as IFRG28 (28 kDa interferon-responsive protein), IFI35 (interferon-induced protein 35), IFI44L (interferon-induced protein 44-like), IFIT1 (interferon-induced protein with tetratricopeptide repeats 1), IFIT2, IRF2 (interferon-regulatory factor 2), IRF7, GIP2 (interferon a-inducible protein 2), GIP3, SERPING1 (serine proteinase inhibitor clade G member 1, C1 inhibitor), OAS1 (29-59-oligoadenylate synthetase 1), OAS2, MX1 (Myxovirus resistance 1), ISG15 (interferon-induced protein 15) and RSAD2 (radical S-adenosyl methionine domain containing 2). These findings have now been replicated in several other studies using independent cohorts (Thurlings et al., 2010; O'Hanlon et al., 2011; Higgs et al., 2011; Vosslamber et al., 2011). Moreover, IFN-bioactivity was measured in RA serum. Comparative analyses on the extent of the IFN response activity in the blood cells of RA and

SLE patients revealed a 5-fold higher level of expression in SLE compared to RA patients (Higgs et al. 2011, Vosslamber et al., unpublished observation).

2.4.1 Gene expression heterogeneity in blood vs. synovial tissue

Synovial tissue heterogeneity is likely to reflect differences in the underlying disease pathogenesis. Because of the migration of immune cells to and from lesional sites via the blood as well as the recirculation of immune cells between central and peripheral lymphoid organs, the PB compartment could be an easy accessible compartment to monitor the (immune)pathophysiology of the synovial tissue. Hence, a critical question to answer is whether molecular heterogeneity at the synovial tissue level is reflected in the blood. The identification of processes and biomarkers in PB may facilitate informative studies of a relation between tissue type and clinical parameter. The notion that molecular heterogeneity is present in both the synovial as well as the PB compartment makes it tempting to speculate on molecular and biological features that reflect the tissue pathology (van Baarsen et al., 2010b). However, paired analysis of peripheral blood and affected synovium from 17 patients with RA revealed that differential tissue pathology was not reflected in the PB by differential expression of single genes. Pathway-level analysis showed that co-ordinately regulated genes involved in protein synthesis in PB were associated with high-inflammation tissue types. The increased protein synthesis activity in PB could provide a framework for further studies to identify PB biomarkers representative for the tissue inflammation status.

2.4.2 A type I IFN response signature in the peripheral blood of a subset of RA patients

The significantly differential expression of the IFN-response genes indicates that this pathway is activated systemically in RA. Van der Pouw Kraan provided evidence that this signature is specific for type I IFNs (IFNα/β) (van der Pouw Kraan et al., 2006). Thus this type I IFN signature may be a direct reflection of increased type I IFN activity or other ligands known to activate the type I IFN/STAT-1 pathway. The fact that the serum IFN bioactivity could be inhibited by neutralizing antibodies directed against IFNα and IFNβ, provides evidence for a role of both type I IFNs in the induction of IFN type I response activity in RA (Mavragani et al., 2009). Upregulation of type I IFN-response genes has now been observed in peripheral blood cells and/or target tissues of (a subset of) patients with autoimmune diseases such as RA, SLE (Baechler et al. 2005), SSc (Tan et al, 2006; Bos et al., 2009), SS (Mavragani & Crow, 2010), multiple sclerosis (Van Baarsen et al., 2006) and type 1 diabetes. These findings suggest that an activated IFN response gene expression program is a common denominator in chronic inflammatory diseases in general.

Interestingly, the increased expression of the type I IFN response genes was characteristic of not all, but approximately half of the RA patients, consistent with the heterogeneous nature of RA. Moreover, the immune defense gene program that was activated in the subgroup of RA patients was reminiscent to that of virus-infected macaques (van der Pouw Kraan et al., 2008). Comparative analysis between paired tissue and peripheral blood profile revealed that there exists no concordance in the presence of IFN-response activity between the two compartments (van Baarsen et al., 2010a)

2.5 Monozygotic twins and first degree relatives

O'Hanlon and colleagues studied gene expression profiles of monozygotic (MZ) twin pairs discordant for RA, SLE and idiotypic inflammatory myopathies, their unaffected twins and healthy controls (O'Hanlon et al., 2011). Probands differed significantly in gene expression for 92 genes involving several pathways including immune responses, signaling pathways, transcription/translation regulators, and metabolic functions. As part of the immune response genes they observed that IFN-response genes (IFI27, OASF, PLSCR1, EIF2AK2, TNFAIP6, and TNFSF10) were up-regulated in probands compared to unrelated controls. In unaffected twins intermediate ordering was observed for 84 of the 104 transcripts whose expression differed significantly between probands and unrelated controls. Suggesting that unaffected twins may be in a transitional or intermediate state of immune dysregulation between twins with an autoimmune disease and unrelated controls, perhaps predisposing them to the development of systemic autoimmune diseases given the necessary and sufficient environmental exposures. Maas and colleagues, reported similar results when comparing gene expression profiles between PBMCs from patients and unrelated unaffected individuals (Maas et al., 2005). A total of 127 genes was shared between patients with autoimmune diseases and unaffected first-degree relatives. This commonality between affected and unaffected first-degree relatives suggests a genetic basis for these shared gene expression profiles.

2.6 B-lymphocytes

Szodoray and colleagues compared gene expression differences in pooled peripheral blood B cells from 8 RA patients to the pool of B cells from 8 healthy controls (Szodoray et al., 2006). A total 536 genes were differentially expressed between rheumatoid and healthy B-cells (e.g. S100A9, S100A9, CNNM4, BARD1, U5-116KD, TLR9, IL5-RA, IL-10, IL12A, PTX3, CRLF1, CHRNB1, DRD2, MMP28, VEGFC and FOXo3a). These genes were involved in diverse processes including cell–cycle regulation, proliferation, apoptosis, autoimmunity, cytokine networks, angiogenesis and neuron-immune regulation. E.g. the overexpression of FoxO3a in B cells from patients with RA is reported by others and may increased survival of blood PMNs and T lymphocytes. Functional pathway analysis demonstrated that many of these genes were regulated by cytokine and growth factor activity and correlated with significantly increased serum levels of IL-1b, IL-5, IL-6, IL-10, IL-12p40, IL-17 and VEGF, whereas 231 genes were downregulated in RA B cells.

2.7 CD4 T-lymphocytes

Gene expression analysis of CD4 T cells from 21 patients with RA revealed marked heterogeneity between patients reflected by differential expression of 29 genes (including IFI27, Col6A1, RASD1, TLR4, APOA1, SPP1) in processes such as Toll-like receptor signaling pathway, Calcium signaling pathway, cell adhesion molecules, PPAR signaling pathway, and fatty acid metabolism. The differential expression of IFI27 between patients is in line with earlier observations of interindividual differences in IFN type I response activity among RA patients (Chen et al., 2010).

3. Clinical relevant gene signatures

The success of novel insight in molecular patterns and biological processes in disease pathogenesis and the ability to categorize patients based on molecular criteria held out the promise that this approach might yield clinical useful information. Hence, the next research challenge is to use this information on molecular interindividual heterogeneity to the benefit of patients. Research in this field has primarily focused on (very) early diagnosis, prognosis and prediction of therapy responsiveness.

3.1 Genes and signatures involved in disease activity

Molecular heterogeneity at the tissue level can be a consequence of disease stage and duration. Van Baarsen and colleagues studied the synovial tissue gene expression profiles in relation to immunohistochemical scores and disease parameters. The results demonstrated an excellent correlation between molecular and immunohistochemical scoring (van Baarsen et al., 2010b). Moreover, the high inflammation tissue type was predominantly observed in patients with high disease activity and short disease duration, suggesting temporal differences in the inflammatory status during the course of the disease (Firestein & Zvaifler, 2002). These findings support the hypothesis that RA progresses from an inflammatory, and T- and B-cell driven disease to a more immune-independent process that may be driven by "transformed" FLS (Firestein & Zvaifler, 2002).

The strong association of FLS subtype with synovial tissue inflammation status suggests that FLS markers correlate with disease parameters. Galligan and colleagues showed several significant correlations; (HLA)-DQA2 with HAQ score; Clec12A with RF; MAB21L2, SIAT7E, HAPLN1 and BAIAP2L1 with CRP level; RGMB and OSAP with ESR. Liu and colleagues (2009) identified 19 genes (e.g. COL4A1, TFCP2, FHL3, SKIL, F2RL, PPP1R12B, LTBR, GADD45A, ACYP1) that enabled prediction of future disease activity (Liu et al., 2009).

3.2 Genes and signatures involved in early vs. late RA

Studies on differences in the PBMC gene expression profiles between early (disease duration less than 2 years) and established RA (with an average disease duration of 10 years) marked 53 genes with a three-fold difference in expression. A total of 9 genes, including colony stimulating factor 3 receptor, cleavage stimulation factor, and TGFβ receptor II, were upregulated in the early RA group. The deregulated genes were involved in immunity and cell cycle regulation. Since a quarter of the early arthritis genes overlapped with an influenza-induced gene set it was suggested that the early arthritis signature may partly reflect the response to an unknown infectious agent (Olsen et al., 2004). Accordingly, van der Pouw Kraan and colleagues observed similarity with a common virus response signature in a subset of RA patients (van der Pouw Kraan et al., 2008). Not surprisingly, the majority of these patients had an activated IFN-response program. Although no formal proof for a direct involvement of an infectious agent in RA, these findings suggest at least the presence of an activated pathogen response program in a subset of the patients. A comparative analysis between synovial tissues of RA patients suggested molecular differences between early (< 9 months) and late (> 4years) RA (Lequerre et al., 2009). However, due to the very limited sample size and role of confounding factors (age, treatment, serology) the authors could not exclude a contribution of these factors for the observed differences.

Tsubaki and colleagues applied laser capture microscopy technology to evaluate the synovial lining cells in early (<12 months) and late RA (>5 years) patients (Tsubaki et al., 2005). First, they demonstrated that tissue heterogeneity within RA can already be observed in the phase of RA. The early RA patients could be divided in at least two different groups based on their gene expression profiles. A subgroup with exclusively early RA synovia was characterized by abundant expression of fibronectin1, B2-microglobulin, syndecan, cathepsin B, STAT-1, integrin-b2 and IFNGR2. The other group with cases of both long standing RA and early RA had an increased expression of CASP9, p53-induced gene 11, cathepsin G, CSF2RB, TNFRSF1A and IL-10RB. where expressed at a lower level. Gene expression profiling of synovial tissue of early versus long-standing rheumatoid arthritis suggest stage specific molecular patterns indicative for involvement of different pathophysiological mechanisms during the disease course of RA. A picture emerges that early RA is characterized by elevated expression of genes involved in immune-defense mechanisms, stress response and apoptosis, whereas long-standing RA showed increased expression of genes involved in proliferative processes.

3.3 Pharmacogenomics in RA towards personalized medicine

Gene expression profiling may also proof valuable for the predicting responses to therapy. In general a substantial percentage of patients do not respond to anti-rheumatic therapies, either DMARDs or biological. In particular expensive therapies with biologicals to target proinflammatory mediators of TNF, T- and B-lymphocytes, which are approved worldwide for the treatment of RA urged the need for predictors for therapy response. Clinical experience showed that the targeted therapies with biologicals are not effective for approximately 30-40% of the patients. Given the destructive nature of RA, the risk of adverse effects, and considerable costs for biologics therapy, there is a strong need to make predictions on success before the start of therapy.

In the late 1990s the term *pharmacogenomics* was introduced to frame gene expression profiling studies to delineate processes and identify biomarkers that correlate with the differential clinical outcome of pharmacological intervention. *Pharmacogenomics* is defined as: "The investigation of variations of DNA (genetics) and RNA (transcriptomics) characteristics as related to drug response". The value of pharmacogenomics in guiding clinical management has been highly appreciated in the field of oncology, as can be exemplified by the use of a gene signature to predict the response outcome of patients with breast cancer (Van 't Veer et al., 2002).

3.3.1 Pharmacogenomics of TNF-blockade

In the field of rheumatology specifically the response to TNF-blockers gained much attention. Currently 5 different TNF blockers are registered for clinical use in RA: A soluble TNF-receptor-Fc fusion protein Enbrel® (Etanercept), and 4 monoclonal antibodies directed against TNF Remicade® (Infliximab), Humira® (Adalumimab), Cinzia® (Certolizumab) and Simponi® (Golimumab).

3.3.2 Pharmacodynamics of TNF-blockade

Initial studies focused on the pharmacological effects of TNF blockade in the peripheral blood compartment in order to gain a comprehensive understanding of the mode of action. Global qualitative and quantitative pharmacogenomic analysis on peripheral blood cells suggest that all RA patients treated revealed an overall similar pharmacological response pattern, indicative of the presence of bioactive TNF in the circulation irrespective of clinical response (Van Baarsen et al., 2010c; Batliwalla et al., 2008). These findings suggest a model for the parallel presence of TNF-dependent and TNF-independent disease pathways in the individual patient, whereby the effect of anti-TNF therapy may be dependent on the relative contribution of the TNF-independent pathways. Meugnier and colleagues studied changes in PBMC gene expression after 12 wk of treatment with either etanercept or adalimumab from responder RA patients (Meugnier et al., 2011). Two hundred fifty-one genes displayed significant changes. Genes encoding S100A12 and A8, CD14 antigen, Selectin P, or ribosomal protein L39, reported to be upregulated in RA patients, were found to be decreased upon TNF-blockade. Pathway level analysis revealed that inflammation, immune response, apoptosis, protein synthesis, and mitochondrial oxido-reduction were the most affected pathways in response to anti-TNF-α treatment. Detailed analyses in search of (subtle) differences in the pharmacodynamic changes between responders and non-responders identified IFN-response genes as an informative sets of genes. The regulation of IFN-response genes by infliximab in RA turned out not to be as consistent as previously described for patients with SOJIA (Palucka et al., 2005), but varies between patients. A decrease in IFN-activity appears to be associated with good clinical responses (van Baarsen et al., 2010d; Sekiguchi et al., 2008). Koczan and colleagues reported that early downregulation of genes involved in different pathways and cellular processes such as TNFα signalling via NFκB, NFκB-independent signalling via cAMP, and the regulation of cellular and oxidative stress response (e.g. NFKBIA, CCL4, IL8, IL1B, TNFAIP3, PDE4B, PPP1R15A and ADM) were associated with a good clinical outcome to etanercept-based on ΔDAS >1.2. (Koczan et al., 2008). These studies demonstrated that observing the dynamics of the TNF-blocker intervention may provide insight into the biology of TNF blockade.

3.3.3 Prediction of response to TNF blockade

In an attempt to predict the response prior to treatment several studies have been performed. Initial analyses of synovial tissue gene expression profiles prior to the start of infliximab therapy suggested that patients with features of an activated immune status in their tissue compartment are more likely to benefit from anti-TNF treatment based on ΔDAS28 response criteria (Van der Pouw Kraan et al., 2008; Lindberg et al., 2006). Similar findings were reported for baseline serum markers associated with responsiveness (Hueber et al., 2009). In contrast, Badot and colleagues identified 439 genes involved in cell division and regulation of immune response (e.g. cytokines, chemokines and their receptors) that were associated with poor response based on EULAR criteria (Badot et al., 2009). A recent study performed in 62 RA patients by Lindberg et al. demonstrated an overrepresentation of lymphoid aggregates in EULAR responders (infliximab), in line with the earlier described relationship between inflammation and clinical outcome (Lindberg et al. 2010). These authors also caution for the confounding effect of cellular complexity, suggesting the use of microdissected cell population for explorative genomic synovial tissue analyses.

In the ideal situation a prediction should be made prior to the start of therapy in an easily accessible biosample, such as peripheral blood. Ultimately, this may lead to apply therapy to each patient that is best suited for the patient, also called "personalized medicine". A number of studies focussed on the delineation of baseline differences in peripheral blood cells (whole blood and PBMC) with the purpose of predicting response (Lequerre et al.2006; Koczan et al., 2008; Sekiguchi et al. 2008; Tanino et al. 2009; Julia et al., 2009a; Bienkoska et al., 2009; Van Baarsen et al., 2010c, 2010d; Stuhlmuller et al., 2010). The results of these studies made clear that identification of predictors in the blood compartment is not trivial. Whereas several groups reported the absence of significant gene expression differences between responders and non-responders others were able to identify such markers. In 2006 Lequerre and colleagues report promising results of a study with 33 patients (13 patients in the test group and 20 patients in a validation group) using a in-house made microarray covering 10,000 unique genes, wherein they identified a gene set (consisting of AKAP9, COX7AL2, ELMOD2, EPS15, FBOX5, HLA-DPB1, LAMR1, MCP, MRLP22, MTCBP1, PFKFB4, PSMB9, PTPN12, QIL1, RASGRP3, RPL35, RSP16, RSP28, SCAM1 and TBL2) that predicts the response to infliximab based on the ΔDAS28>1.2 score after 3 months (Lequerre te al. 2006). A selected set of 8 gene transcripts (MTCBP1, AKAP9, RASGRP3, PTPN12, RSP28, HLA-DPB1, MRPL22 and EPS15) allowed them to predict the response with a sensitivity of 80% and a specificity of 100%. Julia and colleagues performed a gene expression analysis using a 47k gene bead array on whole blood RNA samples from 43 RA patients starting infliximab therapy (training set 29 and validation set 14) (Julia et al., 2009a). The clinical response was determined at week 14 using the EULAR criteria. They found an 8 gene classifier consisting of HLA-DRB3, SH2D1B, GNLY, CAMP, SLC2A3, IL2RB, MXD4 and TLR5 that predicted response with a sensitivity of 91.6% and specificity of 50%. In parallel, they observed a significantly higher number of CD4+CD25+ cells (i.e. regulatory T cells) in the responder group compared to the non responder group at baseline. Tanino and colleagues studied whole blood of 68 patients (training set 42 and validation set 26) using a 44k gene microarrays to study. They measured EULAR response criteria at week 14 and discovered a 10 transcript biomarker set consisting of PSPH, CLGN, C21orf58, TBC1D8, LOC643981, ATP51, ANKRD55, TMEM141 and an EST (A_32_P1144), that had a positive predictive value of 80% and a negative predictive value of 44.4% (Tinino et al., 2009). Bienkowska and colleagues constructed a predictor based on 8 gene (CLTB, MXRA7, CXorf52, COL4A3BP, YIPF6, BOD1L, SFRS2 and PGK1) using PBMC of 46 RA patients prior to the start of adalimumab, etanercept, or infliximab. Response status at 14 weeks was based on EULAR criteria (Bienkowska et al. 2009). The accuracy (86%), sensitivity and specificity of the predictor is confirmed by an independent validation data set of 11 patients. Stuhlmuller and colleagues identified a predictor for adalimumab monotherapy using purified monocytes from 77 RA patients (training set of 7 patients and validation set of 70 patients). Clinical outcome was based on the ACR response >20 criteria. They identified CD11c as predictive marker for adalumimab monotherapy (sensitivity 100% and specificity 91.7%). However, CD11c was not predictive of response to adalumimab in combination with MTX (Stuhlmuller et al. 2010).

An important conclusion is that the study results are inconsistent and that the predictive genes from the different studies showed no overlap. How relevant this is for proper prediction and whether this is the consequence of differences in cell source, technological variation (e.g. array platform), data analysis system used, differences in study populations and/or differences in clinical management of the patients remains to be determined. Clearly there is a high need for independent validation and standardization in protocols and technology to understand the basis for the varying results.

3.4 Pharmacogenomics of anakinra

Anakinra is an IL-1-receptor that neutralizes IL-1 activity. Anakinra has proven effective in reducing joint inflammation, pain and bone destruction. However, as with all therapies in RA a substantial percentage of patients do not respond to anakinra. A gene expression study of PBMC of 32 patients (training set of 14 patients and validation set of 18 patients) using an in-house made microarray with a complexity of 10,000 genes identified a 7 gene set (GTF2F2, CCT3, CROT, HNRPA3, ARL15, TMED5, NRG3) that proofed capable to identify responders and non-responders with a sensitivity of 80% and a specificity of 87.5% based on the ΔDAS28>1.2 criteria (Bansard et al., 2011). Strikingly, there was no overlap between genes that were differentially expressed between anakinra and infliximab specific responders and non-responders. (Lequerre et al. 2006) that would be expected based on the crossregulation of IL-1 and TNF. (Lequerre et al. 2006) These results are promising but require validation in a larger independent cohort.

3.5 Pharmacogenomics of rituximab

B cell depletion therapy via rituximab (an anti-CD20 antibody) was shown to be highly effective for suppression of disease activity in RA (Edwards et al., 2004). CD20 is expressed on immature to mature B cells, as well as memory cells, but not on stem cells or precursor cells and, importantly, antibody producing plasma cells. Currently, rituximab is generally used after failure of at least one TNF antagonist. Clinical studies have demonstrated that not all patients show a favorable response to rituximab therapy. Especially the fact that rituximab directly depletes specific B cell populations in all patients treated, irrespective of clinical outcome, has raised questions regarding the mechanism of action.

3.5.1 Pharmacodynamics of rituximab

Gene expression profiling on whole blood cells of 13 RA patients demonstrated that pharmacological responses under the influence of rituximab treatment are highly heterogeneous between patients (Vosslamber et al. 2011). A difference in the kinetics of only a cluster of type I IFN-response genes during rituximab treatment that distinguishes responders from non-responders was observed. Responders exhibited an increase in IFN-response activity after three months treatment with rituximab, whereas the IFN-response activity remained stable during treatment in the non-responders. Thus, whereas rituximab depletes B cells in all patients treated irrespective of their clinical response, gene expression data show that a drug-induced increase of type I IFN-response activity is associated with clinical response. Gutierrez-Roelens and colleagues showed that immunoglobulin genes and genes involved in chemotaxis, leukocyte activation, and immune responses were dowregulated in the synovium at 3 months after the start of therapy (Gutierrez et al., 2011).

3.5.2 Prediction of response to rituximab

Gene expression studies were also performed to search for molecular biomarkers present in RA patients before the start of treatment in relation to the clinical outcome. Julia and colleagues studied whole blood, T cell and B cell profiles of 9 RA patients (Julia et al., 2009). The clinical outcome was determined using the relative improvement of DAS28 activity (relDAS28) after 24 weeks. Several genes were identified that were differential expressed between responders and non-responders at baseline (eg. ARG1, TRAF-1 and TLR4). In another study it was observed that the clinical outcome (based on ΔDAS28 and EULAR criteria) to rituximab is significantly associated with the IFN-response activity prior to the start of treatment (Vosslamber et al., 2011). Good responders have a low or absent IFN-response activity at baseline, whereas non-responders have an activated type I IFN-systems before the start of treatment. During therapy the IFN-activity increases in the IFN^{low} patients and remains stable in the IFN^{high} patients. The association between baseline type I IFN levels and clinical response is in line with previous findings wherein it was demonstrated in two different cohorts (n=20 and n=31) that patients with a low IFN signature had a significantly greater reduction in the DAS28 and more often achieved a EULAR response at weeks 12 and 24 (Thurlings et al., 2010). The clinical utility of the IFN-signature to predict non-responders was demonstrated in an independent study by Receiver Operating Characteristic (ROC)-curve characteristics analyses (unpublished observation).

Overall the above studies demonstrate that it may be feasible to select gene-expression based prognostic biomarkers for rituximab response outcome from the peripheral blood that have clinical relevance.

4. Gene expression in the preclinical (asymptomatic) phase of RA

One of the main goals in the prevention of the disease lies in early diagnosis followed by timely start of effective treatment in order to induce remission. Ideally, early diagnosis in the asymptomatic/preclinical phase is required. Several studies have documented the appearance of anti-citrullinated protein antibodies (ACPAs) and rheumatoid factor (RF) prior to the onset of RA (Rantapaa-Dahlqvist et al., 2003; Nielen et al., 2004)

The results of those studies indicate that ACPA and/or RF may serve as predictive biomarkers for the development for RA, which would allow the selection of candidates for preventive therapy. However, because RA does not ultimately develop in all ACPA and/or RF-positive individuals, the requirements to drive this process are likely to be different between individuals who are at risk (Klareskog et al., 2004). Hence, either additional factors are needed to result in a chronic inflammatory response ultimately leading to RA or some individuals may have a protective immune profile which suppresses disease development despite the presence of autoantibodies. The pathogenic or protective immune response might be selectively induced in susceptible individuals (Klareskog et al., 2004). It was suggested that increased levels of pro-inflammatory cytokines and/or chemokines are associated with the generation of ACPA as amplifiers of inflammatory responses (Rantapaa-

Dahlqvist, et al., 2007). The chemotactic activity could be related to cell migration. However, the exact nature of the pathogenic and/or protective response remains to be determined.

4.1 Gene expression profiles predict arthritis development, independent of ACPA levels

Gene expression profiling blood samples of persons at risk who do and who do not develop RA, revealed new insights in the pathogenic and protective mechanisms in the pre-clinical phase of RA. Gene expression signatures playing either a pathogenic or a protective role were identified in whole blood transcriptome of ACPA/RF positive patients at risk for RA. A total of 109 ACPA/RF positive arthralgia patients at risk for RA were clinically followed for progression to arthritis up to 5 years following inclusion, and clinical features were compared to whole genome expression profiles (Van Baarsen et al. 2010a).

Initial comparison of whole genome expression profiles of 19 autoantibody positive arthralgia patients at inclusion and healthy subject already revealed a marked increase in several immune-related processes in the arthralgia patients. A total of 554 genes were identified whose transcript levels deviated more than two-fold from the median expression level in at least four patients. Two-way hierarchical cluster analysis on these 554 differentially expressed genes clearly indicated that the autoantibody positive arthralgia patients were separated in different subgroups. Pathway-level analysis revealed that these gene clusters represent genes involved in different modes of immune activation e.g. IFN-response activity, B- cell mediated immunity, and chemokine and cytokine mediated signaling. These results were validated in an independent cohort of 90 arthralgia patients again showing considerable heterogeneity among the at risk individuals.

Interim follow-up analysis revealed that 20 autoantibody positive arthralgia patients out of the 109 patients followed had developed arthritis after a median of 7 months (IQR 4-15; median follow-up of all patients is 30 [IQR 22-39] months) in a median of 3 joints (IQR 3-5). Analyzing the distribution of arthritis converters (follow-up time of 12 months (n=102) and corrected for ACPA levels) over the different subgroups revealed that the subgroup that is characterized by an increased expression of genes involved in IFN-mediated immunity and cytokine-chemokine mediated immunity, is associated with arthritis development (OR 21.0; 95% C.I. 2.8-156.1; P=0.003) while the subgroup that is characterized by a relative increased expression of genes involved in B-cell mediated immunity is associated with absence of arthritis (OR 0.38; 95% C.I. 0.21-0.70; P=0.002).

It is speculated that the IFN response programme could be associated with activation of immature monocyte-derived DCs, which regulate deletion of autoreactive lymphocytes. Subsequently, IFN-matured DCs may activate autoreactive T cells, leading to autoreactive B-cell development, representing the first level of autoimmunity. Loss of tolerance may lead to autoantibody production. The decreased B cell gene expression with concomitant increased chemokine activity in the blood of at risk patients who converted to RA may be a consequence of extravasation of lymphocytes from the blood to sites of inflammation and/or lymphoid organs.

Collectively, these analyses reveal that autoantibody positive arthralgia patients with high expression of genes involved in IFN-mediated immunity or chemokine/cytokine mediated immunity combined with a decreased expression of B-cell markers are more likely to develop arthritis.

5. Gene expression and genetics in RA

Sugino and colleagues studied the correlation between the RA susceptibility genes from genome-wide association studies (GWAS) - namely, CD244, PADI4, SLC22A2, PTPN22, CTLA4, TRF1/C5, CD40, CCL21 and STAT4 (Sugino et al., 2010). Gene expression analysis gene expression analysis in RA patients and healthy individuals from a Asian (Japanese) cohort showed that the expressions of four of these genes (CD244, PADI4, SLC22A2, and PTPN22) were significantly higher in RA patients than in healthy individuals, whereas *STAT4* expression was significantly downregulated in the RA group. Data on the upregulated genes is in agreement with results from *in vitro* studies, which revealed the individual upregulation of CD244, PADI4, SLC22A2, and PTPN22 by the mutant alleles.

6. Systems biology

Unique to transcriptome analyses is the identification of gene signatures that represent biological networks that are relevant in disease pathogenesis and thus provide a starting point for a systems biology approach, i.e. a computational modeling approach aimed to understand the structure and dynamics of cellular and organismal functions. Successive research activities on these networks, together with approaches using complementary platforms such as (epi)genetics, multiplex fluorescence-activated cell sorting and advanced metabolomics/proteomics, will provide a complete insight into the mechanism and other network components of processes and pathways relevant to disease. Thus, besides identifying clinically relevant transcriptome markers, DNA-microarray technology provides a basis for an evidence-based systems biology approach to delineate pathogenic processes and reveal other relevant markers. Meta-analysis methods will be instrumental in helping to select those exploratory markers for further biomarker validation, which will pave the way for clinical development and benefit patients. Wu and colleagues devised a method to construct a systemic network of interactions of the processes ongoing in patients affected by RA (Wu et al., 2010) . The network is based on high-throughput data from gene expression profiling and other technology platforms, refined semi-automatically with carefully curated literature-based information. This global network has then been topologically analysed, as a whole and tissue-specifically, in order to translate the experimental molecular connections into topological motifs meaningful in the identification of tissue-specific markers and targets in the diagnosis, and possibly in the therapy, of RA. They demonstrated some nodes in the network that prove to be topologically important, in particular AKT2, IL6, MAPK1 and TP53. Moreover they suggest CRKL as a novel potentially relevant molecule for the diagnosis or treatment of RA. This type of finding proves that the massive amounts of data from high-throughput technologies like gene expression sources create an excellent basis for in silico analyses able to produce highly refined hypotheses, based on vast experimental data, to be tested further and more efficiently. The network is freely available in a standardised and easily exportable .xml Cell Designer format at 'www.picb.ac.cn/ClinicalGenomicNTW/temp.html' and 'www.celldesigner.org'

Moreover, Xing and colleagues described a data analysis strategy for predicting gene expression measures using a combination of comprehensive genotyping, whole blood gene expression profiles and the component of clinical measures (Xing et al., 2011). They identified a total of 22 genes that may have a role in modulating DAS28 score; 6 genes (including CD86, a T-cell costimulatory molecule) could be an alternative target to TNF-blockers and 59 genes are predicted to affect tender and swollen joints. The genes and pathways identified in the networks ensembles represent are potentially promising targets for future investigations.

7. Concluding remarks

Gene expression profiling approaches have fuelled insight into the complexity of RA pathogenesis and provide a framework to identify pathogenic processes and biomarkers as promising tool for future clinical applications. Molecular profiling of blood cells and tissue samples of RA patients has already revealed important information, such as e.g. an activated IFN-system in a subset of patients, that is likely to contribute to the spectrum of diversity in RA. Future efforts are directed on integration of data from different technology platforms combined with information from literature towards a systems biology approach to construct a systemic network of interactions between molecular interactions that reflect disease processes that are ongoing in RA.

8. References

Aidinis V, Carninci P, Armaka M, et al., Cytoskeletal rearrangements in synovial fibroblasts as a novel pathophysiological determinant of modeled rheumatoid arthritis. PLoS Genet 2005, 1:e48.

Badot V, Galant C, Nzeusseu Toukap A, et al., Gene expression profiling in the synovium identifies a predictive signature of absence of response to adalimumab therapy in rheumatoid arthritis. Arthritis Res Ther. 2009;11(2):R57.

Bansard C, Lequerre T, Derambure C, et al., Gene profiling predicts rheumatoid arthritis responsiveness to IL-1Ra (anakinra). Rheumatology 2011;50:283-292

Batliwalla FM, Baechler EC, Xiao X, et al., Peripheral blood gene expression profiling in rheumatoid arthritis. Genes Immun 2005, 6:388-397.

Batliwalla F, Li W, Bienkowska J, Damle A, Khalili H, Hueber W, Allaire M, Mcrann M, Robinson W, Kern M, Carulli JP, Gregersen PK: Differential peripheral blood gene expression profile of rheumatoid arthritis in response to anti-TNF treatment [abstract]. Arthritis Rheum 2007, 56:S700

Baechler EC, Batliwalla FM, Karypis G, et al., Interferon-inducible gene expression signature in peripheral blood cells of patients with severe lupus. Proc Natl Acad Sci USA 2003, 100:2610-2615

Bienkowska JR, Dalgin GS, Batliwalla F, et al., Convergent Random Forest predictor: methodology for predicting drug response from genome-scale data applied to anti-TNF response. Genomics. 2009 Dec;94(6):423-32.

Bos CL, van Baarsen LGM, Timmer TCG, et al., Molecular subtypes of systemic sclerosis in association with anti-centromer antibodies and digital ulcers. Genes Immun. 2009 Apr;10(3):210-8

Bovin LF, Rieneck K, Workman C, Nielsen H, Sorensen SF, Skjodt H, Florescu A, Brunak S, Bendtzen K: Blood cell gene expression profiling in rheumatoid arthritis. Discriminative genes and effect of rheumatoid factor. Immunol Lett 2004, 93:217-226.

Brazma A, Hingamp P, Quackenbush J, et al., Minimum information about a microarray experiment (MIAME)-toward standards for microarray data. Nat Genet. 2001; 29(4):365-371

Brouty-Bové D, Pottin-Clemenceau C, Doucet C et al., Chemokines and CD40 expression in human fibroblasts. Eur. J. Immunol. 2000;30(3):914-919

Lu C, Xiao C, Chen G, et al., Cold and heat pattern of rheumatoid arthritis in traditional Chinese medicine: distinct molecular signatures indentified by microarray expression profiles in CD4-positive T cell. Rheumatol Int. 2010, [E-pub ahead]

Devauchelle V, Marion S, Cagnard N, et al., DNA microarray allows molecular profiling of rheumatoid arthritis and identification of pathophysiological targets. Genes Immun 2004, 5:597-608.

Edwards JC, Szczepanski L, Szechinski J, et al., Efficacy of B-cell-targeted therapy with rituximab in patients with rheumatoid arthritis. N Engl J Med. 2004, 350:2572-2581.

Firestein GS and Zvaifler NJ. How important are T cells in chronic rheumatoid synovitis?: II. T cell-independent mechanisms from beginning to end. Arthritis Rheum. 2002 Feb;46(2):298-308.

Gallagher J, Howlin J, McCarthy C, et al., Identification of Naf1/ABIN-1 among TNF-alpha-induced expressed genes in human synoviocytes using oligonucleotide microarrays. FEBS Lett. 2003 Sep 11;551(1-3):8-12.

Gallagher J, Howlin J, McCarthy C, et al., Identification of Naf1/ABIN-1 among TNF-alpha-induced expressed genes in human synoviocytes using oligonucleotide microarrays. FEBS Lett 2003, 551:8-12.

Galligan CL, Baig E, Bykerk V, et al., Distinctive gene expression signatures in rheumatoid arthritis synovial tissue fibroblast cells: correlates with disease activity. Genes Immun. 2007 Sep;8(6):480-491

Guttierrez-Roelens I, Galant C, Theate I, et al., Rituximab treatment induces the expression of genes involved in healing processes in the rheumatoid arthritis synovium. Arthritis Rheum. 2011 May;63(5):1246-1254.

Heller RA, Schena M, Chai A, et al. Discovery and analysis of inflammatory disease-related genes using cDNA microarrays. Proceedings of the National Academy of Sciences of the United States of America 1997; 94: 2150–2155

Higgs BW, Liu Z, White B, et al., Patients with systemic lupus erythematosus, myositis, rheumatoid arthritis and scleroderma share activation of a common type I interferon pathway. Ann Rheum Dis. 2011 Jul 28. [Epub ahead of print]

Hirohata S, Yanagida T, Nampei A et al., Enhanced generation of endothelial cells from CD34+ cells of the bone marrow in rheumatoid arthritis: possible role in synovial neovascularization. Arthritis Rheum 2004;50, 3888-3896

Hogaboam CM, Steinhauser ML, Chensue SW et al., Novel roles for chemokines and fibroblasts in interstitial fibrosis. Kidney Int. 1998 54(6):2152-2159

Hueber W, Tomooka BH, Batliwalla F, et al., Blood autoantibody and cytokine profiles predict response to anti-TNF therapy in rheumatoid arthritis. Arthritis Res Ther 2009, 11:R76.

Huber R, Hummert C, Gausmann U, et al., Identification of intra-group, inter-individual, and gene-specific variances in mRNA expression profiles in the rheumatoid arthritis synovial membrane. Arthritis Res Ther. 2008;10(4):R98

Jiang M, Xiao C, Chen G, et al., Correlation between cold and hot pattern in traditional Chinese medicine and gene expression profiles in rheumatoid arthritis. Front Med. 2011 ,5;:219-228.

Jongen-Lavrencic M, Peeters HR, Wognum A, Vreugdenhil G, Breedveld FC, Swaak AJ. Elevated levels of inflammatory cytokines in bone marrow of patients with rheumatoid arthritis and anemia of chronic disease. J Rheumatol. 1997;24, 241-245

Julià A, Barceló M, Erra A, Palacio C, Marsal S. Identification of candidate genes for rituximab response in rheumatoid arthritis patients by microarray expression profiling in blood cells. Pharmacogenomics 2009a, 10.1697-708

Julià A, Erra A, Palacio C, et al., An eight-gene blood expression profile predicts the response to infliximab in rheumatoid arthritis. PLoS One. 2009b Oct 22;4(10):e7556.

Kasperkovitz PV, Timmer T, Verbeet NL, et al., Fibroblast-like synoviocytes show the imprint of synovial tissue heterogeneity in rheumatoid arthritis: Evidence for a link between the presence of myofibroblast-like cells and high inflammatory synovitis. Arthr Rheum. (2005) 52:430-441

Kasperkovitz PV, Verbeet NL, Smeets TJ, et al., Activation of the STAT1 pathway in rheumatoid arthritis. Ann Rheum Dis. 2004; 63(3):233-239

Kato H, Matsumine A, Wakabayashi T, et al., Large-scale expression profiles, differentially repressed in osteoarthritis synovium of the knee joint using cDNA microarray technology. Biomarkers 2007;12:384-402

Klareskog L, Alfredsson L, Rantapaa-Dahlqvist S, et al., What precedes development of rheumatoid arthritis? Ann Rheum Dis 2004; 63 Suppl 2: ii28–31.

Koczan D, Drynda S, Hecker M, et al., Molecular discrimination of responders and nonresponders to anti-TNF alpha therapy in rheumatoid arthritis by etanercept. Arthritis Res Ther. 2008;10(3):R50.

Lee HM, Sugino H, Aoki C, et al., Abnormal networks of immune response-related molecules in bone marrow cells from patients with rheumatoid arthritis as revealed by DNA microarray analysis. Arthritis res Ther. 2011 Jun 16;13(3):R89

Lequerré T, Gauthier-Jauneau AC, Bansard C, et al., Gene profiling in white blood cells predicts infliximab responsiveness in rheumatoid arthritis. Arthritis Res Ther. 2006;8(4):R105

Lequerré T, Bansard C, Vittecoq O, et al., Early and long-standing rheumatoid arthritis: distinct molecular signatures identified by gene-expression profiling in synovia. Arthritis Res Ther. 2009;11(3):R99

Liao H, Wu J, Kuhn E, et al., Use of mass spectrometry to identify protein biomarkers of disease severity in the synovial fluid and serum of patients with rheumatoid arthritis. Arthritis Rheum. 2004, 50: 3792–3803

Lindberg J, af Klint E, Ulfgren AK, et al., Variability in synovial inflammation in rheumatoid arthritis investigated by microarray technology. Arthritis Res Ther 2006a, 8:R47

Lindberg J, af Klint E, Catrina AI, et al., Effect of infliximab on mRNA expression profiles in synovial tissue of rheumatoid arthritis patients. Arthritis Res Ther 2006b, 8:R179.

Lindberg J, Wijbrandts CA, van Baarsen LG, et al., The gene expression profile in the synovium as a predictor of the clinical response to infliximab treatment in rheumatoid arthritis. PLoS One. 2010 Jun 25;5(6):e11310.

Liu Z, Sokka T, Maas K, et al., Prediction of Disease Severity in Patients with early rheumatoid arthritis by gene expression profiling. Human Genomics and Proteomics 2009,484351

Maas K, Chen H, Shyr Y, et al., Shared gene expression profiles in individuals with autoimmune disease and unaffected first-degree relatives of individuals with autoimmune disease. Hum Mol Genet 2005, 14:1305-1314.

Mavragani CP, La DT, Stohl W, et al., Association of the response to tumor necrosis factor antagonists with plasma type I interferon activity and interferon-beta/alpha ratios in rheumatoid arthritis patients: a post hoc analysis of a predominantly Hispanic cohort. Arthritis Rheum. 2010 Feb;62(2):392-401

Mavragani CP, Crow MK. Activation of type I interferon pathway in primary Sjogren's syndrome. J Autoimmun 2010; 35:225-231.

Mesko B, Poliska S, Szegedi A, et al., Peripheral blood gene expression patterns discriminate among chronic inflammatory diseases and healthy controls and identify novel targets. BMC Med Genomics. 2010 May 5;3:15

Meugnier E, Coury F, Tebib J, et al., Gene expression profiling in peripheral blood cells of patients with rheumatoid arthritis in response to anti-TNF-alpha treatments. Physiol Genomics. 2011 Apr 12;43(7):365-371

Nakamura N, Shimaoka Y, Tougan T, et al., Isolation and expression profiling of genes upregulated in bone marrow-derived mononuclear cells of rheumatoid arthritis patients. DNA Research. 2006;13, 169-183

Neumann E, Riepl B, Knedla A, et al., Cell culture and passaging alters gene expression pattern and proliferation rate in rheumatoid arthritis synovial fibroblasts. Arthritis Res Ther. 2010;12(3):R83.

Nielen MM, van Schaardenburg D, Reesink HW et al., Specific autoantibodies precede the symptoms of rheumatoid arthritis: a study of serial measurements in blood donors. Arthr Rheum 2004; 50, 380-386

Nzeusseu TA, Galant C, Theate I, et al., Identification of distinct gene expression profiles in the synovium of patients with systemic lupus erythematosus. Arthritis Rheum 2007, 56:1579-1588.

Ochi T, Hakomori S, Adachi M et al. The presence of a myeloid cell population showing strong reactivity with monoclonal antibody directed to difucosyl type 2 chain in epiphyseal bone marrow adjacent to joints affected with rheumatoid arthritis (RA) and its absence in the corresponding normal and non-RA bone marrow. J Rheumatology 1998;15, 1609-1615

O'Hanlon TP, Rider LG, Gan L, et al., Gene expression profiles from discordant monozygotic twins suggest that molecular pathways are shared among multiple systemic autoimmune diseases. Arthritis Res Ther. 2011 Apr 26;13(2):R69.

Olsen N, Sokka T, Seehorn CL, et al., A gene expression signature for recent onset rheumatoid arthritis in peripheral blood mononuclear cells. Ann Rheum Dis. 2004,63;1387-1392

Palucka AK, Blanck JP, Bennet L, et al., Cross-regulation of TNF and IFN-alpha in autoimmune diseases. Proc. Natl. Acad. Sci USA 2005;102,3372-3377

Pohlers D, Beyer A, Koczan D, et al., Constitutive upregulation of the transforming growth factor-beta pathway in rheumatoid arthritis synovial fibroblasts. Arthritis Res Ther. 2007;9(3):R59.

Rantapaa-Dahlqvist S, de Jong BA, Berglin E, et al. Antibodies against cyclic citrullinated peptide and IgA rheumatoid factor predict the development of rheumatoid arthritis. Arthr Rheum 2003;48, 2741-2749

Rantapaa-Dahlqvist S, Boman K, Tarkowski A, Hallmans G. Up regulation of monocyte chemoattractant protein-1 expression in anti-citrulline antibody and immunoglobulin M rheumatoid factor positive subjects precedes onset of inflammatory response and development of overt rheumatoid arthritis. Ann Rheum Dis 2007; 66: 121–3.

Sekiguchi N, Kawauchi S, Furuya T, et al., Messenger ribonucleic acid expression profile in peripheral blood cells from RA patients following treatment with an anti-TNF-alpha monoclonal antibody, infliximab. Rheumatology (Oxford). 2008 Jun;47(6):780-788.

Sha N, Vannucci M, Brown PJ, et al.,. Gene selection in arthritis classification with large-scale microarray expression profiles. Comp Funct Genomics. 2003;4(2):171-181.

Smith RS, Smith TJ, Blieden TM, et al., Fibroblasts as sentinel cells. Synthesis of chemokines and regulation of inflammation. Am. J. Pathol. 1997; 151(2):317-322

Szodoray P, Alex P, Frank MB, et al., A genome-scale assessment of peripheral blood B-cell molecular homeostasis in patients with rheumatoid arthritis. Rheumatology (Oxford). 2006 Dec;45(12):1466-1476.

Taberner M, Scott KF, Weininger L, et al., Overlapping gene expression profiles in rheumatoid fibroblast-like synoviocytes induced by the proinflammatory cytokines interleukin-1 beta and tumor necrosis factor. Inflamm Res. 2005 Jan;54(1):10-6.

Tan FK, Zhou X, Mayes MD, et al., Signatures of differentially regulated interferon gene expression and vasculotrophism in the peripheral blood cells of systemic sclerosis patients. Rheumatology (Oxford) 2006;45:694–702

Stuhlmüller B, Häupl T, Hernandez MM, et al., CD11c as a transcriptional biomarker to predict response to anti-TNF monotherapy with adalimumab in patients with rheumatoid arthritis. Clin Pharmacol Ther. 2010; Mar;87(3):311-321

Sugino H, Lee HM, Nishimoto N. DNA microarray analysis of rheumatoid arthritis susceptibility genes identified by genome-wide association studies. Arthritis Res Ther. 2010;12(2):401. Epub 2010 Mar 12. Erratum in: Arthritis Res Ther. 2010;12(3):403.

Tanabe M, Ochi T, Tomita T, Suzuki R, Sakata T, Shimaoka Y, Nakagawa S, Ono K., Remarkable elevation of interleukin 6 and interleukin 8 levels in the bone marrow serum of patients with rheumatoid arthritis.J Rheumatolog 1994, 21, 830-835

Tanino M, Matoba R, Nakamura S, et al., Prediction of efficacy of anti-TNF biologic agent, infliximab, for rheumatoid arthritis patients using a comprehensive transcriptome analysis of white blood cells. Biochem Biophys Res Commun. 2009 Sep 18;387(2):261-5.

Takemura S, Braun A, Crowson C, et al. Lymphoid neogenesis in rheumatoid synovitis. J Immunol 2001;167:1072–1080.

Teixeira VH, Olaso R, Martin-Magniette ML, et al., Transcriptome analysis describing new immunity and defense genes in peripheral blood mononuclear cells of rheumatoid arthritis patients. PLoS One. 2009 Aug 27;4(8):e6803.

Thurlings RM, Boumans M, Tekstra J, et al., The relationship between the type I interferon signature and the response to rituximab in rheumatoid arthritis. Arthritis Rheum. 2010, 62:3607-3614

Timmer TC, Baltus B, Vondenhoff M, et al., Inflammation and ectopic lymphoid structures in rheumatoid arthritis synovial tissues dissected by genomics technology: identification of the interleukin-7 signaling pathway in tissues with lymphoid neogenesis. Arthritis Rheum 2007, 56:2492-2502.

Tsubaki T, Arita N, Kawakami T, Shiratsuchi T, et al., Characterization of histopathology and gene-expression profiles of synovitis in early rheumatoid arthritis using targeted biopsy specimens. Arthritis Res Ther. 2005;7(4):R825-36.

Turrel-Davin F, Tournadre A, Pachot A, et al., FoxO3a involved in neutrophil and T cell survival is overexpressed in rheumatoid blood and synovial tissue. Ann Rheum Dis. 2010 Apr;69(4):755-760

Ungethuem U, Haupl T, Witt H, et al., Molecular signatures and new candidates to target the pathogenesis of rheumatoid arthritis Physiol. Genomics 2010;42A:(4) 267-282 van Baarsen LG, van der Pouw Kraan TC, Kragt JJ, et al., A subtype of multiple sclerosis defined by an activated immune defense program. Genes Immun. 2006;7:522–531

van Baarsen LG, Bos WH, Rustenburg F, et al., Gene expression profiling in autoantibody-positive patients with arthralgia predicts development of arthritis. Arthritis Rheum. 2010a;62:694-704

van Baarsen LG, Wijbrandts CA, Timmer TC, et al. Synovial tissue heterogeneity in rheumatoid arthritis in relationship to disease activity and biomarkers in peripheral blood. Arthritis Rheum. 2010b ;62:1602-1607

Van Baarsen LG, Wijbrandts C, Gerlag D, et al., Pharmacogenomics of infliximab treatment using peripheral blood cells of patients with rheumatoid arthritis. Genes Immun.2010c;11:622-629

van Baarsen LG, Wijbrandts CA, Rustenburg F, et al., Regulation of IFN response gene activity during infliximab treatment in rheumatoid arthritis is associated with clinical response to treatment. Arthritis Res Ther. 2010d;12:R11

Van der Pouw Kraan TCTM, Van Galen FA, Huizinga TWJ, et al., Discovery of distinctive gene expression profiles in rheumatoid arthritis using cDNA microarray technology: Evidence for the existence of multiple pathways of tissue destruction and repair. Genes & Immunity 2003a;4, 187-196

Van der Pouw Kraan TCTM, Van Galen FA, Kasperkovitz PV, et al., Rheumatoid arthritis is a heterogeneous disease: Evidence for differences in the activation of the STAT1 pathway between rheumatoid tissues. Arthr. Rheum. 2003b;48, 2132-2145

Van der Pouw Kraan TC, Wijbrandts CA, Van Baarsen LG, et al., Rheumatoid Arthritis subtypes identified by genomic profiling of peripheral blood cells: Assignment of a type I interferon signature in a subpopulation of patients. Ann Rheum Dis 2007;66, 1008-1014

Van der Pouw Kraan TC, Van Baarsen LG, Wijbrandts CA, et al., Expression of a pathogen-response program in peripheral blood cells defines a subgroup of Rheumatoid Arthritis patients. Genes Immun. 2008;9:16-22

Van 't Veer LJ, Dai H, van de Vijver MJ, et al., Gene expression profiling predicts clinical outcome of breast cancer. Nature 2002;415:530-536

Vosslamber S, Raterman HG, van der Pouw Kraan CTM, Schreurs MWJ, von Blomberg BME, Nurmohamed MT, Lems WF, Dijkmans BAC, Voskuyl AE, Verweij CL. Pharmacological induction of IFN type I activity following therapy with rituximab determines clinical response in rheumatoid arthritis. Ann Rheum Dis 2011,70(6):1153-1159

Watanabe N, Ando K, Yoshida S, et al., Gene expression profile analysis of rheumatoid synovial fibroblast cultures revealing the overexpression of genes responsible for tumor-like growth of rheumatoid synovium. Biochem Biophys Res Commun 2002 Jun 28;294(5):1121-1129.

Wu G, Zhu L, Dent JE, Nardini C. A comprehensive molecular interaction map forrheumatoid arthritis. PLoS One. 2010 Apr 16;5(4):e10137. Erratum in: PLoS One.2010;5(4). doi:10.1371/annotation/f67a90fb-3e4e-4484-bffe-fcfafbfe88c7

Xing H, McDonagh PD, Bienkowska J, et al., Causal modeling using network ensemble simulations of genetic and gene expression data predicts genes involved in rheumatoid arthritis. PLoS Comput Biol. 2011 Mar;7(3):e1001105.

Zanders ED, Goulden MG, Kennedy TC, Kempsell KE: Analysis of immune system gene expression in small rheumatoid arthritis biopsies using a combination of subtractive hybridization and high-density cDNA arrays. J Immunol Methods 2000, 233:131-140.

4

Vitamin D and Autoimmune Disease

Ayah M. Boudal[1] and Suzan M. Attar[2]
[1]*Jeddah*
[2]*Department Of Internal Medicine*
King Abdul-Aziz University
Consultant Rheumatology & Internal Medicine
King Abdul-Aziz University Hospital
Kingdom of Saudi Arabia

1. Introduction

During the past decade, important advances in the study of vitamin D have been made as vitamin D insufficiency is emerging as a clinical problem at a global level. In addition to its important role in skeletal development and maintenance, evidence is mounting that vitamin D produce beneficial effect on extraskeletal tissues. Recent evidence shows that vitamin D deficiencies contribute autoimmune diseases susceptibility and severity. This chapter will provide a systematic review of the importance of vitamin D in preexisting autoimmune diseases and whether its deficiency predispose patients to such disorders.

2. Agenda

- Overview of vitamin D: structure, sources and metabolism
- Mechanism of vitamin D modulation of the immune responses, the difference between the bone and autoimmune tissues and the role of the vitamin D receptors.
- The optimum serum level of vitamin D for skeletal health
- Vitamin D and autoimmune disease: list of al the autoimmune diseases in which vitamin D is related to
  - Rheumatoogical
  - Non rheumatoogical
- Vitamin D level and vitamin D supplementation in
  - RA
  - SLE
  - Scleroderma
  - Ankylosing spondylitis
  - Undifferentiated connective tissue disease
- The immunological basis for the vitamin D role in preventing autoimmunity
- Summary
- Appendix: 1 Abbreviation

3. Vitamin D structure

Vitamin D is a secosteroid which carries a structure similar to steroid except that two of the B-ring carbon atoms (C9 and 10) of the typical four steroid rings are broken, in this case by ultraviolet B sunlight. It is considered as a prohormone. The main source of vitamin D is *denovo*synthesis in the skin through ultravioletirradiation of 7-dehydrocholesterol. It is biologically inert and mustbe metabolized to 25-hydroxyvitamin D3in the liver and then to1α, 25-dihydroxyvitamin D3in the kidney before it becomes functional **Figure 1**. (1, 2)

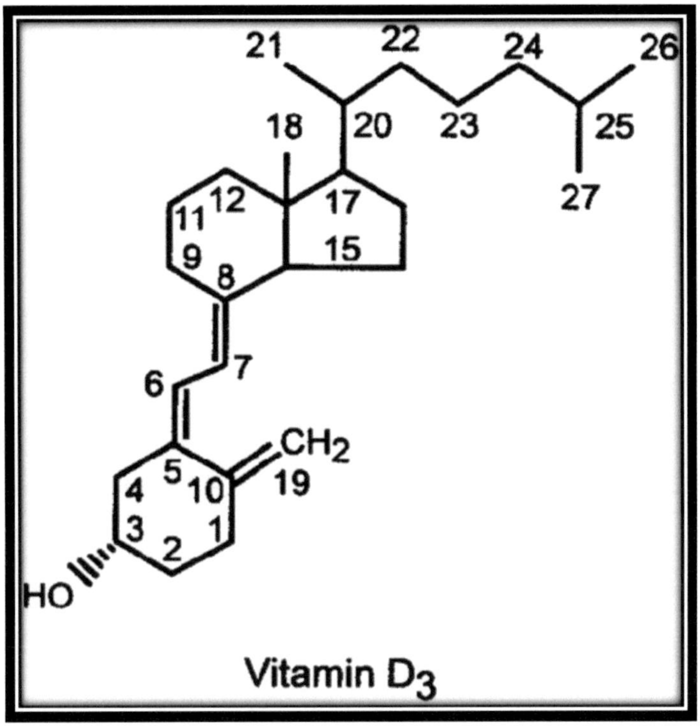

Fig. 1. Structure of vitamin D3, or cholecalciferol

4. Source of vitamin D

The main source of vitamin D is *de novo* synthesis in the skin. Although vitamin D is present in food, dietary intake alone is often insufficient, supplying only 20% of the body's requirements (3). It is not found in plant materials (eg, vegetables, fruits, or grains) and is present in low levels in meats and other animal food sources, except in rare cases such as fish liver oils (2).

5. Metabolism of vitamin D

The terminology related to the biochemistry of vitamin D can be confusing. Vitamin D has 2 forms and several metabolites. The 2 forms are vitamin D2 and vitamin D3, also called ergocalciferol and cholecalciferol, respectively (4).

Both forms of vitamin D undergo identical metabolism (Figure 2). Some evidence indicates that vitamin D2 may be metabolized more rapidly than vitamin D3, but with regular daily intake they can be considered bioequivalent. Both forms of vitamin D are converted to 25-hydroxyvitamin [25(OH)D] in the liver, and the serum level of 25(OH) D is measured to determine the adequacy of vitamin D status. In the kidney, 25(OH)D is hydroxylated to 1, 25-dihydroxyvitamin D [1, 25(OH)2 D], which is the only biologically active form of vitamin D. Acting principally on the duodenum, 1, 25(OH)2 D increases calcium absorption. It also acts on bone cells, both osteoblasts and osteoclasts, to mobilize calcium. The synthesis of 1, 25(OH)2 D is tightly regulated and stimulated primarily by serum parathyroid hormone (PTH) (4).

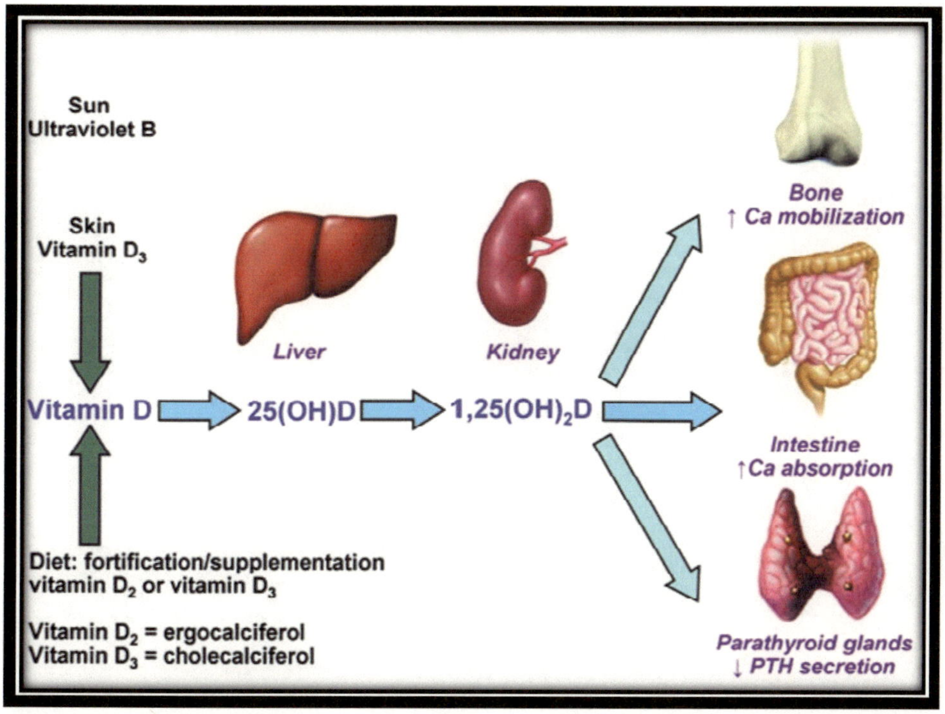

Fig. 2. Vitamin D metabolism. Ca = calcium; 1, 25(OH)2D = 1, 25-dihydroxyvitamin D; 25(OH)D =25-hydroxyvitamin D; PTH = parathyroid hormone.

6. Vitamin D and autoimmune disease

Vitamin D and its prohormones have been the focus of a growing number of studies in past years, demonstrating their function not only in calcium metabolism and bone formation, but also their interaction with the immune system. This is not surprising, since vitamin D receptors (VDR) are expressed in different tissues, such as brain, heart, skin, bowel, gonads, prostate, breasts, and the immune cells(3).

Epidemiological studies have linked vitamin D status with autoimmune disease susceptibility and severity (5). Potentially, vitamin D deficiency could be a clinical problem of global proportions.

7. The mechanisms of vitamin D immunomodulation

Dendritic cells (DCs) are primary targets for the immunomodulatory activity of 1, 25(OH)2D3, as indicated by inhibited DC differentiation and maturation, leading to down-regulated expression of MHC-II, costimulatory molecules (CD40, CD80 and CD86) and decreased production of IL-12. Moreover, 1, 25(OH)2D3 enhances IL-10 production and promotes DC apoptosis. Together, these effects of 1, 25(OH)2D3 inhibit DC-dependent T-cell activation. In particular, the active synthesis of 1, 25(OH)2D3 seems to exert an autoregulatory function by inhibiting the differentiation of monocyte precursors into immature DCs and the subsequent ability of the immature DCs to undergo terminal differentiation in response to maturation stimuli (Fig. 3).

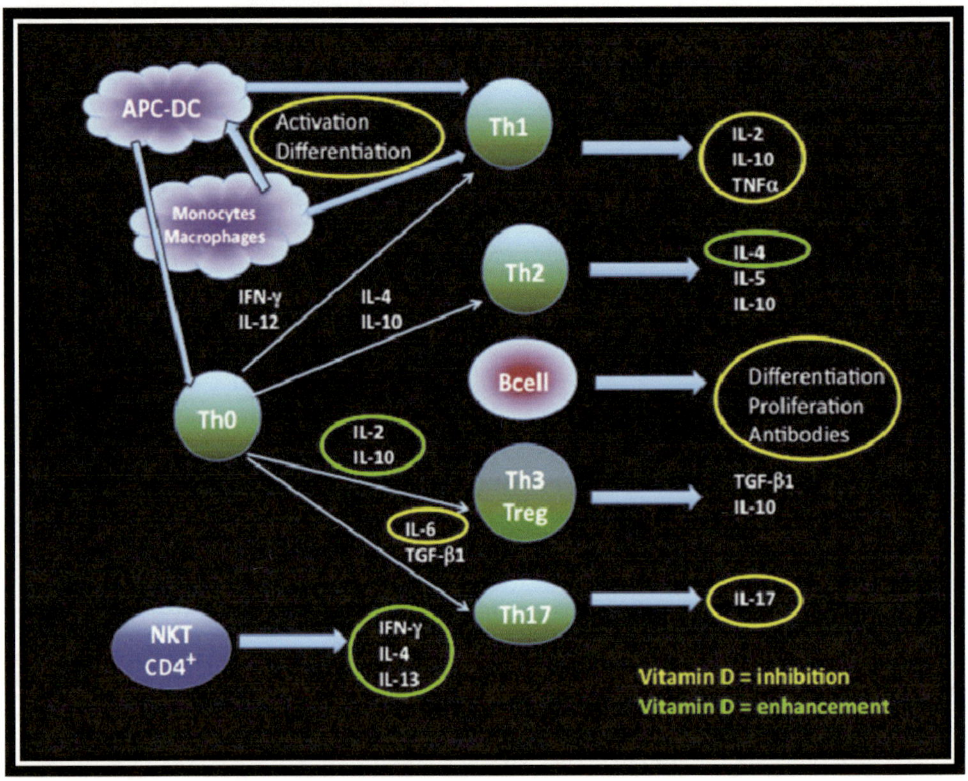

Fig. 3. Mechanisms involved in vitamin D modulation of the immune responses. DCs are primary targets for the immunomodulatory activity of 1, 25(OH)2D3, as indicated by inhibited DC differentiation and maturation, together with inhibition of differentiation of monocyte precursors into immature DCs. 1, 25(OH)2D3 suppresses Th1 (and Th17)driven cytokine responses, induces Treg cells, induces IL-4 production (Th2) and enhances NKT-cell function. Differentiation and maturation of B cells is also inhibited. Th are CD4+ helper cell subsets (Th1, Th2, Th3-Treg, Th17) originating from naıve T cell (Th0). Thin arrows (left) indicate cytokines that induce differentiation of Th0 cells and thicker arrows (right) indicate cytokines produced by activated Th cell subsets. All T cells that have been tested express the VDR. B cells and NKT cells are also reported. The yellow circles indicate the cytokines/activities inhibited by vitamin D. On the contrary, the green circles indicate the cytokines enhanced by vitamin D.

Target cell population	Actions mediated by 1. 25(oH)3 D3
APCs (monocytes, macrophages, dendritic cells)	inhibits the expression of class II MHC molecules inhibits the expression of costimulating molecules (CD40, CD80, and CD86) and other maturation inducing proteins (CD1a, CD83) increases chemotaxis and phagocytosis of monocytes and cytotoxicity against tumor cells and bacteria inhibits the maturation of dendritic cells induces tolerogenic dendritic cells capable of inducing Treg cells inhibits the release of IL-12 p70 inhibitsproinflammatory cytokines (IL-1 and TNF) by monocytes and macrophages.
T lymphocytes	inhibits T cell proliferation, secretion of cytokines, and progression of the cellular cycle from G1a to G1b increases the production of IL-4, IL-5, IL-10 inhibits IL-12, INF-γ, and IL-2 inhibits activation of antigenspecific T lymphocytes inhibits the expression of FasL by activated T lymphocytes
B cells	Expresses vDR Suppresses IgE secretion
NK cells	inhibits INF-γ

Table 1. Actions of vitamin D in the immune system

Tolerogenic DCs induced by a brief treatment with1, 25(OH)2D3or its analogues can induce CD4+ CD25+ T regulatory (Treg) cells that are able to mediate transplantation tolerance and arrest the development of autoimmunity (i. e. autoimmune diabetes). Tolerogenic DCs, however, may not always be necessarily involved in the generation of T-reg cells by VDR agonists and a combination of 1, 25(OH)2D3 and dexamethasone has been shown to induce naïve CD4+ T cells (Th0) to differentiate in vitro into IL-10-producing Treg cells, even in the absence of antigen-presenting cells. VDR agonists not only favour induction of CD4+CD25+ Treg cells and enhance their suppressive activity, but can also promote their recruitment at inflammatory sites. Furthermore, 1, 25(OH)2D3 treatments induced natural killer (NK) T-cell functions *in vitro* and *in vivo*. NKT cells are early innate regulatory cells that can alter the outcome of autoimmunity. Therefore, two types of cells are induced by 1, 25(OH)2D3; the Treg and the NKT cells; induction of these regulatory cells and direct inhibition of Th1 cells are the mechanisms by which 1, 25(OH)2D3 suppresses experimental autoimmunity. In addition, treatment with VDR agonists inhibits the T-cell production of IL-17, a pro-inflammatory cytokine that is produced by pathogenic T cells (Th17) in various models of organ-specific autoimmunity in the brain, heart, synovium and intestines.

nmol/L	ng/mL	Health status
<30	<12	Associated with vitamin D deficiency, leading to rickets in infants and children and osteomalacia in adults
30–50	12–20	Generally considered inadequate for bone and overall health in healthy individuals
≥50	≥20	Generally considered adequate for bone and overall health in healthy individuals
>125	>50	Emerging evidence links potential adverse effects to such high levels, particularly >150 nmol/L (>60 ng/mL)

Table 2. Classification of Vitamin D Status by 25(OH)D Concentration

Interestingly, IL-17 production is sustained by IL-23, an IL-12 family member consisting of p19 and p40 chains, the latter of which is strongly inhibited by VDR agonists. Recently, 1, 25(OH)2D3 treatment induced a significant inhibition of normal lymphoid cell progenitors growth of both T and B lineage and inhibited significantly also the growth of malignant Bcell lineage lymphoid progenitors, without inducing cytotoxic effect. More recently, by testing the effects of 1, 25(OH)2D3 on B-cell responses, it was found that it inhibited the ongoing proliferation of activated B cells and induced their apoptosis, whereas initial cell division was unimpeded.

The generation of plasma cells and post-switch memory B cells was significantly inhibited by 1, 25(OH)2D3 although the up-regulation of genetic programs involved in B-cell differentiation was only modestly affected. B cells expressed mRNAs for proteins involved in vitamin D activity, including 1α-hydroxylase, 24-hydroxylase and the VDR, each of which was regulated by 1, 25(OH)2D3 and/or activation. Interestingly, 1, 25(OH)2D3 up-regulated the expression of p27, but not of p18 and p21, which may be important in regulating the proliferation of activated B cells and their subsequent differentiation in plasma cells.

The net effect of 1, 25(OH)2D3 is enhancement of the innate immune system (protective) and down regulation of the adaptive immune system(acquired). Therefore, 25(OH)D deficiency may theoretically lead to autoimmune diseases.

8. The optimum serum level of vitamin D for skeletal health

Determination of vitamin D status is not based on measurement of serum 1, 25(OH)D concentrations. It is assessed by measuring the prohormone 25(OH)D, which is an indicator of supply rather than function. The most stable and plentiful metabolite of vitamin D in human serum, 25(OH)D, has a half-life of about 3 weeks, making it the most suitable indicator of vitamin D status (4). Using PTH elevation as a biomarker reflecting physiologic low levels of vitamin D, recent reports indicate that vitamin D deficiency would be more accurately defined as a 25D concentration of less than 32 ng/ml (80 nmol/l). The optimal serum concentrations of 25(OH)D begin at 75 nmol/L (30 ng/mL), and the best are between 90-100 nmol/L (36–40 ng/mL) (7). Whether 'normal' serum levels of vitamin D are sufficient for immune homeostasis is not known. In 2009, a standard reference material for 25(OH)D became available that permits standardization of values across laboratories and may improve method-related variability.

9. Vitamin D and autoimmune diseases

Observational studies in humans suggest an association between vitamin D deficiency and many rheumatological and non-rheumatological disorders, listed in Table 3.

Rheumatological	Non Rheumatologicl
1. Rheumatoid Arthritis "RA" (3, 7, 8).	1. Multiple Sclerosis "MS" (7, 8, 12, 14).
2. Undifferentiated Connective tissue (8).	2. Independent Diabetes Mellitus "IDDM" (6, 8, 12).
3. SLE (8).	3. Allergic asthma in children (9, 10).
4. Scleroderma (11).	4. Allergic rhinitis (10).
5. Ankylosing spondylitis (12).	5. Grave's disease (13).
6. Behcet's disease (15).	
7. Psoriasis (16).	
8. Fibromylgia (17)	

SLE: Systemic lupus erythematosis, 25(OH)D: serum vitamin D level

Table 3. Disorders that have been linked to 25(OH)D

10. Vitamin D level and vitamin D supplementation in autoimmune diseases

10.1 Rheumatoid Arthritis (RA)

Rheumatoid arthritis is an immune-mediated disease, mainly driven by Th1 cells. The characteristic features of the disease are erosive arthritis and joint destruction, which lead to severe disability and increased mortality. In various animal models of RA, such as CIA in mice, the disease-modifying effect of VDR ligands has been widely investigated. With 1, 25(OH)2D3 vitamin treatment in the early phase, collagen-induced arthritis was preventable to a certain extent and the progression of arthritis decreased (18).

In the last few years, the possible role of vitamin D in the pathogenesis, activity, and treatment of RA has been raised based on the results and observations of clinical and laboratorial studies(3). There have been 7case control studies evaluating vitamin D in RA patients. Two studies showed lower level of 25(OH)D than controls but 5 did not. In these studies the prevalence of low 25(OH)D was found to be between 30-63%. *The rationale for relating vitamin D deficiency and RA is based on two facts:* evidence indicate that patients with RA have vitamin D deficiency and the presence of 1, 25(OH) and VDR in macrophages, chondrocytes, and synovial cells in the joints of these patients with RA (3).

Low sun exposure and reduced body mass index (BMI) are well established risk factors for vitamin D deficiency in RA patients (19). Few studies have examined dietary or nutritional intake prior to RA onset, and none have assessed the association of vitamin D with disease onset. *Linda et al.* found that greater intake (highest versus lowest tertile) of total daily vitamin D was inversely associated with risk of RA. Inverse associations were apparent for both dietary and supplemental vitamin D. (20). The relationship between polymorphisms of the VDR gene and the onset of RA activity has been demonstrated in a study in which patients with BB or Bb genotypes for VDR had higher indices in the health assessment questioner (HAQ), erythrocyte sedimentation rate (ESR), cumulative dose of corticosteroids, and number of disease-modifying anti-rheumatic drugs (DMARDs) when compared to patients with the BB genotype (3).

In collagen-induced arthritis models, dietarian supplementation or oral administration of vitamin D prevented the development or delayed the progression of arthritis(3). In an open labeled study with 19 patients with RA treated with traditional DMARDs, oral supplementation with high doses of alfacalcidol for three months reduced the severity of the symptoms in 89% of the patients, 45% of which achieved complete remission and 44% had satisfactory results. Higher incidence of side effects, such as hypercalcemia, was not observed (3).

There also seem to be an inverse relationship between disease activity and the concentration of vitamin D metabolites in patients with inflammatory arthritis. A UK study that involved 206 patients demonstrated that at baseline in the pre-treatment patients, there was an inverse association between levels of 25(OH)D and the number of painful joints, DAS28, and HAQ. For each increase in 10 ng/mL in vitamin D serum levels, the DAS28 reduced by 0. 3 points and the levels of CRP by 25%. But at 1 year the only observation is the inverse association with HAQ score (3).

10.2 Systemic Lupus Erythematous (SLE)

Several studies have demonstrated a higher prevalence of vitamin D deficiency in SLE patients when compared to individuals with other rheumatologic diseases and healthy controls(3). *Huisman et al.* observed that 50% of SLE patients had vitamin D deficiency (cut off <50 nmol/L or 20 ng/mL) (21).

Patients with systemic lupus erythematosus have multiple risk factors for 25(OH)D deficiency:(3)

1. Photosensitivity:

Is the characteristic of the disease, and the recommendation to apply sunscreen are responsible for lower sun exposure, decreasing the production of vitamin D in the skin.

2. Chronic treatment with corticosteroids and hydroxichloroquine:

These medications seem to affect vitamin D metabolism, although the evidence for this is not yet clear.

3. Severe renal involvement:

This affects the hydroxylation step of 25(OH)D.

4. African descent:

Severe lupus is more prevalent in people of African descent. It is believed that vitamin D deficiency in this group is a consequence of not only genetic factors, but it is speculated that lower serum concentrations of 25(OH)D, due to the lower cutaneous conversion rate secondary to skin color, would be another important factor.

It has been observed that critical levels of vitamin D (<10 ng/mL) are more common in patients with renal involvement and photosensitive skin lesions (4).

The association between low 25(OH)D and disease activity scores, according to the SLEDAI (Systemic Lupus Erythematosus Disease Activity Index) and ECLAM (European Consensus Lupus Activity Measurement) has been documented (3).

Thudi et al. demonstrated that functional assessment using combined scores (modified HAQ, global VAS by the patient, and fatigue scale) was worse in patients with probable or confirmed diagnosis of lupus and vitamin D deficiency. However, this study did not demonstrate an association between vitamin D deficiency and the levels of auto-antibodies, including anti-DNA (22).

Carvalho et al. investigated the presence of anti-vitamin D antibodies in the serum of SLE patients to better explain vitamin D deficiency in autoimmune diseases. One-hundred and seventy-one SLE patients were investigated and 4% of them had vitamin D antibodies but the levels of 25(OH)D were similar in patients with or without those autoantibodies. Among the clinical and laboratorial associations investigated, the presence of anti-dsDNA was the only one that showed a strong relationship with anti-vitamin D antibodies (23).

10.3 Ankylosing Spondylitis AS

Osteoprosis is frequent in AS and high disease activity which assessed by Bath Ankylosing Spondylitis Disease Activity Index (BASDAI) is associated with an alteration in vitamin D metabolites and increased levels of bone resorption (11).

The inflammatory activity in AS itself plays a major role in the pathophysiology of bone loss, this may be mediated in AS by substances regulating both the inflammatory process and bone turnover. High levels of proinflammatory cytokines such asinterleukin-1 and tumor necrosis factor α (TNFα) are thought to play a major role in chronic inflammation and act on osteroblasts and osteoclasts(12). A prospective study demonstrated a significant loss of bone mass in early AS with a strong association with inflammatory activity (24).

Factors may contribute to the development of osteopenia/osteoporosis in AS: (12)

1. Treatment of AS.
2. Hormone disorder.
3. Decreased mobility or physical activity.

Patients with AS and osteoporosis had significantly higher values for ESR, CRP, and urine-cross-links, and significantly decreased results in 1. 25 D3, 25 D3 and PTH, but no differences in serum calcium, serum calcium corrected for albumin, bone-AP and daily renal calcium excretion were observed (12).

Clinical studies have reported the impact of vitamin D in AS as an endogenous immune modulator, suppressing activated T cells and cell proliferation that may accelerate the inflammation process (25).

10.4 Undifferentiated Connective Tissue Disease (UCTD)

A study by *Zold et al.* demonstrated the presence of a seasonal variation in the levels of 25(OH)D in patients with UCTD and that those levels were lower in this population than in the control population. In this same study, 21. 7% of patients with UCTD and vitamin D deficiency developed established connective tissue disease (especially RA, SLE, Sjgren's syndrome, and mixed connective tissue disease); their mean 25(OH)D was lower than that of patients who remained with undifferentiated disease, 14. 7 ± 6. 45 ng/mL vs 33. 0 ± 13. 4 ng/mL, P =0. 0001 respectively (26). The presence of dermatological symptoms (photosensitivity, erythema, and chronic discoid rash) and pleuritis was associated with low levels of vitamin D.

11. The immunological basis for the vitamin D role in preventing autoimmunity

Prospective studies available for the 4 major autoimmune diseases:RA, SLE, MS, and type 1 DM, have demonstrated the beneficial effects of vitamin D supplementation in modulating the components of the immune system responsible for the inflammation, such as the expression of cytokines, growth factors, nitrous oxide, and metalloproteinase(3). A recent systematic review concluded that total number of studies are small, so no conclusion could be made with regards to the importance of 25(OH)D in preventing autoimmune disease.

12. Summary

The vitamin D endocrine system is recognized as an important immune modulatory factor involved in autoimmune diseases. VDR agonists seem primarily to inhibit DC differentiation, pathogenic pro-inflammatory T cells such as Th1 and Th17 cells and, under appropriate conditions, they seem to favour a deviation to the Th2 pathway. These immunomodulatory and anti-inflammatory activities might be particularly efficient in RA, SLE, Ankylosing spondylitis and UCTD patients and support a therapeutic role of 1, 25(OH)2D in such a disease.

In addition, vitamin D may play an important role in the maintenance of B-cell homeostasis, and the correction of vitamin D deficiency may be useful in the treatment of B cell-mediated autoimmune rheumatic disorders such as SLE.

13. Acknowledgement

The authors would like to thank "**Al-Zaidi Chair of Research in Rheumatic Diseases -Umm Al-Qura University**" who supported the publication of this chapter.

14. References

[1] Holick MF. Vitamin D deficiency. NEngl J Med. 2007 Jul 19; 357(3):266-81.
[2] DeLuca H. Overview of general physiologic features and functions of vitamin D. Am J ClinNutr 2004; 80:1689S-96S. Figure printed with permission
[3] Marques CD, Dantas AT, Fragoso TS, Duarte AL. The importance of vitamin D levels in autoimmune diseases. Bras J Rheumatol 2010; 50:67-80.
[4] Thacher TD, Clarke BL. Vitamine D Insufficiency. Mayo Clin Proc. 2011; 86:50-60. Figure printed with permission
[5] Cutolo M. Vitamin D and autoimmune rheumatic diseases. Rheumatology 2009; 48:210–212. Figure printed with permission
[6] Bischoff-Ferrari HA, Giovannucci E, Willett WC, Dietrich T and Dawson-Hughes B. Estimation of optimal serum concentrations of 25-hydroxyvitamin D for multiple health outcomes. American Journal of Clinical Nutrition. Am J ClinNutr 2006; 84:18-28.

[7] Cantorna MT. Vitamin D and Autoimmunity: Is Vitamin D Status an Environmental Factor Affecting Autoimmune Disease Prevalence?. Proc Soc Exp Biol Med. 2000; 223:230-3.
[8] Cutolo M. Vitamin D or hormonr D deficiency in autoimmune rheumatic disease, including undifferentiated connective tissue disease. Arthritis Research & Therapy 2008; 10:123.
[9] Litonjua AA, Weiss ST. Is vitamin D deficiency to blame for asthma epidemic?. J Allergy ClinImmunol2007; 120:1031-5.
[10] Erkkola M, Kaila M, Nwaru BI, Kronberg-Kippilä C, Ahonen S, Nevalainen J, Veijola R, Pekkanen J, Ilonen J, Simell O, Knip M, Virtanen SM. Maternal vitamin D intake during pregnancy is inversely associated with asthma and allergic rhinitis in 5-year-old children. Clinical & Experimental Allergy 2009; 39:875-882.
[11] Braun-Moscovici Y, Furst DE, Markovits D, Rozin A, Clements PJ, Nahir AM, Balbir-Gurman A. Vitamin D, parathyroid hormone, and acroosteolysis in systemic sclerosis. J Rheumatol. 2008; 35:2201-5.
[12] Lange U, Teichmann J, Strunk J, Müller-Ladner U, Schmidt KL. Association of 1. 25 vitamin D3 deficiency, disease activity and low bone mass in ankylosing spondylitis. Osteoporos Int. 2005; 16:1999-2004.
[13] Ban Y, Taniyama M, Ban Y. Vitamin D receptor gene polymorphism is associated with Graves' disease in the Japanese population. J ClinEndocrinolMetab. 2000; 85:4639-43.
[14] Cantorna MT. Vitamin D and its role in immunology: multiple sclerosis, and inflammatory bowel disease. ProgBiophys Mol Biol. 2006; 92:60-4.
[15] Do JE, Kwon SY, Park S, Lee ES. Effects of vitamin D on expression of Toll-like receptors of monocytes from patients with Behcet's disease. Rheumatology (Oxford). 2008; 47:840-8.
[16] Park BS, Park JS, Lee DY, Youn JI, Kim IG. Vitamin D Receptor Polymorphism is Associated with Psoriasis. J Invest Dermatol. 1999; 112:113-6.
[17] Bhatty SA, Shaikh NA, Irfan M, Kashif SM, Vaswani AS, Sumbhai A, Gunpat. Vitamin D deficiency in Fibromylgia. J Pak Med Assoc. 2010; 60:949-51.
[18] Szodoray P, Nakken B, Gaal J, Jonsson R, Szegedi A, Zold E, Szegedi G, Brun JG, Gesztelyi R, Zeher M, Bodolay E. The complex role of vitamin D in autoimmune diseases. Scand J Immunol. 2008; 68:261-9.
[19] Rossini M, MaddaliBongi S, La Montagna G, Minisola G, Malavolta N, Bernini L, Cacace E, Sinigaglia L, Di Munno O, Adami S. Vitamin D deficiency in rheumatoid arthritis: prevalence, determinants and associations with disease activity and disability. Arthritis Res Ther. 2010; 12:R216.
[20] Merlino LA, Curtis J, Mikuls TR, Cerhan JR, Criswell LA, Saag KG; Iowa Women's Health Study. Vitamin D intake is inversely associated with rheumatoid arthritis: results from the Iowa Women's Health Study. Arthritis Rheum. 2004; 50:72-7.
[21] Huisman AM, White KP, Algra A, Harth M, Vieth R, Jacobs JW, Bijlsma JW, Bell DA. Vitamin D levels in women with systemic lupus erythematosus and fibromyalgia. J Rheumatol. 2001; 28:2535-9.
[22] Thudi A, Yin S, Wandstrat AE, Li QZ, Olsen NJ. Vitamin D levels and disease status in Texas patients with systemic lupus erythematosus. Am J Med Sci. 2008; 335:99-104.

[23] Carvalho JF, Blank M, Kiss E, Tarr T, Amital H, Shoenfeld Y. Anti-vitamin D, vitamin D in SLE: preliminary results. Ann N Y Acad Sci. 2007; 1109:550-7.
[24] Gratacós J, Collado A, Pons F, Osaba M, Sanmartí R, Roqué M, Larrosa M, Múñoz-Gómez J. Significant loss of bone mass in patients with early, active ankylosing spondylitis: a followup study. Arthritis Rheum. 1999; 42:2319-24.
[25] Lange U, Jung O, Teichmann J, Neeck G. Relationship between disease activity and serum levels of vitamin D metabolites and parathyroid hormone in ankylosing spondylitis. Osteoporos Int. 2001; 12:1031-5.
[26] Zold E, Szodoray P, Gaal J, Kappelmayer J, Csathy L, Gyimesi E, Zeher M, Szegedi G, Bodolay E. Vitamin D deficiency in undifferentiated connective tissue disease. Arthritis Res Ther. 2008; 10:R123.

5

Osteoporosis in Rheumatoid Arthritis

Alessandro Geraci
Santa Maria del Prato Hospital, Feltre
Italy

1. Introduction

Rheumatoid arthritis (RA) is the most common form of inflammatory arthritis in adults and is characterized by chronic, progressive, systemic inflammation leading to substantial pain, disability, and other morbidities[1]. Osteoporosis (OP) is more frequent in patients with RA than in the general population due to active systemic inflammation as well as the use of corticosteroids and immobility. OP is characterized by low bone mass, and microarchitectural deterioration of bony tissue, with a consequent increase in bone fragility and susceptibility to fractures. According to the WHO criteria (Tab. 1), osteoporosis can also be defined as a value of bone mineral density (BMD) more than - 2.5 standard deviations below the young normal mean. Subsequent disability may lead to loss of independence and quality of life. Underlining the clinical significance of BMD in RA, the risk of hip[2] and vertebral fractures[3] and the associated morbidity, mortality and healthcare costs are increased in patients with RA (Fig.1).

T - Score	Diagnosis
0 to > -1	Normal bone density
-1 to >-2,5	Osteopenia
< -2,5	Osteoporosis
< -2,5 with fracture	Severe osteoporosis

Table 1. WHO T-score criteria for Bone Mineral Density

Localized bone loss in the form of bone erosions and periarticular osteopenia constitutes an important radiographic criterion for the diagnosis of RA. In addition, generalized bone loss has been demonstrated in RA, systemic lupus erythematosus, and ankylosing spondylitis in several observational and some longitudinal studies using markers of bone turnover, bone histomorphometry, and bone densitometry[4].

---

[1] Pattison DJ, Harrison RA, Symmons DP. The role of diet in susceptibility to rheumatoid arthritis: a systematic review. *J Rheumatol.* 2004;31(7):1310-9.

[2] Cooper C, Coupland C, Mitchell M. Rheumatoid arthritis, corticosteroid therapy and hip fracture. *Ann Rheum Dis* 1995;54:49–52.

[3] Arai, T. & Kragic, D. Van Staa TP, Geusens P, Bijlsma JWJ, Leufkens HGM, Cooper C. Clinical assessment of the long-term risk of fracture in patients with rheumatoid arthritis. *Arthritis Rheum* 2006;54:3104–12.

[4] Eggelmeijer F, Papapoulos SE, Westedt ML, Van Paassen HC, Dijkmans BA, Breedveld FC: Bone metabolism in rheumatoid arthritis; relation to disease activity. *Br J Rheumatol* 1993, 32: 387-391.

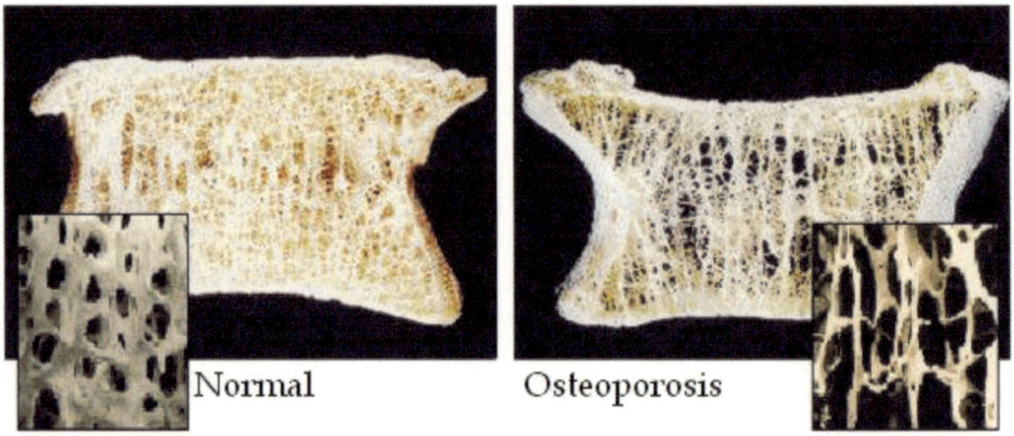

Fig. 1. In osteoporosis, the cortex becomes thinner and more brittle, while the inner trabecular bone develops larger holes

OP occurs in two forms during the course of the AR[5]:

1. periarticular osteopenia in close proximity to inflamed joints, which is a typical phenomenon in early and prolonged rheumatoid disease;
2. generalized osteoporosis, which affects the axial and appendicular bones. Inflammation has the effect of provoking more severe and accelerated bone loss in the hand as compared with hip and spine.

In all inflammatory diseases, use of glucocorticoids (GC) is a common therapy. There is no doubt about the deleterious effect of GC in bone metabolism, suppressing bone formation and enhancing bone resorption. The addition of GC to osteoprogenitor cells *in vitro* actually increases their bone-forming capacity but it also increases apoptosis of mature osteoblasts and osteocytes and therefore affects capacity of bone formation. This potent anti-inflammatory drug reduces production of pro-inflammatory cytokines (IL-1, IL-6, and TNF-α), but provokes bone resorption by increasing the synthesis of RANKL and inhibiting OPG production with consequent induction of osteoclastogenesis[6].

Systemic inflammation and GC use accelerates bone loss independent of other risk factors[7] but other factors must be valorized. Immobilization due to pain from inflamed joints, impairment of physical activity, reduced calcium intake, and poor nutrition associated with enhanced basal energy expenditure are also risk factors related to low BMD, common is this population. In children, delayed puberty and stunted growth can adversely affect bone remodeling[8].

---

5 Sambrook PN: The skeleton in rheumatoid arthritis: common mechanism for bone erosion and osteoporosis? *J Rheumatol* 2000, 27:2541-2542. Gregório LH, Lacativa PG, Melazzi AC, Russo LA.

6 Glucocorticoid-induced osteoporosis. *Arq Bras Endocrinol Metab*. 2006;50(4):793-801.

7 Roldán JF, Del Rincón I, Escalante A. Loss of cortical bone from the metacarpal diaphysis in patients with rheumatoid arthritis: independent effects of systemic inflammation and glucocorticoids. *J Rheumatol*. 2006;33(3):508-16.

8 Viswanathan A, Sylvester FA. Chronic pediatric inflammatory diseases: effects on bone. *Rev Endocr Metab Disord*. 2008;9(2):107-22.

Consequently, increase in bone resorption, both focal and systemic, are common in patients with RA. In patients with active RA compared to matched controls and patients with inactive RA serum osteocalcin which reflects bone formation was found to be significantly lower and crosslinked N-telopeptidases of type 1 collagen (NTX) and deoxypyridinoline (DPD) which reflect bone resorption, were significantly higher. There were positive correlations between these bone markers and disease activity[9].

2. Epidemiology and prevalence

Rheumatoid arthritis is a chronic inflammatory and destructive joint disease that affects 0.5-1% of the world's population and commonly leads to significant disability and consequent impairment of quality of life[10]. It is two or three times more frequent in women than in men and can start at any age, with its peak incidence between the fourth and sixth decades of life[11]. Generalized osteoporosis is an extra-articular complication of rheumatoid arthritis that results in increased risk of fractures and associated morbidity, mortality, and healthcare costs. The incidence of osteoporosis among patients with rheumatoid arthritis is 15-20% at the hip and spine[12]. Haugeberg elegantly showed a twofold increase in osteoporosis in women with RA and a twofold increase of reduced bone mass in men with RA, compared with patients without RA in a population based study[13]. Italian research, performed with patients with established RA, reported disease-related factors, such as long disease duration, high disease activity, joint damage, functional disability and corticosteroid use, as determinants of osteoporosis or reduced BMD[14] . Hence, patients with long-standing RA with destructive disease, functional disability or immobilisation, or who are on longterm corticosteroid treatment are at high risk for osteoporosis[15]. This could be explained by the fact that generalised osteoporosis is more associated with long-standing, destructive and disabling RA,whereas early RA is associated with periarticular osteoporosis. This is further supported by the fact that longer symptom duration is independently associated with more generalised osteoporosis in studies.

---

[9] Seriolo B, Ferretti V, Sulli A, Caratto E, Fasciolo D, Cutolo M. Serum osteocalcin levels in premenopausal rheumatoid arthritis patients. *Ann N Y Acad Sci.* 2002;966:502-7.

[10] Brandão L, Ferraz MB, Zerbini CAF. Avaliação da qualidade de vida na artrite reumatóide: revisão atualizada [Evaluation of quality of life in rheumatoid arthritis]. *Rev Bras Reumatol.* 1997;37(5):275-81.

[11] Gabriel SE. The epidemiology of rheumatoid arthritis. Rheum Dis Clin North Am. 2001;27(2):269-81. Martin JC, Munro R, Campbell MK, Reid DM. Effects of disease and corticosteroids on appendicular bone mass in postmenopausal women with rheumatoid arthritis: comparison with axial measurements. *Br J Rheumatol.* 1999;36(1):43-9.

[12] Lodder MC, Haugeberg G, Lems WF, et al. Radiographic damage associated with low bone mineral density and vertebral deformities in rheumatoid arthritis: the Oslo-Truro-Amsterdam (OSTRA) collaborative study. *Arthritis Rheum.* 2003;49(2):209-15.

[13] Haugeberg G, Uhlig T, Falch JA, Halse JI, Kvien TK. Reduced bone mineral density in male rheumatoid arthritis patients: frequencies and associations with demographic and disease variables in ninety-four patients in the Oslo County Rheumatoid Arthritis Register. *Arthritis Rheum* 2000;43:2776–84.

[14] Sinigaglia L, Nervetti A, Mela Q, Bianchi G, Del Puente A, Di Munno O, et al. A multicenter cross sectional study on bone mineral density in rheumatoid arthritis. Italian Study Group on Bone Mass in Rheumatoid Arthritis. *J Rheumatol* 2000;27:2582–9.

[15] Lems WF, Dijkmans BAC. Should we look for osteoporosis in patients with rheumatoid arthritis? *Ann Rheum Dis* 1998;57:325–7.

Numerous studies have investigated the relation between demographic and disease related variables on the one hand, and bone mass on the other, in patients with RA. These studies tried to identify patients at high risk of osteoporosis[16]. Studies investigating the variables associated with BMD[17] showed some inconsistencies, which might be caused by differences in methodological aspects, such as sample size and patient selection. Moreover, the complex interaction between inflammation, immobility, and corticosteroid use may contribute to the lack of unanimous results.

Only a few studies focusing on BMD in patients with early RA have been performed; however the disease duration in some was up to 5 years[18]. Very little is known about the extent of osteoporosis and the influence of disease-associated factors on BMD in patients with recently diagnosed RA[19]. These data are required in order to unravel the common mechanisms between generalised osteoporosis and RA.

Symptom duration and the presence of RF were the only RAspecific markers for osteoporosis and reduced BMD in this study. It is known that seropositive RA is associated with more aggressive joint disease and is more commonly complicated by extra-articular manifestations than is seronegative RA[20 21]. Previous studies showed an independent association between the presence of RF and osteoporosis or reduced BMD in established and recent onset RA.

3. Etiology and pathophysiology

3.1 Bone remodeling

Throughout life, normal skeletal maintenance occurs by a tightly coupled process of bone remodeling. It consists of a sequential process of bone resorption by osteoclasts followed by deposition of new bone by osteoblasts. Osteoblasts are derived from precursor cells that can also be stimulated to become muscle, fat or cartilage; however, under the right conditions these cells change (or differentiate) to form new bone, producing the collagen that forms the scaffolding or bone matrix. This calcium- and phosphate-rich mineral is added to the matrix to form the hard, yet resilient, tissue that is healthy bone. The osteoclasts remove bone by dissolving the mineral and breaking down the matrix in a process that is called bone resorption. The osteoclasts come from the same precursor cells in the bone marrow that

---

[16] Martin JC, Munro R, Campbell MK, Reid DM. Effects of disease and corticosteroids on appendicular bone mass in postmenopausal women with rheumatoid arthritis: comparison with axial measurements. *Br J Rheumatol* 1997;36:43–9.

[17] Kroot EJ, Nieuwenhuizen MG, Waal Malefijt MC, van Riel PL, Pasker-de Jong PC, Laan RF. Change in bone mineral density in patients with rheumatoid arthritis during the first decade of the disease. *Arthritis Rheum* 2001;44:1254–60.

[18] Shenstone BD, Mahmoud A, Woodward R, Elvins D, Palmer R, Ring F, et al. Bone mineral density in nonsteroid treated early rheumatoid arthritis. *Ann Rheum Dis* 1994;53:681–4.

[19] Keller C, Hafstrom I, Svensson B. Bone mineral density in women and men with early rheumatoid arthritis. *Scand J Rheumatol* 2001;30:213–20.

[20] Egeland T, Munthe E. The role of the laboratory in rheumatology. Rheumatoid factors. *Clin Rheum Dis* 1983;9:135–60. 22.

[21] Van Zeben D, Hazes JM, Zwinderman AH, Cats A, van der Voort EA, Breedveld FC. Clinical significance of rheumatoid factors in early rheumatoid arthritis: results of a follow up study. *Ann Rheum Dis* 1992;9:1029–35.

produce white blood cells. These precursor cells can also circulate in the blood and be available at different sites in need of bone breakdown. Osteoclasts are formed by fusion of small precursor cells into large, highly active cells with many nuclei. Removal and replacement of bone in the remodeling cycleis controlled by local and systemic factors that regulate bone remodeling to fulfill both its structural and metabolic functions. The activation of this process involves an interaction between cells of the osteoblastic lineage and the precursors that will become osteoclasts. The differentiation of myeloid progenitor cells into committed osteoclast lineage is characterized by the appearance of the mRNA and protein for vitronectin receptor, cathepsin K, tartrate-resistant acid phosphatase, and calcitonin receptor[22 23].This process of osteoclastogenesis requires the presence of receptor activator of nuclear factor-κB ligand (RANKL; also known as OPGL, TRANCE, ODF, and SOFA) and the permissive factor, macrophage colony stimulating factor (M-CSF) secreted by the local osteoblast/stromal cells. RANKL binds to its receptor RANK expressed on the surface of osteoclast precursor cells and stimulates their differentiation into mature osteoclasts[24]. The osteoblast/stromal cells also secrete osteoprotegerin (OPG; also known as OCIF, TR-1, FDCR-1, and TNFRSF-11B), a soluble decoy receptor protein that binds to RANKL and prevents its binding to RANK on the preosteoclast cells. The biologic effects of OPG are, therefore, the opposite of those of RANKL, i.e. OPG inhibits osteoclastogenesis and osteoclast function and promotes osteoclast apoptosis[25]. The production and activity of both RANKL and OPG are influenced by several cytokines, inflammatory mediators, and calcitropic hormones that 'converge' onto these proteins. The net RANKL/OPG balance determines the differentiation, activation, and survival of osteoclasts, which in turn determine bone loss[26].

3.2 Focal bone erosion in rheumatoid arthritis: The role of the rank/rankl/OPG system and the TNF-α

Although the mechanisms of cartilage destruction in rheumatoid arthritis (RA) are well described, the mechanisms responsible for bone erosion in this disease have only recently been studied. The role of osteoclasts in bone erosion in RA has been suspected for many years on the basis of indirect evidence, including the identification of multinucleated cells with phenotypic features of osteoclasts at sites of erosion in human RA[27 28].

---

22 Lee SK, Goldring SR, Lorenzo JA: Expression of the calcitonin receptor in bone marrow cell cultures and in bone: a specific marker of the differentiated osteoclast that is regulated by calcitonin. *Endocrinology* 1995, 136:4572-4581.

23 Faust J, Lacey DL, Hunt P, Burgess TL, Scully S, Van G, Eli A, Qian Y, Shalhoub V: Osteoclast markers accumulate on cells developing from human peripheral blood mononuclear precursors. *J Cell Biochem* 1999, 72:67-80.

24 Lacey DL, Timms E, Tan HL, Kelley MJ, Dunstan CR. Osteoprotegerin ligand is a cytokine that regulates osteoclast differentiation and activation. *Cell* 1998, 93:165-176.

25 Simonet WS, Lacey DL, Dunstan CR, Kelley M, Chang MS. Osteoprotegerin: a novel secreted protein involved in the regulation of bone density. *Cell* 1997, 89:309-319.

26 Suda T, Takahashi N, Martin TJ: Modulation of osteoclast differentiation. *Endocr Rev* 1992, 13:66-80.

27 Gravallese EM, Harada Y, Wang JT, Gorn AH, Thornhill TS, Goldring SR. Identification of cell types responsible for bone resorption in rheumatoid arthritis and juvenile rheumatoid arthritis. *Am J Pathol* 1998;152:943–51.

Inflammation modulates bone resorption mainly by two mechanisms. Firstly, pro-inflammatory cytokines have a final common mediator of osteoclast function: receptor activator of nuclear factor-B (RANK) and its functional ligand (RANKL), also known as TRANCE (TNF-related activation induced cytokine)[29 30]. Secondly, osteoclastogenesis can be regulated through the modulation of macrophage colony stimulating factor (M-CSF).

RANKL is a membrane-bound tumor necrosis factor (TNF) receptor expressed on osteoblast precursor cells that recognize RANK on the osteoclast surface through a direct cell-cell interaction. This process is essential for osteoclast differentiation, activation and survival. RANKL is considered the key osteoclastogenic cytokine as the RANKL-RANK interaction stimulates several transcription factors and all three families of MAP kinases[31]. The osteoblast/stromal cells also secrete osteoprotegerin (OPG), a soluble decoy receptor protein that binds to RANKL and prevents its binding to RANK on the preosteoclast cells. The biologic effects of OPG are, therefore, the opposite of those of RANKL; infact, it inhibits osteoclastogenesis and osteoclast function and promotes osteoclast apoptosis[32]. The net RANKL/OPG balance determines the differentiation, activation, and survival of osteoclasts, which in turn determine bone loss[33]. Synovial tissues provide a source of RANKL that could influence osteoclastogenesis. Synovial fibroblasts from patients with RA produce mRNA and protein for RANKL. RANKL is also expressed by T lymphocytes from RA synovial tissues[34]. Adjuvant-induced arthritis (AIA) is an animal model of T lymphocyte mediated inflammatory arthritis characterized by destruction of bone and cartilage similar to that in RA. In this model, activated T cells express RANKL protein on their surface, and through binding of RANKL to RANK on preosteoclasts, these cells promote osteoclastogenesis and subsequent bone loss. Co-culture experiments using RA synovial fibroblasts and peripheral blood mononuclear cells as a source of osteoclast precursors demonstrate that osteoclast-like cells are generated, and the generation of these cells is inhibited by the addition of OPG (Fig.2) Similarly, activated T cells expressing RANKL induce osteoclasts from autologous peripheral blood monocytes, a process that is also inhibited by OPG[35].

---

[28] Suzuki Y, Nishikaku F, Nakatuka M, Koga Y. Osteoclast-like cells in murine collagen induced arthritis. *J Rheumatol* 1998;25:1154–60.

[29] Romas E, Bakharevski O, Hards DK, Kartsogiannis V, Quinn JMW, Ryan PFJ, et al. Expression of osteoclast differentiation factor at sites of bone erosion in collagen-induced arthritis. *Arthritis Rheum 2000*;43:821–6.

[30] Leisen JCC, Duncan H, Riddle JM, Pitchford WC. The erosive front: a topographic study of the junction between the pannus and the subchondral plate in the macerated rheumatoid metacarpal head. *J Rheumatol* 1988;15:17–22.

[31] Mundy GR. Osteoporosis and inflammation. *Nutr Rev*. 2007;65(12 Pt 2):S147-51

[32] Teitelbaum SL. Osteoclasts: what do they do and how do they do it? *Am J Pathol*. 2007;170(2):427-35.

[33] Takayanagi H, Iizuka H, Juji T, Nakagawa T, Yamamoto A. Involvement of receptor activator of nuclear factor kappa-B ligand/osteoclast differentiation factor in osteoclastogenesis from synoviocytes in rheumatoid arthritis. *Arthritis Rheum* 2000;43:259–69.

[34] Kong YY, Feige U, Sarosi I, Bolon B, Tafuri A. Activated T cells regulate bone loss and joint destruction in adjuvant arthritis through osteoprotegerin ligand. *Nature* 1999;402:304–9.

[35] Suzuki Y, Tsutsumi Y, Nakagawa M, Suzuki H, Matsushita K, Beppu MI. Osteoclast-like cells in an in vitro model of bone destruction by rheumatoid synovium. *Rheumatology (Oxford)* 2001;40:673–82.

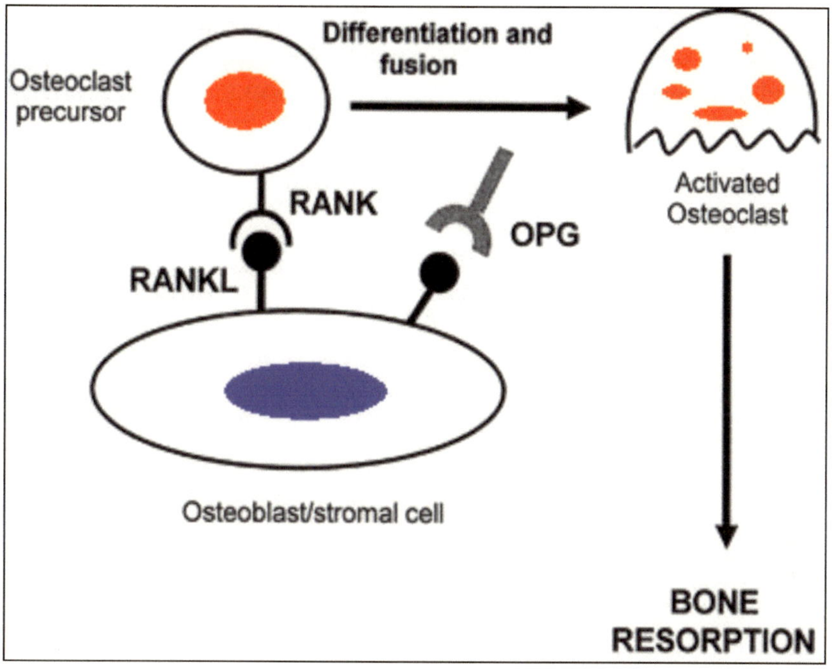

Fig. 2. A schematic overview of the RANK/RANKL/OPG system

Synovial tissues may also provide a source of osteoclast precursor cells, as macrophages isolated from RA synovial tissues differentiate into osteoclasts in the presence of M-CSF plus RANKL. More recent studies have extended these findings. Cells digested from RA synovial tissue samples generate TRAP positivemultinucleated cells that form resorption pits on dentine slices[36] a definitive demonstration that these cells are osteoclasts. Synovial fibroblasts in rheumatoid synovium may also contribute significantly to localized bone loss. These cells produce chemokines such as macrophage inflammatory peptide 1, regulated-upon-activation normal T cell expressed and secreted, IL-8, and IL-16, which promote lymphocyte infiltration and support lymphoproliferation via secretion of various colony-stimulating factors[37]. This results in a large pool of RANKL-expressing lymphocytes supporting osteoclastogenesis and local bone loss. Furthermore, synovial fibroblasts may directly contribute to local bone destruction by expressing RANKL on their surface[38] and by secreting cathepsins. Elevated levels of tumor necrosis factor (TNF)-a have been demonstrated by immunoassays in several inflammatory arthritides. TNF-a promotes expression of adhesion molecules, activation of leukocytes, recruitment of leukocytes, and production of proinflammatory cytokines (e.g. IL-1, IL-6, and IL-8) in RA. There are two mechanisms by which TNF-α acts in osteoclasts, both marrow stromal cells and osteoclast

---

[36] Kontoyiannis D, Kollias G: Fibroblast biology: synovial fibroblasts in rheumatoid arthritis: leading role or chorus line? *Arthritis Res* 2000, 2:342-343.

[37] Ross FP, Chappel J, Alvarez JI, Sander D, Butler WT, Farach-Carson MC. Interactions between the bone matrix proteins osteopontin and bone sialoprotein and the osteoclast integrin alpha v beta 3 potentiate bone resorption: *J Biol Chem* 1993, 268:9901-9907.

[38] Teitelbaum SL. Osteoclasts: what do they do and how do they do it? *Am J Pathol*. 2007;170(2):427-35.

precursors express TNF-α receptors. The main process occurs when stromal cells are exposed to TNF-α and produce RANKL, M-CSF, and IL-1, which promote osteoclast formation and activation. TNF-α and RANKL are synergistic, and minimal levels of one markedly enhances the osteoclastogenic capacity of the other[39] (Fig. 3).

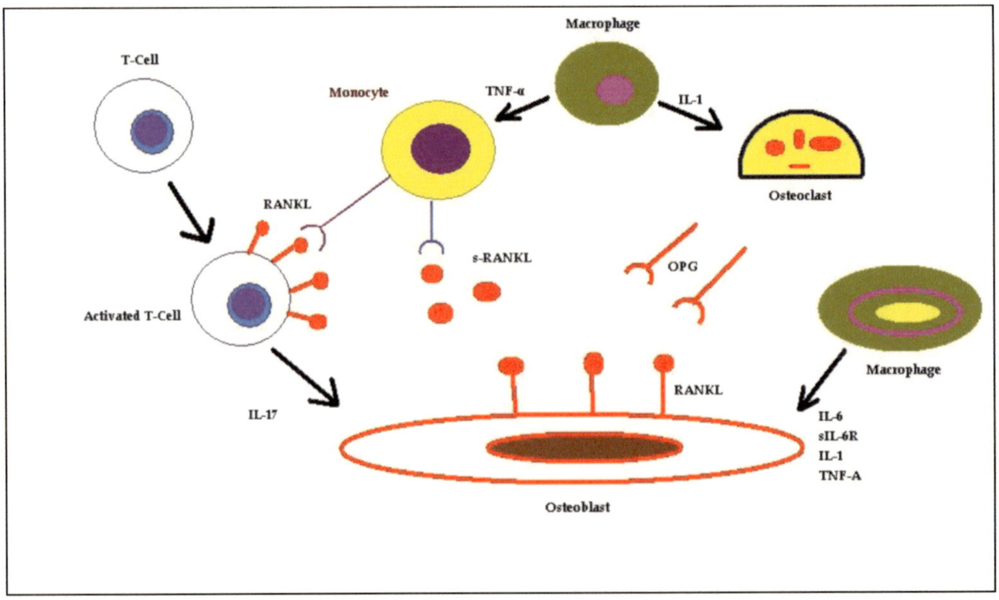

Fig. 3. Activated human T cells induce osteoclastogenesis from human monocytes

TNF-α also has potent antiapoptotic effects on osteoclasts, prolonging their lifespan[40]. The second mechanism occurs when the inflammatory process becomes more aggressive and TNF-α may promote osteoclast formation by directly stimulating its precursors in the absence of stromal cells responsive to the cytokine, perhaps through activation of transforming growth factor (TGF)-β.

3.3 Focal bone erosion in rheumatoid arthritis: The role of the glucocorticoid use

In all inflammatory diseases, use of glucocorticoids (GC) is a common therapy. The use of GC, however, is associated with a variety of adverse effects,1 including the development of osteoporosis and fractures. In patients who have received GCs for longer than six months, the estimated glucocorticoid-induced osteoporosis (GIO) frequency is 50%[41]. The pathogenesis of GIO is multifaceted. Glucocorticoids have indirect effects on osteoporosis by inhibiting calcium absorption from the gastrointestinal track and decreasing the renal tubular reabsorption of calcium and consequentely secondary hyperparathyroidism. GCs

[39] Weitzmann MN, Pacifici R. The role of T lymphocytes in bone metabolism. *Immunol Rev.* 2005;208:154-68.

[40] Van Staa TP, Leufkens HG, Cooper C. The epidemiology of corticosteroid induced osteoporosis: a meta-analysis. *Osteoporos Int.* 2002;13:777- 87.

[41] Pereira RM, Delany AM, Canalis E. Cortisol inhibits the differentiation and apoptosis of osteoblasts in culture. *Bone* 2001;28:484-90.

reduce growth hormone (GH) secretion and may alter the GH/insulin-like growth factor (IGF)-I axis. An important role may be played by skeletal IGF-I because GCs inhibit IGF-I transcription in osteoblasts. Glucocorticoids have direct effects on bone cells. GCs reduce the replication, differentiation and function of osteoblasts[42] and increase the apoptosis rates of mature cells, thereby depleting the osteoblastic cell population and inhibiting the function of mature cells. Furthermore, in the presence of GCs, bone marrow stromal cells do not differentiate into osteoblasts; instead, these cells differentiate toward an adipocyte cell lineage. Moreover, GCs induce apoptosis in osteocytes and affect the functioning of these cells. GCs increase the expression of M-CSF and receptor activator of RANK-L. In addition, GCs decrease the expression of osteoprotegerin in stromal and osteoblastic cells. Through these mechanisms, GCs can induce the formation of osteoclasts and favor bone resorption. GCs also reduce the rate of apoptosis among mature osteoclasts.

4. Diagnosis

The initial evaluation of secondary osteoporosis should include a detailed history of clinical risk factors for fractures and the underlying medical conditions and medications that cause bone loss, a thorough physical. Patients with decreased bone density usually have no specific abnormal physical findings. Those with vertebral compression fractures will have kyposis, protruding abdomen and height loss. Back tenderness is usually only present after an acute fracture. Gait speed and grip strength are often reduced in patients who have or are about to have a hip fracture. Visual acuity should be checked in geriatric patients because it is a risk factor for falling.

Based on these initial findings and the clinical index of suspicion, further laboratory and imaging studies as well as invasive tests are required. examination and laboratory. Optimal evaluation consists of establishing the diagnosis of osteoporosis on the basis of bone mass assessment (BMD), establishing the fracture risk, and determining the need for therapy. Dual-energy x-ray absorptiometry (DXA) is the preferred technique to measure BMD, and is the technique used at most centers[43]. The hip and the spine are the preferred site for BMD measurement due to the high predictive value of hip BMD for fracture risk. The World Health Organization (WHO) has established the following operational definition for osteoporosis based on BMD as measured by DXA (Fig. 4), commonly expressed as a T-score.

The World Health Organization (WHO) has established criteria for making the diagnosis of osteoporosis, as well as determining levels that predict higher chances of fractures. These criteria are based on comparing the BMD of the patient with that of a typical healthy, young female's. BMD values that fall well below the average for the healthy, young female's (stated statistically as 2.5 standard deviations below the average) are diagnosed as osteoporotic. If a patient has a BMD value less than the healthy, young female, but not 2.5 standard deviations below the average, the bone is osteopenic. Osteopenic means decreased bone mineral density, but it's not as severe as osteoporosis.

---

[42] Khan AA, Hanley DA, Bilezikian JP, Binkley N, Brown JP. Standards for performing DXA in individuals with secondary causes of osteoporosis. *Journal of Clinical Densitometry* 2006 9 47–57.
[43] Heaney RP. Thinking straight about calcium. *N Engl J Med* 1993; 328:503-505.

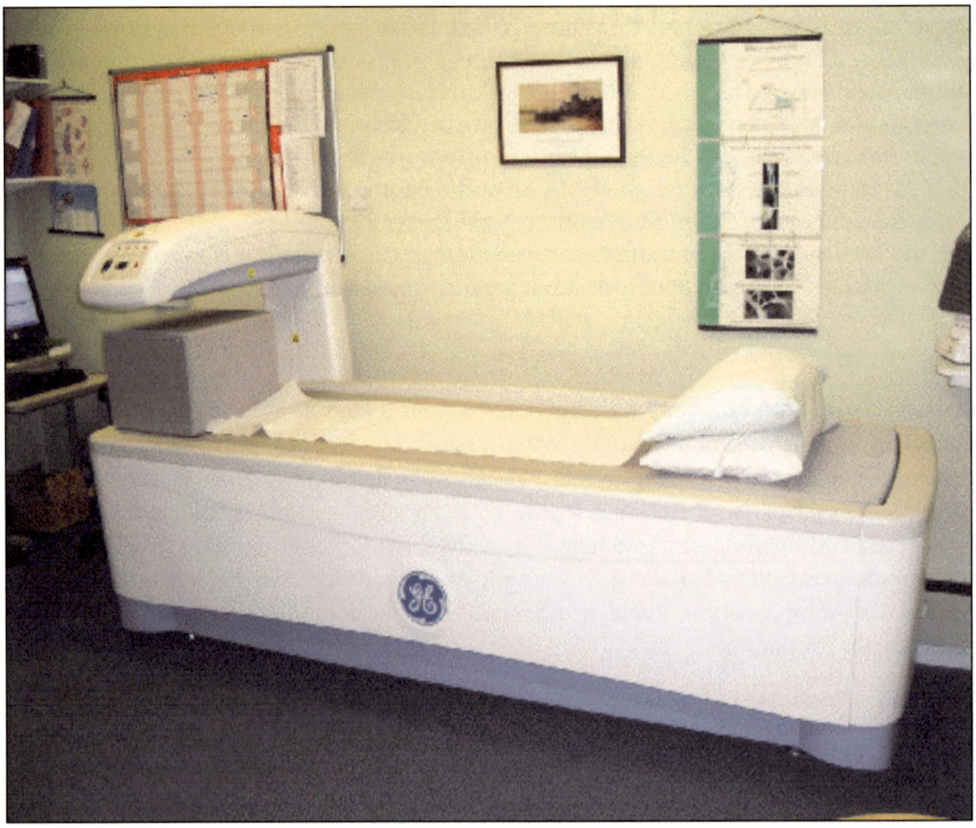

Fig. 4. A scanner used to measure bone density with Dual Energy X-ray absorptiometry.

Although these criteria are widely used, they were based on a Caucasian female, so there will be some differences when these levels are applied to non-Caucasian females or to males in general. Despite this flaw, BMD measurement is a common method that's helpful in all groups. Laboratory evaluation for secondary causes of osteoporosis should be considered when osteoporosis is diagnosed. Serum calcium, phosphorus, alkaline phosphatase, creatinine, vitamin D, complete blood count and thyroid stimulating hormone (TSH) levels are usually sufficient baseline tests. Further laboratory tests can be done as clinically appropriate, such as parathyroid hormone level, urine free cortisol, liver function tests, or serum immune electrophoresis. Biochemical indices of skeletal turnover could potentially be helpful in the diagnosis and monitoring of therapy.

5. Treatment

The treatment of inflammatory bone loss can be aimed at attempts to suppress bone resorption and to increase bone formation.

5.1 Calcium and vitamin D

Both alfacalcidol (25 OH vitamin D3) and calcitriol (1,25 (OH)2 Vitamin D3) are used by some for the treatment of osteoporosis[44]. An adequate intake of calcium and Vitamin D supplementation are recommended as vitamin D. Serum and urinary calcium, serum 25OHD, and PTH concentrations should be used to evaluate hypovitaminosis D, secondary hyperparathyroidism and low net calcium balance. In randomized trials, the use of calcium and vitamin D alone had no significant benefit in bone density. However, these disturbances usually found in inflammatory diseases should be corrected to avoid the interference with anti-osteoporotic treatment efficacy. Calcium intake (from diet, added to supplementation) must be at least 1,200 mg/d, and vitamin D supplementation should be at least 800 UI/d if any of those disturbances are found. In addition, the efficacy of anti-osteoporotic drugs has only been demonstrated in the presence of vitamin D and calcium supplementation. Therapy should be titrated with doses that result in normocalcemia and serum 25-hydroxyvitamin D concentrations of at least 30 ng/ml. In patients with normal renal function, a decrease in serum PTH levels from elevated to normal levels indicates that 25-hydroxyvitamin D deficiency has been corrected. Some anti-epileptic drugs, e.g. phenytoin, phenobarbitone, primidone, and carbamazepine, increase hepatic metabolism of vitamin D, requiring higher vitamin D doses.

5.2 Bisphosphonates

Bisphosphonates have a strong affinity for bone apatite, which is the basis for their clinical use. They are potent inhibitors of bone resorption and produce their effect by reducing the recruitment and activity of osteoclasts and increasing their apoptosis. In general, alendronate (70 mg/week) and risedronate (35 mg/week) are reasonable antiosteoporotic drugs for secondary osteoporosis. However, many patients with osteoporosis secondary to gastrointestinal diseases or concurrent medications not tolerating, or adhering to, oral bisphosphonates and those in whom oral bisphosphonates are contraindicated may benefit from treatment with i.v. ibandronate or zoledronic acid. Many studies have shown that Alendronate and Zoledronate are able to reduce joint swelling and blood inflammatory tests (IL-1, IL-6, TNF-α, b2-microglobulin and erythrocyte sedimentation rate and C-reactive protein values) in various experimental arthritis animal models and in human studies. These medications reduce the macrophage production of TNF-α, IL-1 and nitric oxide (NO) and induce apoptosis of monocyte-macrophage-derived cell lines. These effects are in part dependent on RANKL inhibition and in part dependent on cytoplasmic events which involve protein-kinase C and iron ions. All these effects explain why, although bisphosphonates enhance proliferation of T-lymphocytes, they have been successfully used to treat bone loss secondary to RA[45]. The overall safety profile of bisphosphonates is favorable. Oral bisphosphonates are associated with mild gastrointestinal disturbances, and rarely cause esophagitis and ulcer. A recent study also showed an increase in esophageal cancer among chronic users. Intravenous zolendronate can induce a transient acute phase

[44] Neer RM, Arnaud CD, Zanchetta JR, Prince R, Gaich GA. Effect of parathyroid hormone (1-34) on fractures and bone mineral density in postmenopausal women with osteoporosis. *N Engl J Med.* 2001;344:1434–4.

[45] Ahrader SP, Raggucci KR. Parathyroid hormone (1-84) and treatment of osteoporosis. *Ann Pharmacother.* 2005;39:1511–6.

reaction with fever, bone and muscle pain that ameliorates or disappears after subsequent courses. Osteonecrosis of the jaw has been described in cancer patients receiving high doses of intravenous pamidronate or zoledronate. Atrial fibrillation was noted to occur in a higher frequency after intravenous zolendronate, but a cause-effect relationship was not established and it was not seen in another study.

5.3 Teriparatide

Intermittent administration of PTH (for example, with daily subcutaneous injections) results in an increase of the number and activity of osteoblasts, leading to an increase in bone mass and in an improvement in skeletal architecture at both cancellous and cortical skeletal sites. The 1-34 N-terminal fragment (teriparatide) is used for the management of osteoporosis. Treatment with teriparatide has been shown to reduce significantly the risk of vertebral fractures and to reduce non-vertebral but not hip fractures[46].The recommended dose is 20 µg of teriparatide daily, given as a subcutaneous injection. The effect was initially seen in patients with severe osteoporosis and established vertebral fractures. Efficacy was later shown with osteoporosis even without fractures[47].

5.4 Stronzium ranelate

Strontium ranelate is a recently approved agent in Europe, for the treatment of postmenopausal osteoporosis, to reduce the risk of vertebral and hip fractures (49). There is some evidence that strontium ranelate both inhibits bone resorption and stimulates bone formation, suggesting that the agent may uncouple the bone remodelling process. The recommended daily dose is a one 2-gram sachet once daily by mouth. The absorption of strontium ranelate is reduced by food, milk and its derivative products and the drug should be administered, therefore, between meals. Ideally, it should be taken at bedtime, preferably two hours after eating. Strontium ranelate is not recommended for patients with severe renal impairment (creatinine clearance below 30 mL/min).

5.5 Denosumab

Denosumab, a new drug under evaluation, acts as an anti-RANKL blocking osteoblast differention and slowing bone resorption similar to the OPG. Denosumab is a fully human monoclonal antibody that mimics the activity of osteoprotegerin. It binds to RANKL, thereby preventing RANKL from interacting with RANK and reducing its bone resorption.

5.6 Raloxifene

Raloxifene is part of Selective Estrogen Receptor Modulators (SERMs). They are a class of medications that act on the estrogen receptors throughout the body in a selective manner.

---

[46] Reginster JY, Felsenberg D, Boonen S, Diez-Perez A, Rizzoli R. Effects of long term strontium ranelate treatment on the risk of nonvertebral and vertebral fractures in postmenopausal osteoporosis, results of five year, randomizes, placebo-controlled trial. *Arthritis and Rheumatism*. 2008;58:1687–95.

[47] Gillespie MT. Impact of cytokines and T lymphocytes upon osteoclast differentiation and function. *Arthritis Res Ther*. 2007;9:103.

Normally, bone mineral density (BMD) is tightly regulated by a balance between osteoblast and osteoclast activity in the trabecular bone. Estrogen has a major role in regulation of the bone formation-resorption equilibrium, as it stimulates osteoblast activity[48]. Some SERMs such as raloxifene, act on the bone by slowing bone resorption by the osteoclasts. Raloxifene has the added advantage of reducing the risk of invasive breast cancer.

6. Therapy in glucocorticoid treatment

There are a number of guidelines regarding the management of GIO in patients who are receiving glucocorticoid treatment or that will be starting this therapy. We have analyzed the guidelines established by the American College of Rheumatology (ACR)[49], and the Dutch Society of Rheumatology (DSR)[50]. A Cochrane Database Meta-Analysis concluded that calcium and vitamin D supplementation should be started in all patients who are administered glucocorticoids because of their low toxicity, low cost and the possible benefit in terms of fracture risk[51]. Vitamin D is a hormone that increases intestinal calcium absorption and increases its reabsorption in distal renal tubules. Serum levels of at least 30 ng/mL (82 nmol/L), and optimally of 40–60 ng/mL, of 25-hydroxyvitamin D should be the target treatment regimen for GIO management. To achieve these levels, 1,000 to 2,000 IU of oral vitamin D daily may be necessary[52]. Bisphosphonates are indicated for the prevention and treatment of GIO and most guidelines recommend the use of these drugs. The prevention and treatment goals of bisphosphonate use are stabilized or increased bone mineral density, as well as reduced frequency of fractures. A study using risedronate showed a decrease in vertebral fractures after one year of treatment[53]. Currently, alendronate (70 mg/ week or 10 mg/day) and risedronate (35 mg/week or 5 mg/ day) are the only oral antiresorptive drugs that are recommended in GIO. Recently, zoledronic acid was approved for the prevention and treatment of GIO. In a multicenter, double-blind, double-dummy, randomized controlled trial that included 833 patients, a single 5 mg intravenous infusion of zoledronic caused a greater increase in bone mineral density than oral risedronate at 5 mg daily[54]. Bisphosphonate treatment is recommended while patients

---

[48] Meunier PJ, Vignot E, Garnero P. "Treatment of postmenopausal women with osteoporosis or low bone density with raloxifene. Raloxifene Study Group". *Osteoporos Int* 1999;10 (4): 330–36.

[49] American College of Rheumatology Ad Hoc Committee on Glucocorticoid-Induced Osteoporosis Recommendations for the prevention and treatment of glucocorticoid-induced osteoporosis: 2001 update. Arthritis Rheum. 2001;44:1496-503.

[50] Geusens PP, de Nijs RN, Lems WF, Laan RF, Struijs A, van Staa TP, et al. Prevention of glucocorticoid osteoporosis: a consensus document of the Dutch Society for Rheumatology. Ann Rheum Dis. 2004; 63:324-5.

[51] Berris KK, Repp AL, Kleerekoper M. Glucocorticoid-induced osteoporosis. Curr Opin Endocrinol Diabetes Obes. 2007;14:446-50.

[52] Heaney RP. The vitamin D requirement in health and disease. J Steroid Biochem Mol Biol. 2005;97:13-9, doi: 10.1016/j.jsbmb.2005.06.020.

[53] Wallach S, Cohen S, Reid DM, Hughes RA, Hosking DJ, Laan RF, et al. Effects of risedronate treatment on bone density and vertebral fracture in patients on corticosteroid therapy. Calcif Tissue Int. 2000;67:277-85.

[54] Reid DM, Devogelaer JP, Saag K, Roux C, Lau CS, Reginster JY, et al. Zoledronic acid and risedronate in the prevention and treatment of glucocorticoid-induced osteoporosis (HORIZON): a multicentre, doubleblind, double-dummy, randomised controlled trial. Lancet. 2009;373:1253-63,

are on glucocorticoids; however, in subjects with significant bone loss, therapy may need to be continued following the discontinuation of glucocorticoids. Caution needs to be exercised when considering the use of bisphosphonates in women of childbearing age with GIO,[55 56] given that bisphosphonates have an extended half-life and may cross the placenta with potentially unfavorable effects on fetal skeletal development. A recent review of 51 human cases examining exposure to bisphosphonates before or during pregnancy did not demonstrate skeletal abnormalities or other congenital malformations in the infants. Similarly, a related case-controlled study suggested that preconceptional and first-trimester use of bisphosphonates may pose limited fetal risk[57]. Saag et al., published a randomized multicenter trial to compare use of oral alendronate (10 mg/day) and subcutaneous teriparatide (20 mg/day) over 18 months in patients with established GIO. The study showed that among patients with osteoporosis with a high risk for fracture, the bone mineral density increase in patients receiving teriparatide was greater than in those receiving alendronate[58].

7. Conclusion

Localized bone loss in RA results from the activation of an inflammatory immune response, which increases both the number and the activity of osteoclasts.

Osteoporosis in patients with rheumatoid arthritis is a silent disease that evolves in parallel with the underlying disease and gives a sign to exist only after the fracture. patients with rheumatoid arthritis are subject to chronic systemic inflammation and a chronic intake of corticosteroids. These elements form the basis of the osteoclastic process. The diagnosis and prevention becomes necessary to understand in all its aspects, the patient rheumatic disease and to avoid untoward developments. Therapy to prevent or reverse this bone loss should be directed at the suppression of inflammation, direct inhibition of osteoclastmediated bone resorption, or stimulation of osteoblastic bone formation.

The challenge now is to determine if altering this inflammatory induced bone loss in RA will translate into reduced functional disability. The future is promising in this scientific arena.

8. Acknowledgment

I would like to thank Prof. Vincenzo Miceli that was my first surgical teacher and taught me the professional honesty and the importance of scientific research.

9. References

Ahrader SP, Raggucci KR. Parathyroid hormone (1-84) and treatment of osteoporosis. *Ann Pharmacother.* 2005;39:1511–6.

---

[55] Franchimont N, Canalis E. Management of glucocorticoid induced osteoporosis in premenopausal women with autoimmune disease. Autoimmun Rev. 2003;2:224-8.

[56] Djokanovic N, Klieger-Grossmann C, Koren G. Does treatment with bisphosphonates endanger the human pregnancy? J Obstet Gynaecol Can. 2008;30:1146-8.

[57] Levy S, Fayez I, Taguchi N, Han JY, Aiello J, Matsui D, et al. Pregnancy outcome following in utero exposure to bisphosphonates. Bone. 2009;44:428-30.

[58] Saag KG, Shane E, Boonen S, Marı´n F, Donley DW, Taylor KA, et al. Teriparatide or alendronate in glucocorticoid-induced osteoporosis. N Engl J Med. 2007;357:2028-39.

American College of Rheumatology Ad Hoc Committee on Glucocorticoid-Induced Osteoporosis Recommendations for the prevention and treatment of glucocorticoid-induced osteoporosis: 2001 update. *Arthritis Rheum.* 2001;44:1496-503.

Arai, T. & Kragic, D. Van Staa TP, Geusens P, Bijlsma JWJ, Leufkens HGM, Cooper C. Clinical assessment of the long-term risk of fracture in patients with rheumatoid arthritis. *Arthritis Rheum* 2006;54:3104–12.

Berris KK, Repp AL, Kleerekoper M. Glucocorticoid-induced osteoporosis. *Curr Opin Endocrinol Diabetes Obes.* 2007;14:446-50.

Brandão L, Ferraz MB, Zerbini CAF. Avaliação da qualidade de vida na artrite reumatóide: revisão atualizada [Evaluation of quality of life in rheumatoid arthritis]. *Rev Bras Reumatol.* 1997;37(5):275-81.

Cooper C, Coupland C, Mitchell M. Rheumatoid arthritis, corticosteroid therapy and hip fracture. *Ann Rheum Dis* 1995;54:49–52.

Djokanovic N, Klieger-Grossmann C, Koren G. Does treatment with bisphosphonates endanger the human pregnancy? *J Obstet Gynaecol Can.* 2008;30:1146-8.

Egeland T, Munthe E. The role of the laboratory in rheumatology. Rheumatoid factors. *Clin Rheum Dis* 1983;9:135–60. 22.

Eggelmeijer F, Papapoulos SE, Westedt ML, Van Paassen HC, Dijkmans BA, Breedveld FC: Bone metabolism in rheumatoid arthritis; relation to disease activity. *Br J Rheumatol* 1993, 32: 387-391.

Faust J, Lacey DL, Hunt P, Burgess TL, Scully S, Van G, Eli A, Qian Y, Shalhoub V: Osteoclast markers accumulate on cells developing from human peripheral blood mononuclear precursors. *J Cell Biochem* 1999, 72:67-80.

Franchimont N, Canalis E. Management of glucocorticoid induced osteoporosis in premenopausal women with autoimmune disease. *Autoimmun Rev.* 2003;2:224-8.

Gabriel SE. The epidemiology of rheumatoid arthritis. Rheum Dis Clin North Am. 2001;27(2):269-81. Martin JC, Munro R, Campbell MK, Reid DM. Effects of disease and corticosteroids on appendicular bone mass in postmenopausal women with rheumatoid arthritis: comparison with axial measurements. *Br J Rheumatol.* 1999;36(1):43-9.

Geusens PP, de Nijs RN, Lems WF, Laan RF, Struijs A, van Staa TP, et al. Prevention of glucocorticoid osteoporosis: a consensus document of the Dutch Society for Rheumatology. *Ann Rheum Dis.* 2004; 63:324-5.

Gillespie MT. Impact of cytokines and T lymphocytes upon osteoclast differentiation and function. *Arthritis Res Ther.* 2007;9:103.

Glucocorticoid-induced osteoporosis. *Arq Bras Endocrinol Metab.* 2006;50(4):793-801.

Gravallese EM, Harada Y, Wang JT, Gorn AH, Thornhill TS, Goldring SR. Identification of cell types responsible for bone resorption in rheumatoid arthritis and juvenile rheumatoid arthritis. *Am J Pathol* 1998;152:943–51.

Haugeberg G, Uhlig T, Falch JA, Halse JI, Kvien TK. Reduced bone mineral density in male rheumatoid arthritis patients: frequencies and associations with demographic and disease variables in ninety-four patients in the Oslo County Rheumatoid Arthritis Register. *Arthritis Rheum* 2000;43:2776–84.

Heaney RP. Thinking straight about calcium. *N Engl J Med* 1993; 328:503-505.

Heaney RP. The vitamin D requirement in health and disease. *J Steroid Biochem Mol Biol.* 2005;97:13-9.

Keller C, Hafstrom I, Svensson B. Bone mineral density in women and men with early rheumatoid arthritis. *Scand J Rheumatol* 2001;30:213–20.

Khan AA, Hanley DA, Bilezikian JP, Binkley N, Brown JP. Standards for performing DXA in individuals with secondary causes of osteoporosis. *Journal of Clinical Densitometry* 2006 9 47–57.

Kong YY, Feige U, Sarosi I, Bolon B, Tafuri A. Activated T cells regulate bone loss and joint destruction in adjuvant arthritis through osteoprotegerin ligand. *Nature* 1999;402:304–9.

Kontoyiannis D, Kollias G: Fibroblast biology: synovial fibroblasts in rheumatoid arthritis: leading role or chorus line? *Arthritis Res* 2000, 2:342-343

Kroot EJ, Nieuwenhuizen MG, Waal Malefijt MC, van Riel PL, Pasker-de Jong PC, Laan RF. Change in bone mineral density in patients with rheumatoid arthritis during the first decade of the disease. *Arthritis Rheum* 2001;44:1254–60.

Lacey DL, Timms E, Tan HL, Kelley MJ, Dunstan CR. Osteoprotegerin ligand is a cytokine that regulates osteoclast differentiation and activation. *Cell* 1998, 93:165-176.

Lee SK, Goldring SR, Lorenzo JA: Expression of the calcitonin receptor in bone marrow cell cultures and in bone: a specific marker of the differentiated osteoclast that is regulated by calcitonin. *Endocrinology* 1995, 136:4572-4581.

Leisen JCC, Duncan H, Riddle JM, Pitchford WC. The erosive front: a topographic study of the junction between the pannus and the subchondral plate in the macerated rheumatoid metacarpal head. *J Rheumatol* 1988;15:17–22.

Lems WF, Dijkmans BAC. Should we look for osteoporosis in patients with rheumatoid arthritis? *Ann Rheum Dis* 1998;57:325–7.

Levy S, Fayez I, Taguchi N, Han JY, Aiello J, Matsui D, et al. Pregnancy outcome following in utero exposure to bisphosphonates. *Bone.* 2009;44:428-30.

Lodder MC, Haugeberg G, Lems WF, et al. Radiographic damage associated with low bone mineral density and vertebral deformities in rheumatoid arthritis: the Oslo-Truro-Amsterdam (OSTRA) collaborative study. *Arthritis Rheum.* 2003;49(2):209-15.

Martin JC, Munro R, Campbell MK, Reid DM. Effects of disease and corticosteroids on appendicular bone mass in postmenopausal women with rheumatoid arthritis: comparison with axial measurements. *Br J Rheumatol* 1997;36:43–9.

Meunier PJ, Vignot E, Garnero P. "Treatment of postmenopausal women with osteoporosis or low bone density with raloxifene. Raloxifene Study Group". *Osteoporos Int* 1999;10 (4): 330–36.

Mundy GR. Osteoporosis and inflammation. *Nutr Rev.* 2007;65(12 Pt 2):S147-51.

Neer RM, Arnaud CD, Zanchetta JR, Prince R, Gaich GA. Effect of parathyroid hormone (1-34) on fractures and bone mineral density in postmenopausal women with osteoporosis. *N Engl J Med.* 2001;344:1434–4.

Pattison DJ, Harrison RA, Symmons DP. The role of diet in susceptibility to rheumatoid arthritis: a systematic review. *J Rheumatol.* 2004;31(7):1310-9.

Pereira RM, Delany AM, Canalis E. Cortisol inhibits the differentiation and apoptosis of osteoblasts in culture. *Bone* 2001;28:484-90.

Reginster JY, Felsenberg D, Boonen S, Diez-Perez A, Rizzoli R. Effects of long term strontium ranelate treatment on the risk of nonvertebral and vertebral fractures in postmenopausal osteoporosis, results of five year, randomizes, placebo-controlled trial. *Arthritis and Rheumatism*. 2008;58:1687–95.

Reid DM, Devogelaer JP, Saag K, Roux C, Lau CS, Reginster JY, et al. Zoledronic acid and risedronate in the prevention and treatment of glucocorticoid-induced osteoporosis (HORIZON): a multicentre, doubleblind, double-dummy, randomised controlled trial. *Lancet*. 2009;373:1253-63,

Roldán JF, Del Rincón I, Escalante A. Loss of cortical bone from the metacarpal diaphysis in patients with rheumatoid arthritis: independent effects of systemic inflammation and glucocorticoids. *J Rheumatol*. 2006;33(3):508-16.

Romas E, Bakharevski O, Hards DK, Kartsogiannis V, Quinn JMW, Ryan PFJ, et al. Expression of osteoclast differentiation factor at sites of bone erosion in collagen-induced arthritis. *Arthritis Rheum 2000*;43:821–6.

Ross FP, Chappel J, Alvarez JI, Sander D, Butler WT, Farach-Carson MC. Interactions between the bone matrix proteins osteopontin and bone sialoprotein and the osteoclast integrin alpha v beta 3 potentiate bone resorption: *J Biol Chem* 1993, 268:9901-9907.

Sambrook PN: The skeleton in rheumatoid arthritis: common mechanism for bone erosion and osteoporosis? *J Rheumatol* 2000, 27:2541-2542. Gregório LH, Lacativa PG, Melazzi AC, Russo LA.

Saag KG, Shane E, Boonen S, Marı´n F, Donley DW, Taylor KA, et al. Teriparatide or alendronate in glucocorticoid-induced osteoporosis. *N Engl J Med*. 2007;357:2028-39,

Seriolo B, Ferretti V, Sulli A, Caratto E, Fasciolo D, Cutolo M. Serum osteocalcin levels in premenopausal rheumatoid arthritis patients. *Ann N Y Acad Sci*. 2002;966:502-7.

Shenstone BD, Mahmoud A, Woodward R, Elvins D, Palmer R, Ring F, et al. Bone mineral density in nonsteroid treated early rheumatoid arthritis. *Ann Rheum Dis* 1994;53:681–4.

Simonet WS, Lacey DL, Dunstan CR, Kelley M, Chang MS. Osteoprotegerin: a novel secreted protein involved in the regulation of bone density. *Cell* 1997, 89:309-319.

Sinigaglia L, Nervetti A, Mela Q, Bianchi G, Del Puente A, Di Munno O, et al. A multicenter cross sectional study on bone mineral density in rheumatoid arthritis. Italian Study Group on Bone Mass in Rheumatoid Arthritis. *J Rheumatol* 2000;27:2582–9.

Suda T, Takahashi N, Martin TJ: Modulation of osteoclast differentiation. *Endocr Rev* 1992, 13:66-80.

Suzuki Y, Nishikaku F, Nakatuka M, Koga Y. Osteoclast-like cells in murine collagen induced arthritis. *J Rheumatol* 1998;25:1154–60.

Suzuki Y, Tsutsumi Y, Nakagawa M, Suzuki H, Matsushita K, Beppu Ml. Osteoclast-like cells in an in vitro model of bone destruction by rheumatoid synovium. *Rheumatology (Oxford)* 2001;40:673–82.

Takayanagi H, Iizuka H, Juji T, Nakagawa T, Yamamoto A. Involvement of receptor activator of nuclear factor kappa-B ligand/osteoclast differentiation factor in osteoclastogenesis from synoviocytes in rheumatoid arthritis. *Arthritis Rheum* 2000;43:259–69.

Teitelbaum SL. Osteoclasts: what do they do and how do they do it? *Am J Pathol*. 2007;170(2):427-35.

Van Staa TP, Leufkens HG, Cooper C. The epidemiology of corticosteroid induced osteoporosis: a meta-analysis. *Osteoporos Int*. 2002;13:777- 87.

Van Zeben D, Hazes JM, Zwinderman AH, Cats A, van der Voort EA, Breedveld FC. Clinical significance of rheumatoid factors in early rheumatoid arthritis: results of a follow up study. *Ann Rheum Dis* 1992;9:1029–35.

Viswanathan A, Sylvester FA. Chronic pediatric inflammatory diseases: effects on bone. *Rev Endocr Metab Disord.* 2008;9(2):107-22.

Wallach S, Cohen S, Reid DM, Hughes RA, Hosking DJ, Laan RF, et al. Effects of risedronate treatment on bone density and vertebral fracture in patients on corticosteroid therapy. *Calcif Tissue Int.* 2000;67:277-85.

Weitzmann MN, Pacifici R. The role of T lymphocytes in bone metabolism. *Immunol Rev.* 2005;208:154-68.

6

Infectious Complications of Anti-Tumour Necrosis Factor-α Therapy in Rheumatoid Arthritis

Ioannis D. Xynos and Nikolaos V. Sipsas
Department of Pathophysiology, Medical School, National and Capodistrian University of Athens, Greece

1. Introduction

In the last decade the use of Tumor Necrosis Factor- α inhibitors including infliximab, etanercept, adalimumab; and lately certolizumab and golimumab, has revolutionized the treatment of rheumatoid arthritis (RA). These agents have been effective in reducing inflammatory activity and limiting joint destruction in patients with RA however their application has raised a number a safety concerns. Increased risk of infections is of predominant importance given these factors' major role in altering host defense mechanisms.

2. Infections in rheumatoid arthritis patients

2.1 Background infection risk in patients with RA

As infection adverse effects are common in patients with RA due to the underlying disease itself and/or concurrent medications used in its treatment such as immunosuppressants, it is of great importance to identify whether biological treatments increase this risk further (Furst 2010).

Epidemiological studies prior the introduction of biological treatments have shown that patients with RA are at increased risk of certain types of infections including pulmonary infection, generalized sepsis, osteomyelitis, cellulitis, and septic arthritis with relative risks of infection - related mortality ranging from 5 to 15 (Mitchell, Spitz et al. 1986; Wolfe, Mitchell et al. 1994; Symmons, Jones et al. 1998). Nevertheless, the confounding influence of treatment with glycocorticoids and other disease -modifying antirheumatic drugs (DMRDs) is difficult to interpret. Disease it self leads to alterations in cellular immunity, including a decline in the number and function of T-suppressor and natural killer (NK) cells (Dobloug, Forre et al. 1982; Fox, Fong et al. 1984; Young, Adamson et al. 1984); changes that may predispose patients to infection. Other studies have suggested a genetic component to the risk of infection in RA. For example the incidence of urinary tract infection in patients with rheumatoid arthritis patients has been correlated with the number of risk alleles defined by single nucleotide polymorphisms in the genes for TNF-α, lymphotoxin-α and the Fcγ receptors 2A, 3A and 3B (Hughes, Criswell et al. 2004).

2.2 Bacterial infections

2.2.1 Randomised controlled trials and extension studies of anti-TNF agents

Infliximab

The 1- year anti- TNF trial in Rheumatoid Arthritis with concomitant Therapy (ATTRACT study) reported similar incidences of infections among patients treated with infliximab (3 or 10 mg/kg, given every 4 weeks or every 8 weeks) [1-5 patients (1-6%)] compared to patients receiving methotrexate (MTX) alone [5 patients (6%)]. (Maini, St Clair et al. 1999). The serious infections were described as bacterial infections, bronchitis, cellulitis, peritonitis, pneumonia, pyelonephritis and urinary tract infection, sepsis and tuberculosis, although the relative incidence of each of these infections was not reported. Notably, the frequency of any infection was significantly increased in patients receiving 10 mg/kg of infliximab, but not in those receiving 3 mg/kg. Similar incidence of serious infections was reported when ATTRACT was extended to 2 years (10-13%) (Maini, Breedveld et al. 2004). On the contrary, the incidence of serious infections in the 54 weak active controlled study of patients receiving infliximab for treatment of early onset RA (ASPIRE study) was significantly higher in the group receiving infliximab (3 or 6 mg/kg, given every 8 weeks in combination with MTX than in the group of patients receiving MTX monotherapy (St Clair, van der Heijde et at 2004. More specifically, serious infections included pneumonia, tuberculosis (TB), sepsis, bronchitis and septic bronchitis and occurred more commonly in patients receiving MTX -3 mg/kg infliximab [21 patients (5.6%)] or MTX -6 mg/kg infliximab [19 patients (5.0%)] than in those receiving MTX alone [6 patients (2.1%)] (P=0.02 and P=0.4, respectively). Among the serious infections, pneumonia occurred more frequently in the infliximab-treated patients than in those treated with MTX alone [15/749 (2.0%) versus 0/291 (0.0%)]. According to the authors of the ASPIRE study most of these cases were community-acquired pneumonias that responded appropriately to antibiotic therapy. It has been suggested that the apparent differences in the incidence of severe infections between the ASPIRE and ATTRACT trials may reflect, at least partially, differences in study design. ASPIRE had substantially more patients enrolled (N=291-377 per treatment arm, compared with 81-88 in ATTRACT) and in addition ASPIRE excluded patients that had prior treatment with MTX or anti-TNF while all patients in ATTRACT were receiving MTX at the time of the enrollment (Furst 2010).

Etanercept

With regards to etanercept, a 1 year study comparing MTX with 10 mg or 25 mg etanercept twice weekly reported similar number of patients with one or more infections in all treatment groups (Bathon, Martin et al. 2000). Interestingly, when the number of events that occurred per patient-year was analyzed, the rate of all types of infection was significantly higher among patients who received MTX than among those who received either dose of etanercept (1.9 vs. 1.5 events per patient-year, P=0.006). The frequency of upper respiratory tract infections was similar in the MTX group and the group assigned to receive 25 mg of etanercept, while the rate of infections at other sites in the respiratory tract was higher in the MTX group (1.3 vs. 1.0 events per patient-year, P=0.006). Infections requiring hospitalization or the intravenous administration of antibiotics occurred in less than 3% of patients in each group. There were no opportunistic infections, and no deaths from infections. When this study was extended to 2 years, similar incidences of serious infections in each treatment arm were reported and did not increase in frequency during the second year of the study (Genovese, Bathon et al. 2002). Over the 2-year study period, 21 patients had infections that required hospitalization or use of intravenous antibiotics, including 9 patients in the MTX group, 5 patients in the 10 mg etanercept group, and 7 patients in the 25 mg group. The types of serious infection observed in the second year were similar to those reported in the first year and included cellulitis (1 patient each in all 3 treatment groups), bronchitis (1 patient in the 10 mg group), pneumonia (1 patient in the 10 mg group), and cystitis (2 patients in the 25 mg group); no cases of TB and no opportunistic infections were seen. Similarly, in a double-blind, randomized, clinical efficacy, safety, and radiographic study (TEMPO) involving 686 patients with active rheumatoid arthritis randomly allocated to treatment with etanercept 25 mg (administered subcutaneously twice a week), oral MTX (up to 20 mg every week), or the combination, similar incidences of infections and serious infections have been recorded in all treatment arms with no reports of TB or opportunistic infections (Klareskog, van der Heijde et al. 2004). Those results were sustained into the 2 year follow up of the TEMPO trial showing similar rates of serious infections among all treatment groups (van der Heijde, Klareskog et al. 2006). Again, no cases of TB were reported but there was one case of bronchopulmonary aspergillosis in the combination therapy group. A similarly favorable safety profile for etanercept was reported from the ADORE study, which evaluated the efficacy and safety of combination etanercept and MTX versus etanercept alone in patients with RA with an inadequate response to MTX. The study showed comparable incidence of infections in the two arms and notably no cases of opportunistic infections or TB were reported in the combination group (van Riel, Taggart et al. 2006).

Adalimumab

The safety profile of adalimumab was initially evaluated in 3 double blind placebo controlled short term (24-26 weeks) trials reporting low incidence of serious infections (Furst, Schiff et al. 2003; van de Putte, Atkins et al. 2004; Weinblatt, Keystone et al. 2006). In a subsequent 52 weeks - long study comparing treatment with adalimumab (40mg every other week or 20 mg every week) plus concomitant MTX in patients with active RA who had an inadequate response to MTX, the proportion of patients with serious infections was higher in the group receiving adalimumab (3.8%) than in those receiving MTX (0.5%) ($P \leq 0.02$), and was highest in the patients receiving 40 mg adalimumab every other week (Keystone, Kavanaugh et al. 2004). Adjusting for exposure time, serious infections occurred at a rate of 0.06 patients / patient-year with adalimumab 40 mg every other week, 0.03 patients per patient-year with adalimumab 20 mg weekly, and 0.01 patients per patient-year with MTX alone. One patient treated with adalimumab 40 mg every other week was diagnosed as having primary TB of the cervical lymph nodes, and nodes, was withdrawn from the study and successfully treated. At baseline, this patient had a negative tuberculin purified protein derivative (PPD) test result and a normal chest radiograph. One patient treated with adalimumab 40 mg every other week plus MTX was diagnosed with histoplasmosis infection after 78 days of treatment, and was subsequently withdrawn from the study and successfully treated with antifungal therapy. This patient lived in an area which was endemic for histoplasmosis infection. One patient treated with adalimumab 40 mg every other week was diagnosed as having herpes zoster and developed encephalitis, which resolved but resulted in mild lower extremity weakness. In the 2- year multicenter, double blind, active Comparator-controlled study designed to compare the efficacy and safety of adalimumab plus MTX versus MTX monotherapy or adalimumab monotherapy in patients with early, aggressive RA who had not previously received MTX treatment (PREMIER study), the overall rate of infectious adverse events (AEs) did not differ significantly among the 3 treatment groups (123, 110, and 119 events per 100 patient-years in the combination therapy, adalimumab monotherapy, and MTX monotherapy groups, respectively) (Breedveld, Weisman et al. 2006). The rate of serious infections in the adalimumab monotherapy group was significantly lower than that in the combination treatment group, but not significantly different compared with the MTX monotherapy group. Notably, serious infections were more common in the combination therapy arm with 9 serious infections reported, including 3 pulmonary infections (1 case of pleural TB) and 1 case each of sinus infection, wound infection, septic arthritis, infected hygroma, cellulitis, and urinary tract infection. In the adalimumab monotherapy arm, serious infections included 1 case each of pneumonia, cellulitis, and septic arthritis. In the MTX monotherapy arm, the 7 serious infections consisted of 2 cases of pneumonia and 1 each of septic arthritis, sinusitis, abscess, bacteremia, and parotitis. The long term safety of adalimumab was investigated in the 4-year open-label extension of the ARMADA trial (Weinblatt, Keystone et al. 2006). The rate of serious infections was slightly lower throughout the entire study than in the blinded period alone with the most common serious infections reported being pneumonia, urinary tract infections and septic arthritis. A PPD skin test was performed at the screening visit for all patients. Standard chest radiographs were also taken at the screening visit and at week 24. Notably, at baseline, 11/271 (4.1%) randomized patients had positive PPD results at screening, including 9/209 (4.3%) adalimumab treated patients and 2/62 (3.2%) placebo treated patients. These patients were treated with TB prophylaxis in accordance with routine medical practice. No cases of TB or other opportunistic infections were reported. The safety profile of adalimumab was analyzed further in a cumulative analysis of data from 10050 patients who participated in randomized controlled trials, open label extensions, and two phase IIIb open label trials, representing 12506 patient-years (PYs) of adalimumab exposure (Schiff, Burmester et al 2006). The rate of serious infections in the clinical trial safety database as of April 2005 was 5.1/100 PYs. This rate is nearly identical to that observed in August 2002 (4.9/100 PYs) and was similar to rates reported for the general RA population. Four cases of histoplasmosis were reported, all in endemic areas (0.03/100 PYs). No cases of coccidioidomycosis have been reported in RA clinical trials.

2.2.2 Registry data, observational data and chart reviews

The safety profile of anti-TNF agents in the everyday clinical practice was elucidated further by registry data analysis, observational studies and chart reviews. Data derived from these studies could be highly informative; however the lack of a standard comparator, strict inclusion and exclusion criteria and the inherent differences in patient characteristics with respect to ethnic, geographical and socio-economical characteristics often reduce their credibility and, produce desperate results and do not allow direct comparisons among different studies. Nevertheless, these studies become important when they investigate specific or relatively rare types of infections and raise specific concerns with regards to infections in certain population groups (Furst 2010).

In the German registry study, data of 512 patients receiving etanercept, 346 patients receiving infliximab, 70 patients receiving anakinra, and 601 control patients treated with disease-modifying antirheumatic drugs were analyzed. After adjusting for confounding factors, the relative risks of serious AEs were 2.2 [95% CI (confidence interval) 0.9–5.4] for patients receiving etanercept and 2.1 (95% CI 0.8–5.5) for patients receiving infliximab, compared to those treated with DMARDs. Respiratory tract infections were the most frequent followed by skin and subcutaneous tissue infections, influenza like illness, herpes virus infections, and urinary tract infections. Lower respiratory tract infections were the most common serious infections (Listing, Strangfeld et al. 2005). Updated results from the British Register for Biologic Therapies (BSRBR) (Galloway, Hyrich et al. 2011) also showed in contrary to previous reports (Dixon, Watson et al. 2006) that anti-TNF therapy is associated with a small but significant overall risk of serious infections. The adjusted hazard ratio (adjHR) for serious infections in the anti-TNF cohort was 1.2 (95% CI 1.1, 1.5). The risk did not differ significantly between the three agents adalimumab, etanercept and infliximab and it was highest during the first 6 months of therapy [adjHR (Hazard Ratio) 1.8, 95% CI 1.3-2.6]. This was in accordance with the work of Askling and Dixon who reviewed all available studies on infection risk associated with anti-TNF therapy in RA and found that the risk was highest in the first few months but declined later during the course of treatment (Askling and Dixon 2008). It has been proposed that this variation in risk may reflect biological functions (anti-TNF therapy causing early infections in susceptible individuals), or bias (clinicians having a lower threshold for treating infections early in therapy). In addition the depletion of susceptible individuals (a healthy user effect) by withdrawing patients who develop an infection from the anti-TNF cohort may reduce the apparent risk of the drug through subsequent patient selection bias. Furthermore, as patients become established on anti-TNF therapy, their RA becomes better controlled and other confounding factors such as mobility may improve or their dose of steroids may be reduced thus contributing to the complexity of interpretation (Askling and Dixon 2008; Galloway, Hyrich et al. 2011).

Registries and chart reviews can be particularly useful in identified specific infectious risks for susceptible patients. For example, data from the French registry estimated the relative risk of legionellosis when receiving treatment with a TNF-α antagonist to be between 16.5 and 21.0, compared with the relative risk in France overall (Tubach, Ravaud et al. 2006).

2.2.3 Case reports

Numerous case reports have raised awareness to rare bacterial infections in RA patients treated with anti-TNF. These included reports on reactivation of brucellosis (Jimenez, Colmenero et al. 2005), *Capnocytophaga cynodegmi*-related cellulitis (Gerster and Dudler 2004), *Roseomonas mucosa* induced septic arthritis (Sipsas, Papaparaskevas et al. 2006), and *Propionebacterim acnes*-related endogenous endophthalmitis (Montero, Ruiz-Moreno et al. 2006).

2.2.4 Meta-analyses

One solution to the lack of precision in the estimates of harm derived from individual randomized trials is to pool their results using meta-analysis. Results however from the two existing meta-analyses studies on anti-TNF therapy and risk of infection are disparate. A meta-analysis of nine randomized, controlled studies including 3493 patients with RA who received anti-TNF antibody treatment (infliximab and adalimumab) and 1512 patients who received placebo reported a doubled risk of serious infection [odds ratio (OR) 2.0, 95% CI 1.3–3.1] and a tendency towards a dose–response association (Bongartz, Sutton et al. 2006). On the contrary, a second meta-analysis of five published, placebo-controlled trials involving a total of 2945 randomized patients, who received at least one dose of abatacept (0.5, 2 or 10 mg/kg) (n=1960) or placebo (n=985) for a duration of treatment ranging between 24 and 48 weeks did not reveal a statistically significant increased risk of serious infection for abatarcept (Salliot, Dougados et al. 2009). The 49 serious infections reported in the abatacept cohort were mainly broncho-pulmonary, streptococcal and pyogenic septicaemia, staphylococcal arthritis, abscesses, gastrointestinal infections (6 of whom 3 diverticulitis), dermatological infections (six of whom one was a cellulitis) and pyelonephritis. One case of unconfirmed TB and one case of pulmonary aspergillosis were reported. The last patient (who had a history with TB and pulmonary fibrosis) died with aspergillosis and *Pseudomonas aeruginosa* septicaemia.

2.3 Tuberculosis and opportunistic infections

As shown earlier, the incidence of TB in pre-registration clinical trials has been low. It was only after licensing of these medications that post-marketing surveillance registers showed results suggestive a strong association between ant-TNF treatment and TB. Keane *et al* analysed data from the US Food and Drug Administration's (FDA) Adverse Event Reporting System (AERS) for reports of TB with infliximab from its licensure in 1998 through May 29, 2001 (Keane, Gershon et al. 2001). There were 70 reported cases of TB after treatment with infliximab for a median of 12 weeks. In 48 patients, TB developed after three or fewer infusions and 40 of the patients had extrapulmonary disease (17 had disseminated disease, 11 lymph-node disease, 4 peritoneal disease, 2 pleural disease, and 1 each meningeal, enteric, paravertebral, bone, genital, and bladder disease). An estimated rate of 24.4 cases of tuberculosis per 100 000 in the USA compared with a background rate in American patients with RA who had not received the drug of 6.2 cases per 100000 was calculated. The rather atypical presentation of the disease (e.g. extrapulmonary dissemination), the temporal relation between development of active tuberculosis and the start of therapy, the age of the patients (median, 57 years), the small number of cases with reported recent exposure to TB, and the low incidence of TB in the countries from which the reports were received suggested reactivation of the disease (Keane, Gershon et al. 2001).

As of March, 2002, 121000 patients had been treated with etanercept worldwide with about 94% of the use in the USA. In a search of the FDS's AERS database reported up to March 2002, Mohan and co-workers detected 25 cases of tuberculosis that occurred during or after etanercept therapy (Mohan, Cote et al. 2004). Patients with etanercept-associated TB were fewer but clinically similar to those with infliximab-associated TB (Keane, Gershon et al. 2001). The numbers of patients who had been exposed to etanercept and infliximab were roughly similar, yet the TB rate for US patients using etanercept was lower than that for patients using infliximab (~10 vs. ~41 cases/100000 patient-years of exposure). It has been proposed that this difference might be due to the divergent ways in which the 2 agents neutralize TNF-α, the use of MTX concurrently with infliximab (as indicated for RA in the infliximab package insert), differences in proportions of international patients treated with the 2 agents, or other factors (Gardam, Keystone et al. 2003; Mohan, Cote et al. 2004). Overall, in a large systematic review of infectious complications of TNF antagonists extracted from 35275 distinct reports from the AERS database between for January 1998–September 2002, granulomatous infections were reported at rates of ~239 per 100000 patients who received infliximab and ~74 per 100,000 patients who received etanercept (P <0.001) (Wallis, Broder et al. 2004). TB was the most frequently reported disease, occurring in ~144 and ~35 per 100,000 infliximab-treated and etanercept-treated patients, respectively P<0.001. Candidiasis, coccidioidomycosis, histoplasmosis, listeriosis, nocardiosis, and infections due to nontuberculous mycobacteria were reported with significantly greater frequency among infliximab-treated patients. 72% of these infection occurred 90 days after starting infliximab treatment, and 28% occurred after starting etanercept treatment P<0.001. These data indicated a relative risk of granulomatous infection that was >3 among patients who received infliximab compared to those who received etanercept. The clustering of reports shortly after initiation of treatment with infliximab was consistent with reactivation of latent infection.

Geographical associations between anti-TNF therapy and specific granulomatous diseases have been suggested. For example, disseminated histoplasmosis has been reported more frequently in endemic regions in the US (Lee, Slifman et al. 2002). In a review of the FDA passive surveillance database, nine cases of invasive disseminated histoplasmosis associated with infliximab and 1 associated with etanercept were reported. In patients treated with infliximab, manifestations of histoplasmosis occurred within 1 week to 6 months after the first dose and typically included fever, malaise, cough, dyspnea, and interstitial pneumonitis. All patients had received concomitant immunosuppressive medications in addition to infliximab or etanercept, and all resided in histoplasmosis endemic regions of central US (Lee, Slifman et al. 2002). Similarly, anti-TNF therapy was shown to be associated with increased reports of leishmaniasis in endemic areas in Europe (Xynos, Tektonidou et al. 2009).

A major factor that has influenced data relating to the risk of TB associated with biological treatments has been the introduction of vigorous screening of patients participating in clinical trials; hence rates for newer biological agents such as abatarcept may be biased. Screening for TB exposure with PPD skin testing or newer interferon-based serum tests (although their optimal use in this setting is not yet clear) should be performed before beginning therapy with anti-TNF agents (Winthrop and Chiller 2009). Anergy is known to occur in patients with RA or Crohn's disease, and the possibility of false-negative skin tests should be taken into consideration. Nevertheless from a therapeutic point of view, since the implementation of strict guidelines (e.g. BTS recommendations, 2005) with regards to screening patients for exposure risks and treating latent TB prior to initiation of any biological treatment, the risk of tuberculosis has decreased. This is depicted in the data from the Spanish Registry showing that these strategies have resulted in dropping the rates of active TB in RA patients by 83% reaching those observed for RA patients not treated with TNF antagonists (Carmona, Gomez-Reino et al. 2005).

2.3.1 TNF-α pathophysiology and infections

TNF is essential for granuloma formation and maintenance which are key components of host defences against intracellular pathogens (Furst, Wallis et al. 2006). TNF can support host immunity through the secretion of chemokines, up-regulation of adhesion molecules and the induction of macrophage apoptosis. While TNF blockers may therefore interfere with these important immune functions, other less predictable immune effects have been seen with these agents. In particular, TNF-blockers have been shown to diminish interferon (IFN)-γ effects and stimulate apoptosis of key immune cells, including monocytes, $CD4^+$ T helper cells and Mtb-reactive $CD8^+$ T cells. Anti-TNF therapy is also associated with increased regulatory T cell (T_{reg}) function, which has been linked with susceptibility to TB (Harris and Keane 2010). TNF-α neutralization in mice has resulted in fatal reactivation of persistent tuberculosis characterized by a moderately increased tissue bacillary burden and severe pulmonic histopathological deterioration that was associated with changes indicative of squamous metaplasia and fluid accumulation in the alveolar space (Mohan, Scanga et al. 2001).

2.4 Postoperative infections

Although several studies have attempted to address the risk of postoperative infection, limited statistical precision has been a major concern. The largest study reported a 50% (but not statistically significant) increased risk of surgical site infections for those patients who continued therapy peri-operatively (den Broeder, Creemers et al. 2007). Nevertheless, considering the morbidity of orthopedic surgical site infections (especially prosthesis infections) as compared to a transient surge in disease activity, withholding anti-TNF agents peri-operatively appears to be the most reasonable and prudent approach at present (Bongartz 2007).

2.5 Viral infections

Reactivation of Hepatitis B (HBV) infection is a well described complication of immunosuppression in the setting of organ transplantation or cancer chemotherapy, occurring in up to 50% of patients where concomitant anti-viral treatment is not applied (Shale, Seow et al. 2010). The use of anti-TNF medications has been reported in isolated case reports, case series and chart reviews with a variety of outcomes ranging from apparent viral clearance to fatal hepatitis. In a comprehensive review of these cases by Zingarelli *at al* involving 27 HBV-infected patients treated with anti-TNF agents, HBV reactivation was documented in 14% of patients treated with lamivudine compared with 73% of patients not receiving HBV prophylaxis (Zingarelli, Frassi et al. 2009) thus suggesting that the use of prophylactic lamivudine could help reducing the risk of HBV reactivation. More recently, interesting data with regards to the relative safety of anti-TNF agents in HBV carriers were presented by Charpin *et al* (Charpin, Guis et al. 2009). Their cohort included 21 patients with serologically cured HBV infection, that is HBsAg –ve plus anti-HBc +ve patients and results were suggestive that anti-TNF therapy appeared to be safe during the a limited follow up period of three years. Nevertheless, about 30% of patients involved in this study had significant lower antibody titers over the follow up period which may be relevant during long-term follow up (Jansen 2010). Similar findings we reported by others over a shorter follow up period of 2 years (Vassilopoulos, Apostolopoulou et al. 2010) yet the decrease in antibody titers observed in the later study was comparable to that observed in a control group of patients treated with MTX alone, indicating no apparent specific effect of anti-TNF on HBV protective immunity.

Anti-TNF therapy for RA in the setting of Hepatitis C (HCV) infection could be of particular interest in light of the existing evidence suggesting a role for inflammatory cytokines including TNF-α in the mediating hepatocyte destruction in chronic CMV (Parke and Reveille 2004). It may therefore carefully assumed that anti-TNF agents may be safer in patients infected with HCV rather than HBV (Shale, Seow et al. 2010) and furthermore this notion has been tested in a phase 2 randomised, double-blind, placebo-controlled study where etanercept given for 24 weeks as adjuvant therapy to interferon and ribavirin was shown to significantly improve virological response among patients with chronic HCV and was associated with decreased incidence of most adverse effects associated with interferon and ribavirin (Zein 2005). Although overall experience to date with anti-TNF agents in the chronic HCV setting suggests an acceptable short-term safety profile (Marotte, Fontanges et al. 2007), long-term issues remain to be clarified.

The safety of anti-TNF therapy in HIV is a controversial subject. TNF inhibition in the setting of HIV induced immunosuppression does not appear appealing in view of the potential role for TNF-α in the host defence against infections. Notably, in an early report, the use of etanercept in HIV positive patient with psoriasis and CD4 count of $<200/mm^3$ was associated with polymicrobial infections prompting termination of the treatment (Aboulafia, Bundow et al. 2000). Subsequent reports though have shown a favourable safety profile (Kaur, Chan et al. 2007; Cepeda, Williams et al. 2008), yet clinical decisions should be taken cautiously; careful consideration of the risks and benefits for the individual patient would be needed and close clinical and virological monitoring should always be warranted.

The safety of TNF inhibitors in patients with herpes virus (HSV) infections has also been considered. In particular the risk of herpes zoster infection in patients with RA is twice as much even in the absence of therapy (Wolfe, Michaud et al. 2006; Smitten, Choi et al. 2007) and severe herpes zoster infections have been reported in randomised controlled trials and their open-label follow up studies in patients with RA receiving the TNF inhibitors infliximab or adalimumab (Lipsky, van der Heijde et al. 2000; Furst, Schiff et al. 2003; Keystone, Kavanaugh et al. 2004; Maini, Breedveld et al. 2004). A study by Strangfeld *et al* (Strangfeld, Listing et al. 2009) addressed the question whether this association actually represents a true association between TNF inhibitors reactivation of latent viral infections or simply reflects the increased risk of herpes zoster infection in RA patients (Bongartz and Orenstein 2009). In this prospective cohort the investigators identified 86 episodes of herpes zoster among 5040 patients from the German biologics register RABBIT, receiving anti-TNF agents or conventional DMARDs. Adjusted for age, RA severity and glucocorticoid use, a significant increased risk was observed for treatment with the monoclonal antibodies (HR, 1.82 [95% CI, 0.73-2.55]), although this risk was lower than the threshold (of 2.5) for clinical significance. No significant associations were found for etanercept use (HR 1.36, 95% CI 0.73-2.55) or for anti-TNF treatment (HR 1.63, 95% CI 0.97-2.74) as a class. Equally important, the incidence rate of multidermatomal and ophthalmic zoster was higher in patients taking TNF inhibitors implying severe disease often requiring hospitalisation (Bongartz and Orenstein 2009). Nevertheless, anti-TNF therapy can generally be restarted following temporary interruption and conventional anti-viral therapy until the skin lesions are completely healed (Wendling, Streit et al. 2008). Isolated varicella infections have also been reported in RA patients receiving anti-TNF therapy (Vonkeman, ten Napel et al. 2004; Choi, Kim et al. 2006; Lee, Kim et al. 2007). Notably the rash in one of these cases was atypical (Choi, Kim et al. 2006) stressing the need for high index of suspicion upon diagnosing primary varicella infection in susceptible patients with atypical skin lesions.

Finally, although a prospective study involving 15 patients with refractory forms of RA under treatment with infliximab (3 mg/kg) did not show evidence of lymphotropic herpesviruses reactivation (CMV, HHV-6, HHV-7, HHV-8, EBV) in RA patients (Torre-Cisneros, Del Castillo et al. 2005), two isolated case reports have associated infliximab with HHV8 related Kaposi's sarcoma (Cohen, Horster et al. 2003) and cytomegalovirus (CMV) retinitis (Haerter, Manfras et al. 2004).

2.6 Response to vaccination

As patients with RA receiving conventional DMARDs and biologics are at increased risk of vaccine preventable diseases such as respiratory tract infections caused by *H. Influenza* and *S. Pneumoniae*, safety and efficacy evaluation of vaccines in this setting is of paramount importance. The use of TNF inhibitors in particular has raised specific concerns with regards to their potential influence on antibody responses to vaccination. The potential influence of anti-TNF inhibition on the efficacy of influenza vaccination was evaluated in a prospective cohort study involving 149 patients with RA including 50 patients treated with TNF blockers (etanercept or infliximab) in combination with MTX, 62 patients receiving TNF blockers alone or with other DMARDs and 37 patients treated with MTX alone plus 18 healthy controls (Kapetanovic, Saxne et al. 2007). Vaccination with trivalent vaccine resulted in better serological response in RA patients treated with MTX without TNF inhibitors compared with those receiving TNF inhibitors alone or in combination with MTX and/or other DMRDS. Nevertheless, the immune response according to the authors was sufficiently large to warrant influenza vaccination to all RA patients regardless of treatment. Similar results were reported by others (Fomin, Caspi et al. 2006). Equally reassuring were results from studies investigating the efficacy of pmeumococcal vaccine in RA patients receiving anti-TNF therapy. In one study, immune response to 23-valent pneumococcal vaccine was better in patients treated with TNF inhibitors without MTX compared to those treated with TNF inhibitors in combination with MTX or MTX alone. Response rates were 50, 31 and 13% for the TNF inhibition without MTX, TNF inhibition with MTX and MTX groups respectively (Kapetanovic, Saxne et al. 2006). In a different prospective cohort of RA patients receiving either adalimumab or placebo, investigators reported that following pneumococcal vaccination, the percentage of patients achieving a vaccine response were similar in the adalimumab and placebo groups [37.4% and 40.4%, respectively; 95% CI -16.2%, 10.3%]. Equally similar was the percentage of patients with protective antibody titres in both treatment groups (adalimumab: 85.9%, placebo: 81.7%) (Kaine, Kivitz et al. 2007). Thus, anti-TNF therapy should not deter physicians from offering patients with RA vaccination against *H. Influenza* and *S. Pneumoniae.*

3. Conclusions and future directions

TNF-α blockade strategies have revolutionized the treatment RA, raising though safety concerns with regards to increased risk for infections. Although pre-registration clinical trials for TNF inhibitors showed no clear increased risk for infections, long term clinical trials and post registrations studies have shown a small but consistent increase in infection risk in patients treated with anti-TNF therapy compared to those treated with conventional DMARDs. Common infections involve sites as the respiratory tract, skin and soft tissue and the urinary tract. The risk of *M. tuberculosis* infection also appear to be increased with the use of these agents and is highest during the first 6 months of therapy, most probably reflecting reactivation of latent TB. Screening patients for exposure risks and latent TB prior to the initiation of anti-TNF therapy and administration of standard chemo-prophylaxis has decreased the incidence of new TB cases. Other opportunistic infections such as histoplasmosis, coccidioidomycosis and leishmaniasis may occur following geographical criteria, indicating increased incidence of these illnesses in endemic areas. In view of the increased infectious risk associated with these agents, we should reiterate the importance of efficient pre-treatment screening and close monitoring of patients throughout their treatment. Physicians should be aware of infectious diseases endemic to their geographic area and be vigilant for unusual presentation of symptoms and signs of infectious illnesses. They should stop biologic therapy when these occur, treat those infectious complications promptly and report such cases to regulatory or public health authorities where appropriate. As new biological agents are developed and reach the market place, large scale post marketing surveillance with registry studies and other observational studies will be needed to establish the long term safety profile of these novel therapies.

4. References

Aboulafia, D. M., Bundow, D., Wilske, K., & Ochs, U. I. (2000). Etanercept for the treatment of human immunodeficiency virus-associated psoriatic arthritis. *Mayo Clin Proc*, 75(10), 1093-1098.

Askling, J., & Dixon, W. (2008). The safety of anti-tumour necrosis factor therapy in rheumatoid arthritis. *Curr Opin Rheumatol*, 20(2), 138-144.

Bathon, J. M., Martin, R. W., Fleischmann, R. M., Tesser, J. R., Schiff, M. H., Keystone, E. C., Genovese, M. C., Wasko, M.C., Moreland, L. W., Weaver, A.L., Markenson, J., & Finck, B. K. (2000). A comparison of etanercept and methotrexate in patients with early rheumatoid arthritis. *N Engl J Med*, 343(22), 1586-1593.

Bongartz, T. (2007). Elective orthopedic surgery and perioperative DMARD management: many questions, fewer answers, and some opinions. *J Rheumatol*, 34(4), 653-655.

Bongartz, T., & Orenstein, R. (2009). Therapy: The risk of herpes zoster: another cost of anti-TNF therapy? *Nat Rev Rheumatol*, 5(7), 361-363.

Bongartz, T., Sutton, A. J., Sweeting, M. J., Buchan, I., Matteson, E. L., & Montori, V. (2006). Anti-TNF antibody therapy in rheumatoid arthritis and the risk of serious infections and malignancies: systematic review and meta-analysis of rare harmful effects in randomized controlled trials. *JAMA*, 295(19), 2275-2285.

Breedveld, F. C., Weisman, M. H., Kavanaugh, A. F., Cohen, S. B., Pavelka, K., van Vollenhoven, R., Sharp, J., Perez J. L., & Spencer-Green, G. T. (2006). The PREMIER study: A multicenter, randomized, double-blind clinical trial of combination therapy with adalimumab plus methotrexate versus methotrexate alone or adalimumab alone in patients with early, aggressive rheumatoid arthritis who had not had previous methotrexate treatment. *Arthritis Rheum*, 54(1), 26-37.

Carmona, L., Gomez-Reino, J. J., Rodriguez-Valverde, V., Montero, D., Pascual-Gomez, E., Mola, E. M., Carreno , L., & Figueroa, M. (2005). Effectiveness of recommendations to prevent reactivation of latent tuberculosis infection in patients treated with tumor necrosis factor antagonists. *Arthritis Rheum*, 52(6), 1766-1772.

Cepeda, E. J., Williams, F. M., Ishimori, M. L., Weisman, M. H., & Reveille, J. D. (2008). The use of anti-tumour necrosis factor therapy in HIV-positive individuals with rheumatic disease. *Ann Rheum Dis*, 67(5), 710-712.

Charpin, C., Guis, S., Colson, P., Borentain, P., Mattei, J. P., Alcaraz, P., Balandraud, N., Thomachot, B., Roudier J., & Gerolami, R. (2009). Safety of TNF-blocking agents in rheumatic patients with serology suggesting past hepatitis B state: results from a cohort of 21 patients. *Arthritis Res Ther*, 11(6), R179.

Choi, H. J., Kim, M. Y., Kim, H. O., & Park, Y. M. (2006). An atypical varicella exanthem associated with the use of infliximab. *Int J Dermatol*, 45(8), 999-1000.

Cohen, C. D., Horster, S., Sander, C. A., & Bogner, J. R. (2003). Kaposi's sarcoma associated with tumour necrosis factor alpha neutralising therapy. *Ann Rheum Dis*, 62(7), 684.

den Broeder, A. A., Creemers, M. C., Fransen, J., de Jong, E., de Rooij, D. J., Wymenga, A., de Waal-Malefijt. M., & van den Hoogen, F. H. (2007). Risk factors for surgical site infections and other complications in elective surgery in patients with rheumatoid arthritis with special attention for anti-tumor necrosis factor: a large retrospective study. *J Rheumatol*, 34(4), 689-695.

Dixon, W. G., Watson, K., Lunt, M., Hyrich, K. L., Silman, A. J., & Symmons, D. P. (2006). Rates of serious infection, including site-specific and bacterial intracellular infection, in rheumatoid arthritis patients receiving anti-tumor necrosis factor therapy: results from the British Society for Rheumatology Biologics Register. *Arthritis Rheum*, 54(8), 2368-2376.

Dobloug, J. H., Forre, O., Kvien, T. K., Egeland, T., & Degre, M. (1982). Natural killer (NK) cell activity of peripheral blood, synovial fluid, and synovial tissue lymphocytes from patients with rheumatoid arthritis and juvenile rheumatoid arthritis. *Ann Rheum Dis*, 41(5), 490-494.

Fomin, I., Caspi, D., Levy, V., Varsano, N., Shalev, Y., Paran, D., Levartovsky, D., Litinsky, I., Kaufman, I., Wigler, I., Mendelson E., & Elkayam, O. (2006). Vaccination against influenza in rheumatoid arthritis: the effect of disease modifying drugs, including TNF alpha blockers. *Ann Rheum Dis*, 65(2), 191-194.

Fox, R. I., Fong, S., Tsoukas, C., & Vaughan, J. H. (1984). Characterization of recirculating lymphocytes in rheumatoid arthritis patients: selective deficiency of natural killer cells in thoracic duct lymph. *J Immunol*, 132(6), 2883-2887.

Furst, D. E. (2010). The risk of infections with biologic therapies for rheumatoid arthritis. *Semin Arthritis Rheum*, 39(5), 327-346.

Furst, D. E., Breedveld, F. C., Kalden, J. R., Smolen, J. S., Burmester, G. R., Dougados, M., Emery, P., Gibofsky, A., Kavanaugh, A. F., Keystone, E. C., Klareskog, L., Russell, A. S., van de Putte, L. B., & Weisman, M. H. (2003). Updated consensus statement on biological agents for the treatment of rheumatoid arthritis and other immune mediated inflammatory diseases (May 2003). *Ann Rheum Dis*, 62 Suppl 2, ii2-9.

Furst, D. E., Schiff, M. H., Fleischmann, R. M., Strand, V., Birbara, C. A., Compagnone, D., Fischkoff, S. A., & Chartash, E. K. (2003). Adalimumab, a fully human anti tumor necrosis factor-alpha monoclonal antibody, and concomitant standard antirheumatic therapy for the treatment of rheumatoid arthritis: results of STAR (Safety Trial of Adalimumab in Rheumatoid Arthritis). *J Rheumatol*, 30(12), 2563-2571.

Furst, D. E., Wallis, R., Broder, M., & Beenhouwer, D. O. (2006). Tumor necrosis factor antagonists: different kinetics and/or mechanisms of action may explain differences in the risk for developing granulomatous infection. *Semin Arthritis Rheum*, 36(3), 159-167.

Galloway, J. B., Hyrich, K. L., Mercer, L. K., Dixon, W. G., Fu, B., Ustianowski, A. P., Watson, K. D., Lunt, M., & Symmons, D. P. (2011). Anti-TNF therapy is associated with an increased risk of serious infections in patients with rheumatoid arthritis especially in the first 6 months of treatment: updated results from the British Society for Rheumatology Biologics Register with special emphasis on risks in the elderly. *Rheumatology (Oxford)*, 50(1), 124-131.

Gardam, M. A., Keystone, E. C., Menzies, R., Manners, S., Skamene, E., Long, R., & Vinh, D. C. (2003). Anti-tumour necrosis factor agents and tuberculosis risk: mechanisms of action and clinical management. *Lancet Infect Dis*, 3(3), 148-155.

Genovese, M. C., Bathon, J. M., Martin, R. W., Fleischmann, R. M., Tesser, J. R., Schiff, M. H., Keystone, E. C., Wasko, M. C., Moreland, L. W., Weaver, A. L., Markenson, J., Cannon, G. W., Spencer-Green, G., & Finck, B. K. (2002). Etanercept versus methotrexate in patients with early rheumatoid arthritis: two-year radiographic and clinical outcomes. *Arthritis Rheum*, 46(6), 1443-1450.

Gerster, J. C., & Dudler, J. (2004). Cellulitis caused by Capnocytophaga cynodegmi associated with etanercept treatment in a patient with rheumatoid arthritis. *Clin Rheumatol*, 23(6), 570-571.

Haerter, G., Manfras, B. J., de Jong-Hesse, Y., Wilts, H., Mertens, T., Kern, P., & Schmitt, M. (2004). Cytomegalovirus retinitis in a patient treated with anti-tumor necrosis factor alpha antibody therapy for rheumatoid arthritis. *Clin Infect Dis*, 39(9), e88-94.

Harris, J., & Keane, J. (2010). How tumour necrosis factor blockers interfere with tuberculosis immunity. *Clin Exp Immunol*, 161(1), 1-9.

Hughes, L. B., Criswell, L. A., Beasley, T. M., Edberg, J. C., Kimberly, R. P., Moreland, L. W., Seldin, M. F., & Bridges, S. L. (2004). Genetic risk factors for infection in patients with early rheumatoid arthritis. *Genes Immun*, 5(8), 641-647.

Jansen, T. L. (2010). When rheumatology meets hepatology: are anti-TNFs safe in hepatitis B virus carriers? *Arthritis Res Ther*, 12(1), 103.

Jimenez, F. G., Colmenero, J. D., & Irigoyen, M. V. (2005). Reactivation of brucellosis after treatment with infliximab in a patient with rheumatoid arthritis. *J Infect*, 50(4), 370-371.

Kaine, J. L., Kivitz, A. J., Birbara, C., & Luo, A. Y. (2007). Immune responses following administration of influenza and pneumococcal vaccines to patients with rheumatoid arthritis receiving adalimumab. *J Rheumatol*, 34(2), 272-279.

Kapetanovic, M. C., Saxne, T., Nilsson, J. A., & Geborek, P. (2007). Influenza vaccination as model for testing immune modulation induced by anti-TNF and methotrexate therapy in rheumatoid arthritis patients. *Rheumatology (Oxford)*, 46(4), 608-611.

Kapetanovic, M. C., Saxne, T., Sjoholm, A., Truedsson, L., Jonsson, G., & Geborek, P. (2006). Influence of methotrexate, TNF blockers and prednisolone on antibody responses to pneumococcal polysaccharide vaccine in patients with rheumatoid arthritis. *Rheumatology (Oxford)*, 45(1), 106-111.

Kaur, P. P., Chan, V. C., & Berney, S. N. (2007). Successful etanercept use in an HIV-positive patient with rheumatoid arthritis. *J Clin Rheumatol*, 13(2), 79-80.

Keane, J., Gershon, S., Wise, R. P., Mirabile-Levens, E., Kasznica, J., Schwieterman, W. D., Siegel, J. N., & Braun, M. M. (2001). Tuberculosis associated with infliximab, a tumor necrosis factor alpha-neutralizing agent. *N Engl J Med*, 345(15), 1098-1104.

Keystone, E. C., Kavanaugh, A. F., Sharp, J. T., Tannenbaum, H., Hua, Y., Teoh, L. S., Fischkoff, S. A., & Chartash, E. K. (2004). Radiographic, clinical, and functional outcomes of treatment with adalimumab (a human anti-tumor necrosis factor monoclonal antibody) in patients with active rheumatoid arthritis receiving concomitant methotrexate therapy: a randomized, placebo-controlled, 52-week trial. *Arthritis Rheum*, 50(5), 1400-1411.

Klareskog, L., van der Heijde, D., de Jager, J. P., Gough, A., Kalden, J., Malaise, M., Martin Mola, E., Pavelka, K., Sany, J., Settas, L., Wajdula, J., Pedersen, R., Fatenejad, S., & Sanda, M. (2004). Therapeutic effect of the combination of etanercept and methotrexate compared with each treatment alone in patients with rheumatoid arthritis: double-blind randomised controlled trial. *Lancet*, 363(9410), 675-681.

Lee, J. H., Slifman, N. R., Gershon, S. K., Edwards, E. T., Schwieterman, W. D., Siegel, J. N., Wise, R. P., Brown, S. L., Udall, Jr J. N., & Braun, M. M. (2002). Life-threatening histoplasmosis complicating immunotherapy with tumor necrosis factor alpha antagonists infliximab and etanercept. *Arthritis Rheum*, 46(10), 2565-2570.

Lipsky, P. E., van der Heijde, D. M., St Clair, E. W., Furst, D. E., Breedveld, F. C., Kalden, J. R., Smolen, J. S., Weisman, M., Emery, P., Feldmann, M., Harriman, G. R., & Maini, R. N. (2000). Infliximab and methotrexate in the treatment of rheumatoid arthritis. Anti-Tumor Necrosis Factor Trial in Rheumatoid Arthritis with Concomitant Therapy Study Group. *N Engl J Med*, 343(22), 1594-1602.

Listing, J., Strangfeld, A., Kary, S., Rau, R., von Hinueber, U., Stoyanova-Scholz, M., Gromnica-Ihle, E., Antoni, C., Herzer, P., Kekow, J., Schneider, M., & Zink, A. (2005). Infections in patients with rheumatoid arthritis treated with biologic agents. *Arthritis Rheum*, 52(11), 3403-3412.

Maini, R., St Clair, E. W., Breedveld, F., Furst, D., Kalden, J., Weisman, M., Smolen, J., Emery, P., Harriman, G., Feldmann, M., & Lipsky, P. (1999). Infliximab (chimeric anti-tumour necrosis factor alpha monoclonal antibody) versus placebo in rheumatoid arthritis patients receiving concomitant methotrexate: a randomised phase III trial. ATTRACT Study Group. *Lancet*, 354(9194), 1932-1939.

Maini, R. N., Breedveld, F. C., Kalden, J. R., Smolen, J. S., Furst, D., Weisman, M. H., St Clair, E. W., Keenan, G. F., van der Heijde, D., Marsters, P. A., & Lipsky, P. E. (2004). Sustained improvement over two years in physical function, structural damage, and signs and symptoms among patients with rheumatoid arthritis treated with infliximab and methotrexate. *Arthritis Rheum*, 50(4), 1051-1065.

Marotte, H., Fontanges, E., Bailly, F., Zoulim, F., Trepo, C., & Miossec, P. (2007). Etanercept treatment for three months is safe in patients with rheumatological manifestations associated with hepatitis C virus. *Rheumatology* (Oxford), 46(1), 97-99.

Mitchell, D. M., Spitz, P. W., Young, D. Y., Bloch, D. A., McShane, D. J., & Fries, J. F. (1986). Survival, prognosis, and causes of death in rheumatoid arthritis. *Arthritis Rheum*, 29(6), 706-714.

Mohan, V. P., Scanga, C. A., Yu, K., Scott, H. M., Tanaka, K. E., Tsang, E., Tsai, M. M., Flynn, J. L., & Chan, J. (2001). Effects of tumor necrosis factor alpha on host immune response in chronic persistent tuberculosis: possible role for limiting pathology. *Infect Immun*, 69(3), 1847-1855.

Montero, J. A., Ruiz-Moreno, J. M., Rodriguez, A. E., Ferrer, C., Sanchis, E., & Alio, J. L. (2006). Endogenous endophthalmitis by Propionibacterium acnes associated with leflunomide and adalimumab therapy. *Eur J Ophthalmol*, 16(2), 343-345.

Parke, F. A., & Reveille, J. D. (2004). Anti-tumor necrosis factor agents for rheumatoid arthritis in the setting of chronic hepatitis C infection. *Arthritis Rheum*, 51(5), 800-804.

Salliot, C., Dougados, M., & Gossec, L. (2009). Risk of serious infections during rituximab, abatacept and anakinra treatments for rheumatoid arthritis: meta-analyses of randomised placebo-controlled trials. *Ann Rheum Dis*, 68(1), 25-32.

Schiff, M. H., Burmester, G. R., Kent, J. D., Pangan, A. L., Kupper, H., Fitzpatrick, S. B., & Donovan, C. (2006). Safety analyses of adalimumab (HUMIRA) in global clinical trials and US postmarketing surveillance of patients with rheumatoid arthritis. *Ann Rheum Dis*, 65(7), 889-894.

Shale, M. J., Seow, C. H., Coffin, C. S., Kaplan, G. G., Panaccione, R., & Ghosh, S. (2010). Review article: chronic viral infection in the anti-tumour necrosis factor therapy era in inflammatory bowel disease. *Aliment Pharmacol Ther*, 31(1), 20-34.

Sipsas, N. V., Papaparaskevas, J., Stefanou, I., Kalatzis, K., Vlachoyiannopoulos, P., & Avlamis, A. (2006). Septic arthritis due to Roseomonas mucosa in a rheumatoid arthritis patient receiving infliximab therapy. *Diagn Microbiol Infect Dis*, 55(4), 343-345.

Smitten, A. L., Choi, H. K., Hochberg, M. C., Suissa, S., Simon, T. A., Testa, M. A., & Chan, K. A. (2007). The risk of herpes zoster in patients with rheumatoid arthritis in the United States and the United Kingdom. *Arthritis Rheum*, 57(8), 1431-1438.

St Clair, E. W., van der Heijde, D. M., Smolen, J. S., Maini, R. N., Bathon, J. M., Emery, P., Keystone, E., Schiff, M., Kalden, J. R., Wang, B., Dewoody, K., Weiss, R., & Baker, D. (2004). Combination of infliximab and methotrexate therapy for early rheumatoid arthritis: a randomized, controlled trial. *Arthritis Rheum*, 50(11), 3432-3443.

Strangfeld, A., Listing, J., Herzer, P., Liebhaber, A., Rockwitz, K., Richter, C., & Zink, A. (2009). Risk of herpes zoster in patients with rheumatoid arthritis treated with anti-TNF-alpha agents. *JAMA*, 301(7), 737-744.

Symmons, D. P., Jones, M. A., Scott, D. L., & Prior, P. (1998). Longterm mortality outcome in patients with rheumatoid arthritis: early presenters continue to do well. *J Rheumatol*, 25(6), 1072-1077.

Torre-Cisneros, J., Del Castillo, M., Caston, J. J., Castro, M. C., Perez, V., & Collantes, E. (2005). Infliximab does not activate replication of lymphotropic herpesviruses in patients with refractory rheumatoid arthritis. *Rheumatology* (Oxford), 44(9), 1132-1135.

Tubach, F., Ravaud, P., Salmon-Ceron, D., Petitpain, N., Brocq, O., Grados, F., Guillaume, J. C., Leport, J., Roudaut, A., Solau-Gervais, E., Lemann, M., Mariette, X., & Lortholary, O. (2006). Emergence of Legionella pneumophila pneumonia in patients receiving tumor necrosis factor-alpha antagonists. *Clin Infect Dis*, 43(10), e95-100.

van de Putte, L. B., Atkins, C., Malaise, M., Sany, J., Russell, A. S., van Riel, P. L., Settas, L., Bijlsma, J. W., Todesco, S., Dougados, M., Nash, P., Emery, P., Walter, N., Kaul, M., Fischkoff, S., & Kupper, H. (2004). Efficacy and safety of adalimumab as monotherapy in patients with rheumatoid arthritis for whom previous disease modifying antirheumatic drug treatment has failed. *Ann Rheum Dis*, 63(5), 508-516.

van der Heijde, D., Klareskog, L., Rodriguez-Valverde, V., Codreanu, C., Bolosiu, H., Melo-Gomes, J., Tornero-Molina, J., Wajdula, J., Pedersen, R., & Fatenejad, S. (2006). Comparison of etanercept and methotrexate, alone and combined, in the treatment of rheumatoid arthritis: two-year clinical and radiographic results from the TEMPO study, a double-blind, randomized trial. *Arthritis Rheum*, 54(4), 1063-1074.

van Riel, P. L., Taggart, A. J., Sany, J., Gaubitz, M., Nab, H. W., Pedersen, R., Freundlich, B., & MacPeek, D. (2006). Efficacy and safety of combination etanercept and methotrexate versus etanercept alone in patients with rheumatoid arthritis with an inadequate response to methotrexate: the ADORE study. *Ann Rheum Dis*, 65(11), 1478-1483. 10.1136/ard.2005.043299

Vassilopoulos, D., Apostolopoulou, A., Hadziyannis, E., Papatheodoridis, G. V., Manolakopoulos, S., Koskinas, J., Manesis, E. K., & Archimandritis, A. I. (2010). Long-term safety of anti-TNF treatment in patients with rheumatic diseases and chronic or resolved hepatitis B virus infection. *Ann Rheum Dis*, 69(7), 1352-1355.

Vonkeman, H., ten Napel, C., Rasker, H., & van de Laar, M. (2004). Disseminated primary varicella infection during infliximab treatment. *J Rheumatol*, 31(12), 2517-2518.

Wallis, R. S., Broder, M. S., Wong, J. Y., Hanson, M. E., & Beenhouwer, D. O. (2004). Granulomatous infectious diseases associated with tumor necrosis factor antagonists. *Clin Infect Dis*, 38(9), 1261-1265.

Weinblatt, M. E., Keystone, E. C., Furst, D. E., Kavanaugh, A. F., Chartash, E. K., & Segurado, O. G. (2006). Long term efficacy and safety of adalimumab plus methotrexate in patients with rheumatoid arthritis: ARMADA 4 year extended study. *Ann Rheum Dis*, 65(6), 753-759.

Weinblatt, M. E., Keystone, E. C., Furst, D. E., Moreland, L. W., Weisman, M. H., Birbara, C. A., Teoh, L. A., Fischkoff, S. A., & Chartash, E. K. (2003). Adalimumab, a fully human anti-tumor necrosis factor alpha monoclonal antibody, for the treatment of rheumatoid arthritis in patients taking concomitant methotrexate: the ARMADA trial. *Arthritis Rheum*, 48(1), 35-45.

Wendling, D., Streit, G., Toussirot, E., & Prati, C. (2008). Herpes zoster in patients taking TNFalpha antagonists for chronic inflammatory joint disease. *Joint Bone Spine*, 75(5), 540-543.

Winthrop, K. L., & Chiller, T. (2009). Preventing and treating biologic-associated opportunistic infections. *Nat Rev Rheumatol*, 5(7), 405-410.

Wolfe, F., Michaud, K., & Chakravarty, E. F. (2006). Rates and predictors of herpes zoster in patients with rheumatoid arthritis and non-inflammatory musculoskeletal disorders. *Rheumatology (Oxford)*, 45(11), 1370-1375. 10.1093/rheumatology/kel328

Xynos, I. D., Tektonidou, M. G., Pikazis, D., & Sipsas, N. V. (2009). Leishmaniasis, autoimmune rheumatic disease, and anti-tumor necrosis factor therapy, Europe. *Emerg Infect Dis*, 15(6), 956-959.

Young, C. L., Adamson, T. C., 3rd, Vaughan, J. H., & Fox, R. I. (1984). Immunohistologic characterization of synovial membrane lymphocytes in rheumatoid arthritis. *Arthritis Rheum*, 27(1), 32-39.

Zein, N. N. (2005). Etanercept as an adjuvant to interferon and ribavirin in treatment-naive patients with chronic hepatitis C virus infection: a phase 2 randomized, double-blind, placebo-controlled study. *J Hepatol*, 42(3), 315-322.

Zingarelli, S., Frassi, M., Bazzani, C., Scarsi, M., Puoti, M., & Airo, P. (2009). Use of tumor necrosis factor-alpha-blocking agents in hepatitis B virus-positive patients: reports of 3 cases and review of the literature. *J Rheumatol*, 36(6), 1188-1194.

7

Pamidronate Treatment in Charcot Neuro-Osteoarthropathy: Change in Biochemical Markers of Bone Turnover and Radiographic Outcome After Treatment

Ivonne Vázquez, Mireia Moreno and Marta Larrosa
Hospital of Sabadell, Corporació Sanitària i Universitària Parc Taulí (UAB), Rheumatology Service
Spain

1. Introduction

Charcot neuro-osteoarthropathy (CNO) is a disabling, rapidly progressive destructive arthropathy and a devastating condition in patients with sensitive neuropathy secondary to different diseases such as diabetes mellitus, syringomyelia, polyomielitis, multiple sclerosis or leprosy (Storey, 2004). Diabetes is nowadays the most common cause of neuroarthropathy, with the joints of foot being most frequently affected (Shae & Boulton, 1995). The reported incidence and prevalence of CNO varies between 0,1-0,4% of diabetic population, but the real prevalence of CNO in patients with diabetes mellitus is unknown because many cases are undiagnosed due to a lack of recognition of the clinical symptoms of acute presentation (Bailer & Root, 1947; Fabrin et al., 2000; Klenerman, 1996; Rajbhandari et al., 2002; Sinha et al., 1972). Both type 1 and type 2 diabetic patients are at risk. The majority of patients with CNO are between the fifth and sixth decades although type 1 diabetes present CNO at a younger age and most patients have had diabetes for at least 10 years (Clouse et al., 1974; Cofield et al., 1983; Petrova et al., 2004). Bilateral involvement has been described in up to 30% of patients with CNO affecting the feet (Shae & Boulton, 1995). The basic physiopathologic mechanism of CNO is poorly understood although repetitive trauma and autonomic nervous dysfunction are probably implicated (the neurotraumatic and neurovascular theories). Probably there is a triggering factor including trauma or infection which triggers the onset of an inflammatory cascade which leads to an increased osteoclastic activity in some predisposed patients.

Although there is no clear evidence, the RANK/RANKL/OPG system may play an important role in the osteolysis seen in the acute CNO. The initial trigger leads to a production of proinflammatory cytokines, including tumor necrosis factor alpha (TNFα) and interleukin-1β(IL-1β). The expression of these cytokines could increase the expression of receptor activator of nuclear factor-κB (RANKL), the ligand of receptor activator of NF-kB (RANK), that when activated, stimulates the production of nuclear transcription factor NF-kB (NF-kB). When NF-kB is expressed in osteoclast precursors cells, it leads to their differentiation to mature osteoclasts and, in consequence, bone resorption (Jeffcoate et al.,

2005; Jeffcoate, 2008; Molines et al., 2010). In this sense, Mabilleau et al. studied isolated peripheral blood monocytes from diabetic Charcot patients, diabetic controls and healthy controls and demonstrated that resorption in acute CNO is related to an increase in RANKL-mediated osteoclastic activity (Mabilleau et al., 2008).

The usual initial presentation of acute CNO is a swelling, tender and warm involved joint and there is usually a temperature difference greater than 2°C when compared with the contralateral joint (Jude & Boulton, 2001; Petrova & Edmonds, 2008). The whole clinical picture can simulate an infection in its appearance. The chronic CNO is painless, without a temperature difference and characterized by established deformity.

The aim of this chapter is to review the usefulness of biochemical bone markers and the image features for both diagnosis and for follow-up after treatment of CNO with bisphosphonates (pamidronate).

2. Imaging and biochemical markers of turnover in diagnosis of Charcot neuro-osteoarthropathy

Although the diagnostic is based on clinical findings, conventional radiography, radionucleide scintigraphy and magnetic resonance imaging (MRI) are the more common modalities used for helping to the diagnosis of CNO.

2.1 Plain radiography

X-plain radiographs are usually the first exam used and they are useful for anatomical information. However they are neither sensitive nor specific to differentiate acute CNO changes from osteomyelitis.

In early stages, the presence of effusion with minimal subluxation and fracture-bone fragmentation should alert to the physician to the possibility of CNO. These initial changes may progress to collapse, resorption and subchondral bone fragmentation, bone proliferation with sclerosis and osteophytosis, intra-articular bone fragments, complete subluxation, massive soft tissue enlargement and effusion and fracture of neighboring bones (Resnick & Niwayama).

The Eichenholtz classification (Eichenholtz, 1966) modified by Shibata et al. (Shibata et al., 1990) describe a correlation between clinical findings and radiographic features (table 1).

Stage 0	early phase	acute symptoms	no changes
Stage 1	development stage	acute symptoms	osteopenia, bone destruction, debris formation, fragmentation of the subchondral bone , capsular distention, subluxations ,dislocations
Stage 2	coalescence stage	decreased symptoms	resorption of debris, bony sclerosis , fusion of bone fragments
Stage 3	reconstruction stage	resolved	bony remodeling, rounding of fragments

Table 1. Eichenholtz classification modified by Shibata.

Medical literature focused on radiology findings describe two patterns of CNO: a hypertrophic pattern characterized by joint destruction and bone fragmentation, debris formation, sclerosis and osteophytosis, such as osteoarthritis and an atrophic pattern showing osseous resorption and joint disorganization that may appear similar to septic arthritis, so, differential diagnosis between atrophic CNO and septic arthritis may be difficult. Frequently, patients present a combination of hypertrophic and atrophic patterns (Aliadabi et al., 2003; Jones et al., 2000).

In the diabetic population, destructive or resorptive bony abnormalities can predominate depending on the location of CNO. At the mid-foot or tarsometatarsal joints (Lisfranc) [the most common localization representing about 60%(Brodsky)], bone fragmentation, sclerosis with fracture-dislocation and complete disintegration of one or more tarsal bone are frequently found. This may lead to a collapse of the longitudinal arch and increased load bearing on the cuboid, resulting in a "rocker-bottom" deformity. If the metatarsophalangeal joints are affected, bone resorption is the predominant feature, leading to a disappearance, partial or complete, of the metatarsal heads and proximal phalanges. Finally, the hindfoot and ankle, although less frequent, it may be affected with fragmentation, eburnation and dislocation of the affected bones.

In summary, the five D's describe the radiological features of CNO: joint distension, dislocations, debris, disorganization and increased density (Rajbhandari et al., 2002), being the presence of multiples fractures the most suggestive radiologic pattern of CNO.

2.2 Radionucleide scintigraphy

Three imaging phases ^{99}Technetium bone scan (^{99}Tc-scan) are highly sensitive (91%) for osseus pathology but lacks specificity (54%) for the diagnosis of CNO (Aliadabi et al., 2003; Sella, 2009; Schauwecker et al., 1988). The scintigraphy is positive in all 3 phases, reflecting an increased bone turnover, a similar situation to that found in other conditions such as osteomyelitis. In these cases, in order to improve the specificity of the test to rule out infection the labeled white cell scans (^{99}Tc-WBC, HMPAO, ^{111}In-WBC) can be used. These scintigraphy techniques show increased activity at the site of infection, reaching a specificity of 60-86% depending on the studies and on the radiotracer used to label white cells (Sella, 2009).

A fourth phase or 24-hour phase image ^{99}Tc-scan can be used to improve the localization of the affected site when there is too much background activity.

The ^{67}Ga/bone imaging study is not reliable for diagnosing osteomyelitis because ^{67}Ga also accumulates in sterile CNO (Glynn, 1981; Knight et al. 1988).

Given its high sensitivity, the scintigraphy may be useful in early diagnosis although can not rule out the presence of a coexisting infection. However it has two major limitations: sometimes may not differentiate bone infection from that of adjacent soft tissues due to low resolution, and the presence of peripheral ischemia can limit sensitivity.

2.3 Magnetic resonance imaging

The role of MRI for diagnostic imaging of the diabetic foot is increasing due to its advantages over scintigraphy and radiographs but its use is still unclear.The T_1-weighted sequences show anatomical references, both normal or abnormal, while T_2- and STIR- (short tau inversion recovery) weighted sequences are better to demonstrate edema and inflammatory changes in the soft tissues and bone.

Some possible algorithms have been proposed (Giurato & Uccioli, 2006) but it is usually considered that MRI is not necessary in patients with evidence of CNO on plain radiographs and no clinical signs of infection (Giurato & Uccioli, 2006; Marcus et al., 1996).

CNO may present with two types of changes on MRI, depending on the evolution time of the process. Acute CNO shows a low signal intensity within bone marrow on T_1-weighted sequences and high signal intensity on T_2- and STIR-weighted sequences, findings that are similar to those observed in osteomyelitis. In a chronic CNO, besides cortical fragmentation, joint deformity and dislocation, typically appears a low signal intensity in the bone marrow on both T_1- and T_2-weighted sequences consistent with osteosclerosis on plain radiography. Another finding in chronic CNO is cyst-like lesions in the bone marrow which appear as well-defined clearly marginated low signal lesions on T_1-weighted images and as high signal intensity on T_2-weighted images (Beltran et al. 1990; Marcus et al., 1996).

MRI may also be useful to early diagnosis when patients present acute symptoms and no changes in plain radiographs can be detected (stage 0 of Eichenholtz classification). In these cases, MRI may detect early events, such as bone edema, occult fractures and joint effusion (Chantelau & Poll, 2006; Edmonds et al., 2006; Greenstein et al., 2002).

Bone and soft tissue infection involving the foot is particularly common in patients with diabetes mellitus, and in these patients, CNO often coexists. The differentiation between these two entities is difficult. There are some MRI features that help to differentiate acute CNO from osteomyelitis: bone marrow signal damage and edema pattern, distribution of the changes, presence of deformity and soft tissue changes (ulcers, abscess or sinus tracts) (Lederman & Morrison, 2005; Lederman et al., 2002; Tan & Teh, 2007). Ahmadi et al., in a retrospective review of contrast-enhanced MRI study of 128 neuropathic feet joints in 63 diabetic patients with a suspicion of osteomyelitis, found that the presence of sinus tract, the presence of soft-tissue fluid collection and extensive bone marrow abnormality were MRI features commonly present in a superimposed infection (Ahmadi et al., 2006) (table 2).

Several studies demonstrate that MRI has a high sensitivity (77-100%) and specificity (80-100%) for osteomyelitis. Furthermore, in osteomyelitis MRI has a positive predictive power of 93% and almost a negative predictive power of 100% according to studies that compared MRI results to bone biopsy, which is considered the gold standard for diagnosing osteomyelitis (Levine et al., 1994; Marcus et al., 1996). However there are no studies assessing neither the sensitivity nor specificity of MRI detecting osteomyelitis in CNO patients.

The use of gadolinium in CNO is controversial (Marcus et al.,1996; Morrison et al., 1993) although may be useful to complete the soft tissue study (abscesses, sinus tracts, cellulitis).

In summary, MRI is a useful, non-invasive tool for the early diagnosis of CNO and may have utility for detecting a superimposed infection, being the soft tissue alteration the most specific finding.

	Osteomyelitis	Charcot Neuro-osteoarthropathy	
	Bone features		
Bone marrow	Low intensity T_1- High intensity T_2- and STIR-	**Acute CNO**	**Chronic CNO**
		Low intensity T_1- High intensity T_2- and STIR-	Low intensity T_1- Low intensity T_2- and STIR-
	Diffuse edema	Periarticular and subcondral edema	
Distribution	Focal bone involvement Weight bearing regions	Several bone affected Predominant midfoot involvement	
Deformity	Not common	Common	
	Soft tissue features		
	Frequently involved: sinus tracts, cellulitis, abscess	Infrequently involved	

Table 2. Differential MRI patterns between osteomyelitis and Charcot neuro-osteoarthropathy.

2.4 Biochemical markers of bone turnover

Biochemical markers of bone turnover are often altered in CNO. There are few studies done, most of them evaluating the changes of these markers after treatment, mainly bisphosphonates. Some studies on bone turnover markers show an increase of these parameters in acute CNO, indicating an unspecific increased in bone activity. Gough et al. measured the pyridoline cross-linked carboxy-terminal telopeptide domain of type 1 collagen (1CTP) and carboxy-terminal propeptide of type 1 collagen (P1CP), both validated as markers of bone resorption and formation respectively, in diabetic patients with acute CNO, chronic CNO, diabetic controls and non-diabetic controls subjects (Gough et al., 1997). Serum 1CTP was significantly raised in the dorsal venous arch of the acute CNO feet compared to chronic CNO, diabetic controls and non-diabetic controls. The authors did not find any significant difference in serum P1CP levels in any group. These levels of 1CTP and P1CP suggest an increase in osteoclastic activity without concomitant increase of osteoblastic function. Selby et al. found an increase in bone-specific alkaline phosphatase (bone formation marker) with no significant changes among the others biochemical parameters studied: osteocalcin, urinary hydroxyproline, urinary desoxypyridinoline (Selby et al., 1998). Increased levels of urinary cross-linked N-telopeptides of type 1 collagen (NTX) have been also demonstrated in CNO patients (Edelson et al., 1996).

In summary, there are few studies focused on bone markers in CNO. The data suggest an increase of them in acute CNO especially of resorption parameters. However, it seems that the role of bone markers for the diagnosis is yet to be determined.

3. Imaging and biochemical markers of bone turnover after medical treatment of Charcot neuro-osteoarthropathy

Although the cornerstone of treatment of CNO is immobilization, there are some studies that demonstrate the clinical benefit of bisphosphonates. The improvement with bisphosphonates appears to be sooner compared to patients with conventional therapy (immobilization) (Anderson et al., 2004). Most studies use pamidronate, although alendronate has been demonstrated to be useful in one study (Pitocco et al., 2005). The optimal treatment regimen of pamidronate remains to be defined. Multiples observational studies have been published using different doses and duration, and all of them have demonstrated some clinical improvement (Navqi et al., 2008; Selby et al., 1994; Young, 1999). Furthermore, some reports have also shown an improvement in radiological changes (Guis et al., 1999) and/or decrease of biochemical bone turnover markers.

Jude et al. published the first trial of pharmacologic treatment, a randomized, double-blinded, placebo-controlled study in 39 active CNO patients (Jude et al., 2001). Twenty-one patients recieved a single infusion of 90 mg of pamidronate and this group showed a significantly reduction in all biochemical markers analized (bone-specific alkaline phosphatase (BSAP) and urine deoxypyridoline cross-linked (D-pyr)) that persisted until 24 weeks in the case of BSAP. However, after 12 months follow-up, both biomarkers rose toward baseline levels.

Comparable results were obtained in 11 patients during treatment with alendronate 70 mg once a week over 6 months, in a randomized controlled double blind study. A clinical improvement was observed and, 1CTP and urinary hydroxyproline levels, as indicators of bone resorption, showed a significant decrease in the treated group after treatment (Pitocco et al., 2005).

Some case reports have demonstrated healing or stabilization of changes on plain radiography after intravenous pamidronate (Guis et al., 1999; Naqvi et al., 2008; Young, 1999).

In a short communication, Mc Gill et al. reported that bone uptake scintigraphy and skin temperature improved over 12 months with immobilization (McGill et al., 2000), but there are no studies evaluating changes in neither MRI nor bone scintigraphy after bisphosphonate treatment.

Bem and collages determined quantitative bone scan parameters (ratio of foot and whole-body uptake and blood flow velocity) and markers of bone turnover (1CTP and BSAP) in 42 CNO patients (21 with acute and 21 with non-acute CNO) (Bem et al., 2010). The authors observed that there was a significant correlation between bone scintigraphy parameters and bone turnover markers. In addition, in acute CNO, there was a significant reduction of both scintigraphy parameters and levels of 1CTP and BSAP after treatment with calcitonin.

Schlossbauer and col. published the first report on quantitative assessment of signal alterations on constrast-enhanced MRI in CNO stage 0, before and after treatment with pressure-relieving means (Schlossbauer et al., 2008). In this study they analyzed the clinical symptoms of 13 patients with acute CNO and compared with MRI findings at baseline and after 4-month follow-up. They found a significant correlation between bone marrow edema and soft tissue edema and pain, with a significant decrease of these parameters after treatment. Thus, they concluded that MRI in early stage of CNO provides valuable information on the activity of the disease.

Our group published an open, prospective therapeutical study with a 12-month follow-up including 7 consecutive patients (four diabetic, two with syringomielia and one with an autonomic neuropathy) with active CNO seen over a period of 3 years (Moreno et al., 2007).

Patients included in this protocol received three intravenous infusions of pamidronate at 0, 2 and 4 months and traditional immobilization methods. Two diabetic patients had a concomitant septic arthritis in the affected joint and they received also antibiotic treatment. Biochemical markers of bone remodeling, radiological exam and ^{99}Tc-scan were performed before and after 12 months treatment. The bone remodeling markers study included blood alkaline phosphatase (ALP) and BSAP, urinary crosslinks NTX, pyridoline (pyr) and D-pyr. Clinical symptoms improved after the first infusion. Although in most cases the bone basal remodeling markers were within normal range values, a clear decrease in almost all of these remodeling markers was observed after treatment in all patients, reaching statistical significance for NTX and urinary pyr, suggesting that the blocking of the osteoclastic activity may play an important role in the physiopathology of CNO, as observed in previous studies. All patients, except one with a siringomyelia, showed signs of radiological healing with a marked sclerosis and reconstruction of the cortical bone (figure 1). In one case pamidronate was administered very early, avoiding the progression and preventing the occurrence of radiological changes during the follow-up period (figure 2). Quantitative scintigraphy was performed only in 3 cases, showing a decrease in radiotracer uptake after treatment although it did not become completely normal. In agreement with previous studies, pamidronate improved not only clinical signs but also stopped the progression of disease in most cases.

Before treatment After treatment

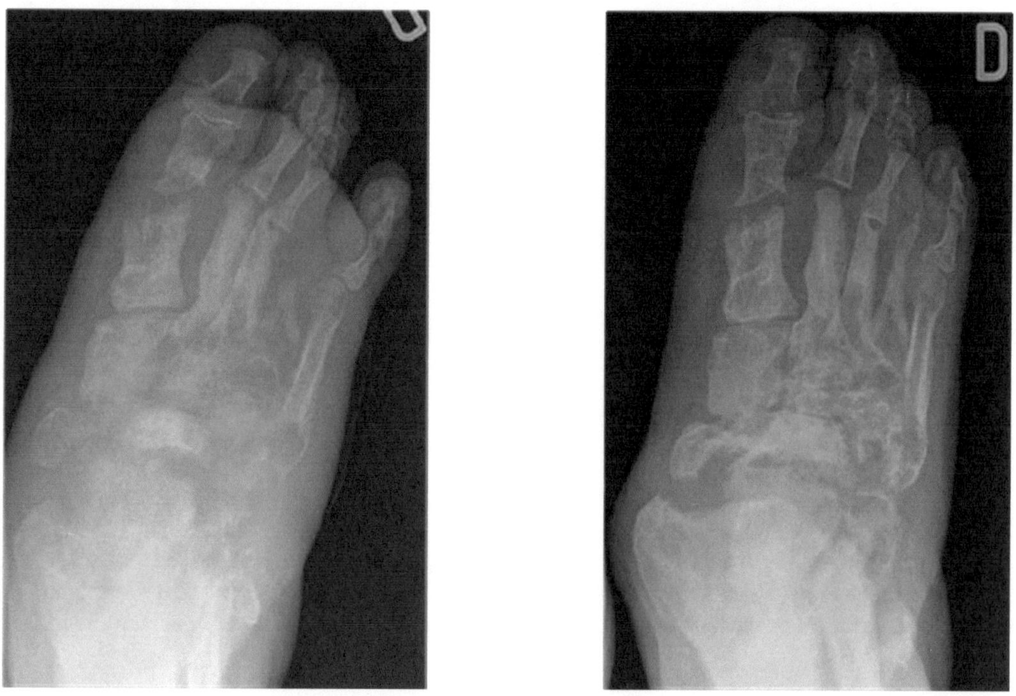

Fig. 1. Patient with a Charcot foot and concomitant septic arthritis. Note before pamidronate treatment the presence of bone fragmentation, subluxation, loss of defined contours and eburnation and after 6-months treatment sclerosis and defined contours.

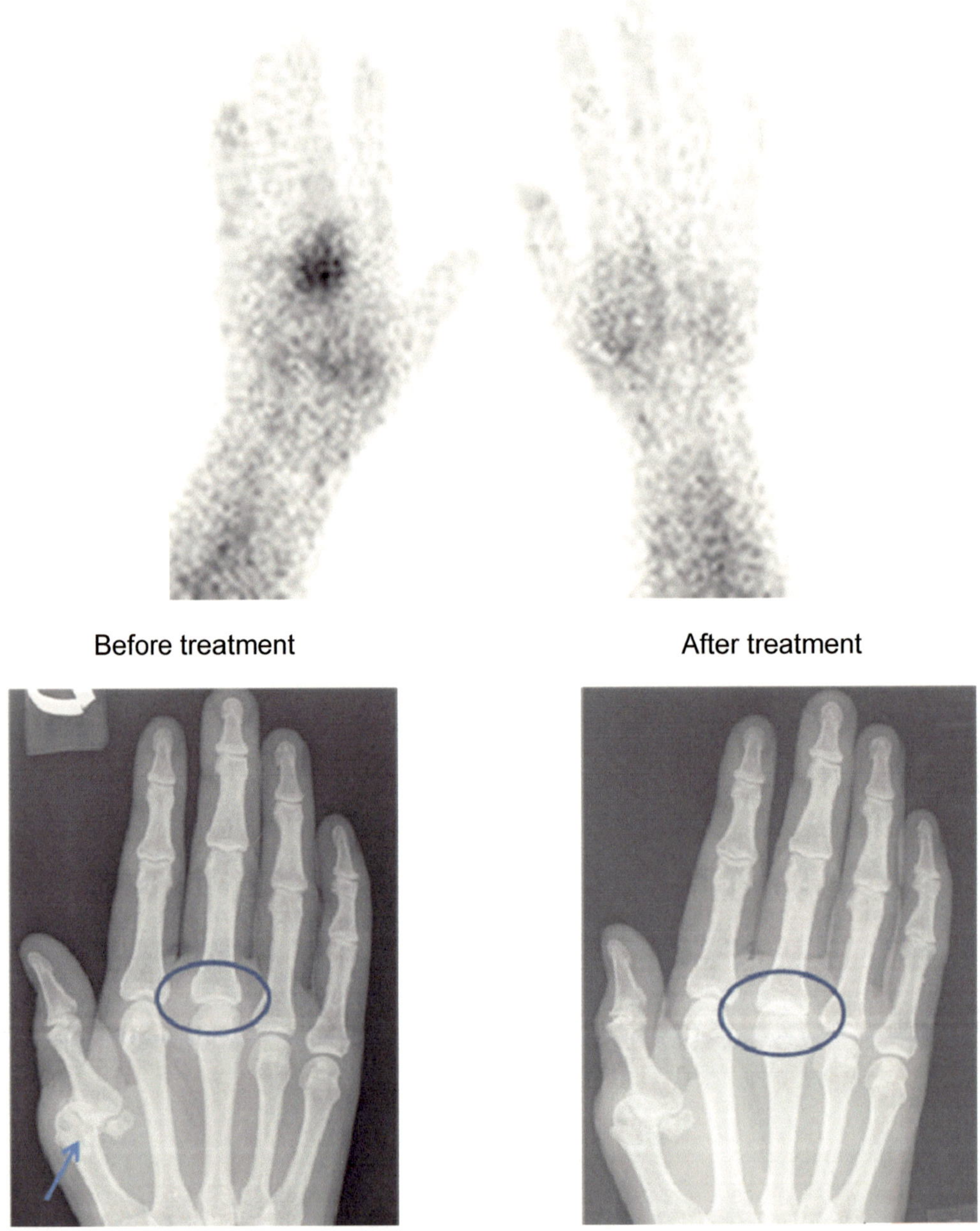

Fig. 2. Patient with a known CNO secondary to syringomielia involving 1st right MCP (arrow). She developed a 3rd MCP swelling joint, early detected with scintigraphy. Initial radiography did not show any changes. Treatment was administered very early avoiding established deformities.

4. Conclusions

- early diagnosis in CNO is difficult and needs a high index of suspicion

- ^{99}Tc bone scan scintigraphy and MRI are useful in order to establish early diagnosis
- ^{99}Tc bone scan scintigraphy and MRI can help to detect superimposed infection, a condition quite common in diabetic patients
- biomarkers of bone turnover are increased in acute phase, especially resorptive ones. However, their utility for monitoring treatment response remains to be established
- bisphosphonate treatment appears to be effective not only for clinical improvement but also for disease outcome
- early diagnosis and treatment may be important to avoid late structural damage

5. References

Ahmadi ME, Morrison WB, Carrino JA, Schweitzer ME, Raikin SM & Ledermann HP. (2006). Neuropathic arthropathy of the foot with and without superimposed osteomyelitis: MR imaging characteristics. *Radiology*, Vol. 238, No. 2, (February), pp. 622-631.

Aliababi P, Nikpoor N & Alparslan L. (2003). Imaging of neuropathic arthropathy. *Seminars Musculoskelet Radiol*, Vol. 7, No. 3, (September), pp. 217-225.

Anderson JJ, Woelffer KE, Holtzman JJ & Jacobs AM. (2004). Bisphosphonates for the treatment of Charcot neuroarthropathy. *J Foot Ankle Surg*, Vol. 43, No. 5, (September-October), pp. 285-289.

Bailer CC & Root HF. (1947). Neuropathic foot lesions in diabetes mellitus. *N Engl J Med*, 13, Vol. 236, No. 11. (March), pp. 397-401.

Beltran J, Campanini DS, Knight C & McCalla M. (1990). The diabetic foot: magnetic resonance imaging evaluation. *Skeletal Radiol*, Vol. 19, No. 1, pp. 37-41.

Bem R, Jirkovská A, Dubsky M, Fejfavorá V, Buncová M, Skibová J & Jude EB. (2010). Role of quantitative bone scanning in the assessment of bone turnover in patients with Charcot foot. *Diabetes Care*, Vol. 33, No. 2, (February), pp. 348-349.

Brodsky JW. The diabetic foot. In MJ Coughlin, RA Mann and Saltzman CL (Eds). Surgery of the foot and ankle, 1281-1368.

Chantelau E, & Poll LW. (2006). Evaluation of the diabetic Charcot foot by MR imaging or plain radiography-an observational study. *Exp Clin Endocrinol Diabetes*, Vol. 114, No. 8, (September), pp. 428-431.

Clouse ME, Gramm HF, Legg M & Flood T. (1974). Diabetic osteoarthropathy. Clinical and roentgenographic observations in 90 cases. *Am J Roentgenol Radium Ther Nucl Med*, Vol. 121, (May) pp. 22-34.

Cofield RH, Morrison MJ & Beabout JW. (1983). Diabetic neuroarthropathy in the foot: patient characteristics and patterns of radiographic change. *Foot Ankle Int*, Vol. 4, (July-August), pp. 15-22.

Eichenholtz S (1966). Charcot Joints. Springfield, IL: Charles C Thomas.

Edelson GW, Jensen JL & Kaczynski R. (1996). Identifying acute Charcot arthropathy through urinarycross-linked N-telopeptides. *Diabetes*, Vol. 45 (suppl. 2), abstract 108A.

Edmonds ME, Petrova NL, Edmonds A et al. (2006). What happens to the initial bone marrow oedema in the natural history of Charcot osteoarthropathy (abstract)? *Diabetologia*, Vol. 49 (suppl.), pp. 684.

Fabrin J, Larsen K & Holstein PE. (2000). Long-term follow up in diabetic Charcot feet with spontaneous onset. *Diabetes Care*, Vol. 23, No. 6, (June), pp. 796-800.

Giurato L & Uccioli L. (2006) The diabetic foot: Charcot joint and osteomyelitis. *Nucl Med Commun*, Vol. 27, No. 9, (September), pp. 745-749.

Glynn TP jr. (1981). Marked gallium accumulation in neurogenic arthropathy. *J Nucl Med*, Vol. 22, No. 11, (November) pp. 1016-1017.

Gough A, Abraha H, Li F, Purewal TS, Foster AVM, Watkins PJ, Moniz C & Edmonds ME. (1997). Mesurement of markers of osteoclast and osteoblast activity in patients with acute and chronic diabetic charcot neuroarthropathy. *Diabet Med*, Vol. 14, No. 7, pp. 527-531.

Greenstein AS, Marzo-Ortega H, Emery P, O'Connor P & McGonagle D. (2002). Magnetic resonance imaging as a predictor of progressive joint destruction in neuropathic joint disease. *Arthritis Rheum*, Vol. 46, No. 10, (October), pp. 2814-2815.

Guis S, Pellissier JF, Arniaud D, Turck F, Witjas T, Roux H & Mattei JP. (1999). Healing of Charcot's joint by pamidronate infusion. *J Rheumatol*, Vol. 26, No. 8, (August), pp. 1843-1845.

Jeffcoate WJ, Game F & Cavanagh PR. (2005). The role of proinflammatory cytokines in the cause of neuropathic osteoarthropathy (acute Charcot foot) in diabetes. *Lancet*, Vol. 366, (December) pp. 2058-2061.

Jeffcoate WJ. (2008). The causes of the Charcot Syndrome. *Clin Podiatr Med Surg*, Vol. 25, No. 1, (January), pp. 29-42.

Jones EA, Manster BJ, May DA & Disler DG. (2000). Neuropathic osteoarthropahty: diagnostic dilemmas and differential diagnosis. *Radiographics*, Vol. 20, (October), pp. S279-293.

Jude EB & Boulton AJM. (2001). Update on Charcot neuroarthropathy. *Curr Diab Rep*, Vol. 1, No. 3 (December) pp. 228-232.

Jude EB, Selby PL, Burgess J, Lilleystone P, Mawer EB, Page SR, Donohoe M, Foster AVM, Edmonds ME & Boulton AJM. (2001). Bisphosphonates in the treatment of Charcot neuroarthropathy: a double-blind randomised controlled trial. *Diabetologia*, Vol. 44, No. 11, (November), pp. 2032-2037.

Klenerman L. (1996). The Charcot neuroarthropathy joint in diabetes. *Diabet Med*, Vol. 13, pp. S52-S54.

Knight D, Gray HW, McKillop JH & Bessent RG. (1988). Imaging for infection: caution required with the Charcot joint. *Eur J Nucl Med*, Vol. 13, No. 10, pp 523-526.

Ledermann HP, Morrison WB & Schweitzer ME. (2002). MR image analysis of pedal osteomyelitis: distribution, patterns of spread, and frequency of associated ulcerations and septic arhtiritis. *Radiology*, Vol. 223, No. 3, (June), pp. 747-755.

Ledermann HP & Morrison WB. (2005). Differential diagnosis of pedal osteomyelitis and diabetic neuroarthropathy: MR imaging. *Semin Musculoskelet Radiol*, Vol. 9, No. 3, (September), pp. 272-283.

Levine SE, Neagle CE, Esterhai JL, Wright DG & Dalinka MK. (1994). Magnetic resonance imaging for diagnosis of osteomyelitis in the diabetic patient with a foot ulcer. *Foot Ankle Int*, Vol. 15, No. 3, (March), pp. 151-156.

Mabilleau G, Petrova NL, Edmonds ME & Sabokbar A. (2008). Increased osteoclastic activity in acute Charcot's osteoarthropathy: the role of receptor activator of nuclear factor-kappa B ligand. *Diabetologia*, Vol. 51, (June), pp. 1035-1040.

Marcus CD, Ladam-Marcus VJ, Leone J, Malgrange D, Bonnet-Gausserand FM & Menanteau BP. (1996). MR Imaging of osteomyelitis and neuropathic osteoarthropathy in the feet of diabetics. *Radiographics*, Vol. 16, No. 6, (Noember), pp. 1337-1348.

McGill M, Molyneaux L, Bolton T, Ioannou K, Uren R & Yue DK. (2000). Response of Charcot's arthropathy to contact casting: assessment by quantitative techniques. *Diabetologia*, Vol. 43, No 4, (April), pp. 481-84.

Molines L, Darmon P & Raccah D. (2010). Charcot's foot: newest findings on its pathophysiology, diagnosis and treatment. *Diabetes Metab*, Vol. 31, (September), pp. 251-255.

Moreno M, Gratacós J, Casado E, Galisteo C, Orellana C & Larrosa M. (2007). Utilidad del pamidronato en el tratamiento de la artropatía de Charcot. *Reumatol Clin*, Vol. 3, No. 6, pp. 257-261.

Morrison WB, Schweitzer ME, Bock GW, Mitchell DG, Hume EL, Pathria MN & Resnick D. (1993). Diagnosis of osteomyelitis: utility of fat-suppressed contrast-enhanced MR imaging. *Radiology*, Vol. 189, No. 1, (October), pp. 251-257.

Naqvi A, Cuchacovich R, Saketkoo L & Espinoza LR. (2008). Acute Charcot arthropathy successfully treated with pamidronate: long-term follow-up. *Am J Med Sci*, Vol. 335, No. 2, (February), pp. 145-148.

Petrova NL, Foster AVN & Edmonds ME. (2004). Difference in presentation of Charcot osteoarthropathy in type 1 compared with type 2 diabetes. *Diabetes Care*, Vol. 27, No. 5, (May) pp. 1235-1236.

Petrova NL & Edmonds ME. (2008). Charcot neuro-osteoarthropathy current standards. *Diabetes Metab Res Rev*, Vol. 24 (supl 1), (May-June), pp. S58-61.

Pitocco D, Ruotolo V, Caputo S, Mancini L, Collina CM, Manto A, Caradonna P & Ghirlanda G. (2005). Six-months treatment with alendronate in acute Charcot neuroarthropathy: a randomized controlled trial. *Diabetes care*, Vol. 28, (May), pp. 1214-1215.

Rajbhandari SM, Jenkins RC, Davies C & Tesfaye S. (2002). Charcot neuroarthropathy in diabetes mellitus. *Diabetologia*, Vol. 45, No. 10, (August) pp. 85-96.

Resnick D, Niwayama G (1988). *Diagnosis of bone and Joint disorders*, (second edition). Volume 5. W. B. Saunders Company, 0-7216-1482-5, United States of America.

Schlossbauer T, Mioc T, Sommerey S, Kessler SB, Reiser MF & Peifer KJ. (2008). Magnetic resonance imaging in early stage charcot arthropathy: correlation of imaging findings and clinical symptoms. *Eur J Med Res*, Vol. 22, No. 13(9), (September), pp. 409-414.

Selby PL, Young MJ & Boulton AJM. (1994). Bisphosphonates: a new treatment for diabetic Charcot neuroarthropathy? *Diabet Med*, Vol. 11, No. 1, pp. 28-31.

Selby PL, Jude EB & Burgess J, Page S, Edmonds ME, Foster A, Mawer EB, Adams JE & Boulton AJM. (1998). Bone turnover markers in acute Charcot neuroarthropathy. *Diabetologia*, Vol. 41 (supl1): A 275.

Sella EJ. (2009). Current concepts review: diagnostic imaging of the diabetic foot. *Foot Ankle Int*, Vol. 30, No. 6, (June) pp. 568-576.

Schauwecker DS, Park HM, Burt RW, Mock BH & Wellman HN. (1988). Combined bone scintigraphy and indium-111 leucocyte scans in neuropathic foot disease. *J Nucl Med*, Vol. 29, No. 10, (October), pp. 1651-1655.

Shaw JE & Boulton AJM. (1995). The Charcot foot. *Foot*, Vol. 5, pp. 65-70.
Shibata T, Tada K & Hashizume C. (1990). The results of arthrodesis of the ankle for leprotic neuroarthropathy. *J Bone Joint Surg Am*, Vol. 72, No. 5, (June), pp. 749-756.
Sinha SB, Munichoodappa CS & Kozak GP. (1972). Neuroarthropathy (Charcot joints) in diabetes mellitus. Clinical study of 101 cases. *Medicine (Baltimore)*, Vol. 51, pp. 191-210.
Storey G. (1964). Charcot Joints. *Brit J. Vener Dis*, Vol. 49, (June), pp. 90-117.
Tan PL & Teh J. (2007). MRI of the diabetic foot: differentiation of infection from neuropathic change. *Br J Radiol*, Vol. 80, No. 959, (November), pp. 939-948.
Young MJ. (1999). The management of neurogenic arthropathy: a tale of two charcots. *Diabetes Metab Res Rev*, Vol. 15, No. 1, (January-February), pp. 59-64.

Part 2

Sjögren's Syndrome: Clinical and Immunological Aspects

Diagnostic and Prognostic Features of Sjögren's Syndrome

Muhammad S. Soyfoo[1] and Elie Cogan[2]
[1]*Departments of Rheumatology*
[2]*Internal Medicine*
Erasme Hospital, Université Libre de Bruxelles,
Belgium

1. Introduction

Sjögren's syndrome (SS) is a chronic autoimmune disease characterized by the lymphocytic infiltration of salivary and lacrymal glands leading to xerostomia and keratoconjunctivitis sicca (KCS). The prevalence of SS is variable but recent studies have estimated it to be between 0.1-0.6%(Goransson et al., 2011; Trontzas & Andrianakos, 2005). As such, SS occurs in middle-aged patients with a high female predominance of 9 to 1 (Fox, 2005). SS is classified either as primary (pSS) when occurring alone or secondary (sSS) to other autoimmune diseases such as rheumatoid arthritis or systemic lupus erythematosus. Besides the involvement of exocrine glands entailing the classical sicca syndrome, systemic manifestations resulting from the lymphocytic infiltration of organs can be present in up to 20% of cases. There are actually no specific diagnostic criteria for SS, but for clinical studies and teaching purposes, SS is classified according to the American-European classification criteria, which include subjective and objective criteria of xerostomia and KCS as well as the presence of autoimmune antibodies and histopathological salivary gland involvement. Because of the lack of a "gold standard" for SS, the standard of reference being actually used is clinical diagnosis made by an experienced clinician. The lack of specific diagnostic tests combined with the high frequency of sicca symptoms in the general population makes the diagnosis of SS even more complicated. This holds true especially in early disease where the symptoms and signs are usually mild and might explain the time delay for the diagnosis of SS. The importance of making the diagnosis of pSS is cardinal because of the increased risk of developing lymphoma and serious systemic complications. In an endeavor to increase the likelihood of diagnosis of SS, newer diagnostic tools have been devised such as ultrasound sonography of salivary glands, magnetic resonance imaging of parotid glands as well as epigenetic biomarkers.

2. Pathophysiology of Sjögren's syndrome

Even if tremendous progress in the field of research has been made to unveil the different mechanistic processes underlying the development of SS, the initial triggering events of the disease have yet to be unearthed. Central to the pathophysiology of SS is chronic perpetual stimulation of the autoimmune system. Both B and T cells are implicated in the pathogenesis of the SS, even though the mechanisms underlying humoral and cellular abnormalities are not yet known (Delaleu et al., 2008; Mariette & Gottenberg, 2010).

It is actually believed that a combination of several factors is responsible for triggering disease initiation and perpetuation. In genetically predisposed individuals, psychological or physical stress and hormonal factors can lead to the activation of epithelial cells and to the up regulation of toll-like receptors. Initiation of disease is promoted by altered glandular architecture such as extracellular matrix modification favoring infiltration by cytokines, chemokines and lymphocytes. Up regulation of toll-like receptors leads to T cell activation and ensuing secretion of pro-inflammatory cytokines. Furthermore, activated epithelial cells not only can act as antigen presenting cells leading to the activation of T and B cells, but also activate dendritic cells through up regulation of proapoptotic molecules harboring the formation of exosomes and thereby also further activating B cells. In advanced stages of the disease process, enhanced B-cell activating factor (BAFF) activation and secretion leads to disproportionate activation of B cells thereby favoring aberrant lymphocyte homing, increased glandular destruction, formation of germinal centers and ensuing lymphoma (Figure 1)(Manoussakis & Kapsogeorgou, 2010).

3. Clinical characteristics of SS

The most frequent symptoms of SS include the triad of fatigue, polyarthralgia and sicca symptoms. Because of the higher frequency of these symptoms in the general population, many patients are often diagnosed as having fibromyalgia.

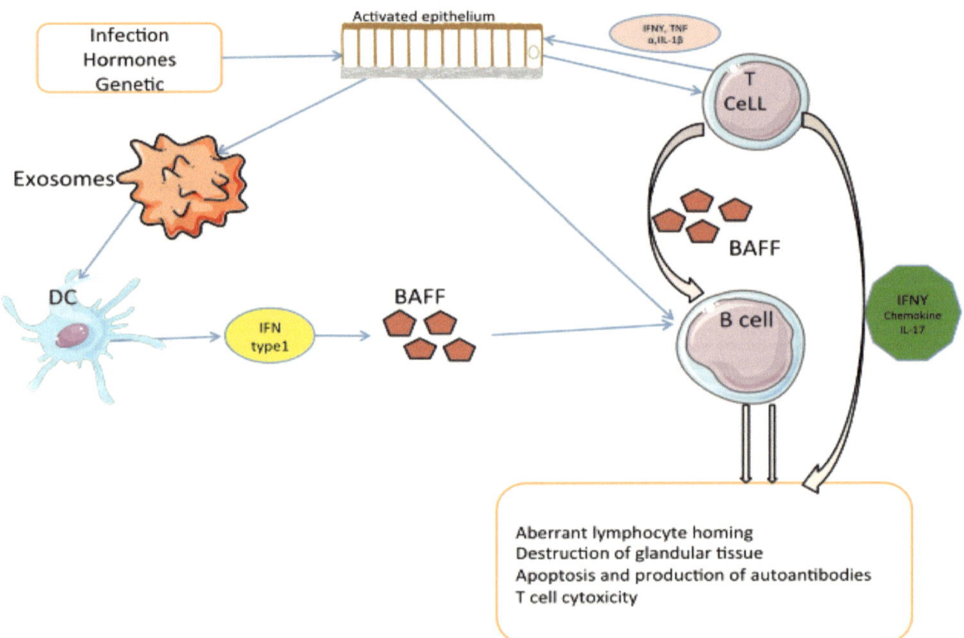

Fig. 1. Mechanisms underscoring the pathogenesis of SS. In the setting of appropriate genetic background, the conjuncture of viral aggression, hormones and environmental factors is thought to initiate epithelium activation which in turn, leads to T cell activation and hence pro-inflammatory cytokines secretion thereby further perpetuating activation of epithelial cells. This results in exosomes formation, dendritic cells (DC) activation and secretion of type I IFN and BAFF leading to B cell stimulation and proliferation, leading to

aberrant lymphocyte homing, T cell cytotoxicity, apoptosis and autoantibodies formation and further glandular destruction. BAFF: B-cell activating factor; Dc dendritic cells; IFN: interferon; IL-1β: interleukin-1β; TNF-α: tumor necrosis factor α.

The most prominent clinical feature of SS is the sicca syndrome of xerostomia and keratoconjunctivitis sicca (KCS) resulting from lymphocytic infiltration of salivary and lachrymal glands. The sicca syndrome is often extended to other organs and might result in skin dryness, vaginal dryness resulting in dyspareunia, and respiratory tract dryness.

3.1 Xerostomia

More than 90% of patients with SS complain of symptoms resulting from functional alteration of salivary glands. Patients often complain of unpleasant taste, difficulties in eating dry food, the need to drink more water or difficulties in controlling dentures. In the early stages of SS, the mouth may appear to be moist, but with disease progression, pooling of saliva in the floor of the mouth disappears, thereby unveiling the lines of contact between frothy saliva and oral soft tissue. With disease progression and especially in advanced stages of SS, the oral mucosa becomes extremely dry and tends to form wrinkles. The surface of the tongue becomes red and lobulated with partial or complete depapillation. The symptoms of xerostomia extend to a painful syndrome with the sensation of permanent burns, soreness, taste alteration, "clicking quality" in the speech of patients with SS, tongue fissuring, dysphagia and angular cheilitis. Gross accumulation of plaque might prevail. Infections by staphylococcus aureus or pneumococcus can result in acute sialadenitis. With further disease progression, teeth decay, periodontal infections, increased incidence of candidiasis infections and ultimately loss of teeth are possible complications (Fox, 2005, Kassan & Moutsopoulos, 2004).

3.2 Keratoconjunctivitis sicca

Ocular dryness in SS, also known as keratoconjunctivitis sicca (KCS), is often less prominent than xerostomia. A detailed anamnestic investigation is necessary to detect ocular dryness symptoms. The main complaint of KCS is foreign-body sensation, but other symptoms such as grittiness, thick rope like secretions at the inner canthus, photosensitivity, burns, and sensation of having a veil before the eyes, absence of tears after irritation or emotion are all frequent features of KCS. Ocular dryness is due to the lymphocytic infiltration of lacrimal glands leading to diminished lacrimal flow and tear composition, thereby altering corneal and conjunctival epithelia, characterizing the known condition of keratoconjunctivitis sicca (KCS). In more severe disease, functional disability with visual impairment occurs. Complications of KCS include corneal ulcerations that can lead to perforations and iridocyclitis (Fox, 2005).

3.3 Systemic manifestations

3.3.1 Musculoskeletal manifestations

Approximately 70% of patients with SS complain of articular manifestations. The main articular features are predominantly arthralgia while arthritis is less frequent (Fauchais et al., 2010). Polyarthralgia is relapsing and remitting. Symmetric, non-erosive, polyarthritis affecting the small joints can also be observed and can even precede the sicca syndrome. The frequency of arthritis in SS has been shown to be nearing 17%. More recently, it has been observed that subclinical synovitis might be more important with the use of ultrasonography and that the frequency of arthritis is around 25%(Iagnocco et al., 2010).

Myalgias are also a frequent feature, accompanied with asthenia, fatigue and muscle tenderness, realizing a fibromyalgia-like syndrome (Mavragani & Moutsopoulos, 2010).

3.3.2 Respiratory manifestations

Diminished secretion from nasal epithelial cells results in nasal crusting, epistaxis and recurrent sinusitis. Due to xerotrachea, patients complain of a dry non-productive cough and dyspnea. In more than 50% of SS patients, dry irritating cough was present without any radiographic abnormalities. Bronchial hyperreactivity due to lymphocytic infiltration might result in small airways obstruction and contribute to the development of cysts and bullae (Parke, 2008).

Interstitial lung disease (ILD) is a classic feature of SS. The clinical manifestations include cough, dyspnea on exertion, bilateral pulmonary infiltrates on plain chest radiographs and other abnormalities on computer tomography scanner such as wall thickening at the segmental bronchi. With disease progression, fibrosis and neutrophilic alveolitis are present (Parambil et al., 2006).

Lymphocytic interstitial pneumonia (LIP), previously considered as a hallmark of lung involvement for SS, forms part of the spectrum of ILD. As such, LIP is the corollary of bronchus associated lymphoid tissue proliferation (BALT). LIP is found in approximately 1% of patients who have SS. Even if LIP is steroid- responsive, approximately 5% of patients who have LIP progress to develop overt lymphoma, and the 5-year mortality for these patients can rise up to 50% (Parambil et al., 2006).

Patients with SS are at increased risk of developing lymphoma, usually low grade MALT lymphoma. Up regulation of the proliferation of BALT might result into malignant transformation with the development of primary pulmonary lymphoma. Typically these patients present with few clinical symptoms such as cough, mild weight loss, and dyspnea on exertion. Strikingly, these minimal symptoms are unparalleled by the severe radiographic changes encompassing micronodules, nodular bilateral and confluent infiltrates, thickening of bronchial walls, air bronchograms and ground glass images (Parke, 2008).

Pulmonary hypertension is a very rare finding in patients with SS. Only 17 cases have been documented in the literature. Prolonged vasospasm and vasculature remodeling have been assigned to contribute to the development of this pathology (Launay et al., 2007).

3.3.3 Renal manifestations

Tubulointerstitial nephritis is the most predominant clinical manifestation of renal involvement in SS. This is characterized by distal tubular acidosis (type 1) and less frequently proximal tubular acidosis (type II) (Fanconi syndrome) (Bossini et al., 2001). Renal biopsy typically reveals interstitial lymphocytic infiltration. Most of the patients present with hyposthenuria and hypokalemic, hyperchloremic distal renal tubular acidosis reflecting interstitial infiltration and destruction by lymphocytes. Distal tubular acidosis might be clinically silent but significant untreated renal tubular acidosis can lead to renal stones, nephrocalcinosis, and compromised renal function.

Glomerulonephritis is very rare in SS. When it occurs it is often due to cryoglobulinemia. Histopathological examination of the kidney shows proliferative glomerulonephritis (Aasarod et al., 2000).

3.3.4 Cutaneous features

Besides the classical features of dry skin, other skin manifestations might also be present. Purpura might be present in up to 30% of patients presenting as petechiae frequently localized on the lower limbs. They follow a remitting and relapsing course and are associated with worse prognosis of SS. Vasculitis is detected in approximately 10% of patients with pSS (Ramos-Casals et al., 2004). It is characterized by a high predominance of leucocytoclastic vasculitis, with life threatening vasculitis being related to cryoglobulinemia. These symptoms usually resolve with corticosteroids. Other manifestations of vasculitis in SS include recurrent urticaria and skin ulcerations. Cryoglobulinemia can be present in SS patients, and can present with a clinical picture of purpura. Other skin manifestations include erythema nodosa, vitiligo, and digital ulcers (Kittridge et al; 2011). One of the most characteristic non-vasculitic cutaneous manifestations of SS are polycyclic, photosensitive cutaneous lesions. These lesions are clinically similar to those observed in cutaneous lupus erythematosus.

3.3.5 Neurological manifestations

The spectrum of neurological disorders associated with SS is broad ranging from peripheral neuropathy to central nervous involvement. The frequency of neurological involvement in SS is relatively low (<5%). In up to 80% of cases, neurological involvement might even precede the diagnosis of SS (Segal et al., 2008).

3.3.5.1 Central nervous system involvement

CNS involvement in SS is very much identical to that of systemic lupus erythematosus. As such, the clinical manifestations include hemiparesis, cranial neuropathy and more often optic nerve neuropathy, brainstem and cerebellar disorders, movement disorders, epilepsia. Spinal cord syndromes encompass transverse myelitis, Brown-Sequard syndrome and progressive myelitis. Due to the presence of optic neuropathy and myelitis, a diagnosis of multiple sclerosis is often evoked. Furthermore, MRI imaging discloses hyperintense lesions in the white matter. Neuromyelitis optica (also known as Devic's disease) is often associated with SS and is characterized by recurrent episodes of myelitis and optic neuropathy.

The clinical features of neuropsychiatric syndrome include often cognition, anxiety, mood changes, and depression and sleep disorders (Lafitte et al., 2001).

3.3.5.2 Peripheral nervous system involvement

Peripheral neuropathy is much more frequent than CNS involvement ranging up to 30% of cases. In most of the cases (93%), peripheral neuropathy precedes the diagnosis of SS. Sensory neuronopathy is considered to be distinctive of SS but sensorimotor neuropathy, sensory neuropathy, autonomic neuropathy, monoeuritis multiplex are amongst other features of peripheral nervous system involvement.

Trigeminal neuropathy is one of the most common vignettes of neurological involvement in SS, which can be either uni or bilateral, but, in essence, is a pure form of sensory neuropathy. It is characterized by painful paresthesias of the face and hypoesthesia (Lafitte et al., 2001).

3.3.6 Gastrointestinal features

The manifestations of gastrointestinal tract are not very specific and include esophageal dysmotility and gastro-intestinal reflux. Patients often complain of dysphagia, nausea and epigastric pain. Subclinical pancreatic involvement is present in approximately 25% of cases.

There are no specific liver abnormalities, which can be attributed to SS, but autoimmune hepatitis and primary biliary cirrhosis can be associated diseases (Mavragani and Moutsopoulos, 2010, Fox, 2005).

3.3.7 Thyroid disease

Hashimoto's thyroiditis is a commonly present in SS. Thirty to fifty percent of patients with SS has anti-thyroid antibodies and elevated basal thyroid stimulating hormone levels (Ramos-Casals et al., 2000).

3.3.8 Laboratory manifestations

3.3.8.1 Non-specific laboratory manifestations

Several hematological features such as anemia, leucopenia and thrombopenia can exist. Mild anemia of chronic disease is present in up to 25% of cases but might also result from hemodilution due to polyclonal hypergammaglobulinemia (Tzioufas & Voulgarelis, 2007). Leucopenia < 4000/mm3 is present in 30% of cases. Hypergammaglobulinemia is most frequent occurring in 80% of cases. In certain cases of major hypergammaglobulinemia, a hyperviscosity syndrome can be present (Fox RI, 2005).

Erythrocyte sedimentation rate is often elevated because of polyclonal hypergammaglobulinemia. In most of the cases serum IgG are increased, while IgA and IgM are normal. If hypogammaglobulinemia exists, lymphoma should be excluded. In 10% of cases, a monoclonal protein is observed. Type II and type III cryoglobulinemia are present in 5% of SS patients (Ramos-Casals et al., 1998). β2-microglobulinemia is significantly increased in the sera of patients suffering from SS. There is significant positive correlation between β2-microglobulinemia levels and disease activity (Skopouli et al., 2000, Gottenberg et al., 2005, Theander et al., 2006, Pertovaara & Korpela, 2011). Serum free light chains have been found to be increased in SS and correlate with disease activity (Gottenberg et al., 2007). Rheumatoid factor is found in 50% of cases in primary SS.

3.3.8.2 Autoimmune laboratory manifestations

Anti nuclear antibodies are frequently observed in the serum of SS patients. Anti-SSA autoantibodies are found in 30 to 50% of sera of patients with SS, while anti-SSB autoantibodies are found in 20 to 30% of cases. In the majority of cases the presence of anti-SSB autoantibodies is associated with the presence of anti-SSA antibodies. Extraglandular manifestations are usually predominant in patients presenting with these autoantibodies. Antibodies against α-fodrin have been exclusively (>95%) found in the sera of SS patients in only one German study while other studies have shown a relatively low sensitivity of 30% (Willeke et al., 2007). Because of the absence of adequate commercially available kit, this test is not routinely performed (Witte, 2005). Recently, new autoantibodies directed against the muscarinic receptors M3 and the proteasomes have been described in patients with SS (Feist et al., 1999, He et al., 2011). Abnormalities complement C4 levels are often associated with the presence of cryoglobulinemia.

3.3.9 Lymphoma

Patients with SS have a 20 to 40-fold risk of developing non-Hodgkin lymphoma (NHL) as compared to the general population (Voulgarelis et al., 1999,Theander et al., 2006, Voulgarelis & Moutsopoulos, 2008). NHL has a prevalence of about 4% in SS and occurs classically following a median of 7.5 years after its initial diagnosis (Skopouli et al., 2000). Various histologic subtypes of NHL for patients with SS have been described, including follicle center lymphomas, lymphoplasmacytoid lymphomas, diffuse large B-cell lymphomas (DLBCLs), and - in particular - mucosa-associated lymphoid tissue (MALT) lymphomas.

Extranodal marginal zone (MZ) B-cell lymphomas of the MALT type are the most frequent type of lymphomas in SS. Generally, MALT lymphomas follow an indolent course, frequently located in both mucosal and non mucosal extranodal sites, a common denominator being the presence of epithelium suggesting that the intrinsic feature of these cells is homing to epithelia rather than mucosa (Pelstring et al., 1999). Most of the organs in which MALT lymphomas arise are devoid of lymphoid tissue, and in the majority of cases MALT acquisition precedes lymphoma development. All of these lymphomas appear to derive from neoplastic transformation of MZ B lymphocytes in spite of the fact that they are associated with several infectious agents or autoimmune disorders such as SS or Hashimoto thyroiditis (Royer et al., 1997). The histological features of MALT lymphoma closely mimic those of Peyer's patch lymphoid tissue and include: (1) reactive lymphoid follicles, with or without colonization by neoplastic cells; (2) MZ and/or monocytoid B-cells (centrocyte-like cells) that infiltrate the overlying epithelium (lymphoepithelial lesions); (3) small B-lymphocytes; and (4) plasma cells, which might or not be of malignant origin.

In most cases MZ lymphomas of the MALT type in patients with SS are either primary low-grade or localized (stage I and II) with extranodal manifestations. The clinical course of the majority of NHL lymphoma is indolent and the clinical characteristics include small tumor burden and good performance status. The salivary glands are the most commonly affected site, but other extranodal sites - such as the stomach, nasopharynx, skin, liver, kidney, and lung - can also be involved. Twenty per cent of patients display involvement of more than one extranodal site at diagnosis, indicating that these lymphomas migrate preferentially to other mucosal sites, thereby emphasizing the importance for complete staging procedures in patients with SS with MALT lymphomas. Even if the lymphoma rarely involves peripheral lymph nodes, it frequently disseminates to locoregional lymph nodes. Presenting symptoms are the result of major gland enlargement, mainly bilateral parotid gland enlargement. The clinical picture in these patients is not characterized by the classical presence of B symptoms (fever, night sweats and weight loss) and bone marrow infiltration is rare. However, in disseminated disease more than one extranodal site is usually involved. The clinical and biological factors heralding imminent lymphoma are low C4/C3 levels, palpable purpura, high β2-microglobulin levels, CD4 lymphocytopenia, parotid gland swelling and persistent enlargement and hypocaptation on salivary scintigraphy, presence of germinal centers in salivary glands, mixed monoclonal cryoglobulinemia, leg ulcers, peripheral neuropathy, splenomegaly and the presence of serum or urine monoclonal bands (Theander et al., 2006, Skopouli et al., 2000). More recently, it has been shown that hypocomplementemia and lymphocytopenia at diagnosis of SS were the strongest predictors of developing lymphoma (Solans-laqué et al., 2011). Consequently, the presence of NHL should be considered at the initial assessment of a patient with SS depicting clinical signs such as significant enlargement of the salivary glands, lymphadenopathy, splenomegaly, skin vasculitis, and peripheral neuropathy.

In certain cases, lymphomas in patients with SS might progress towards a less differentiated cell type. The transition from benign chronic lymphoepithelial sialadenitis (LESA) to indolent extranodal MZ lymphomas of the MALT type and - possibly - to high-grade lymphoma (e.g. DLBCL), is generally considered to represent a multi-step, antigen-driven process. Transformation of MALT lymphoma to DLBCL is heralded by the emergence of an increased number of transformed blasts that form sheets or clusters and finally form a confluence effacing the preceding MALT lymphoma. Most high-grade lymphomas in salivary glands are DLBCLs. It is not known how many of the DLBCLs arise from pre-existing MALT lymphomas and how many are of nodal type or represent transformation of follicular lymphomas. There are several lines of evidence from immunohistochemical, karyotypic, and genotypic studies that the supervening large-cell lymphomas arise from the same clone as the low-grade lymphomas. As such, it can be implied that most of the high-grade lymphomas could represent a blastic variance of either MZ B-cell or follicular-center-cell lymphomas. The clinical manifestation during transformation to high-grade lymphoma is purported by further nodal and extranodal dissemination. Whilst MALT lymphoma in patients with SS carries a good prognosis, the histologic transformation to high grade lymphoma is not with a median overall survival estimated to be only 1.8 years (Voulgarelis et al., 1999).

In summary, NHLs in SS are dichotomized into two categories: the first relating to the majority of patients who develop an indolent extranodal MZ lymphoma and the second, less frequent, relating to those developing high-grade aggressive lymphomas, such as *de novo* or secondary DLBCLs.

4. Diagnostic tools for SS

4.1 Sialometry and sialochemistry

Salivary flow rates can be measured clinically for whole saliva or for separate secretions from the parotid or submandibular and sublingual glands, with or without stimulation. Patients with clinically overt SS have reduced flow. However, flow rates depend on many factors, such as age, sex, medication, and time of day. For analytical purposes, whole saliva is of limited value as it detects neither dysfunction of any of the separate salivary glands nor gland specific sialochemical changes (Kalk et al., 2001). In patients with SS, lower submandibular/sublingual flow rates were observed as compared to controls. Measuring submandibular/sublingual flow rates may contribute to an early diagnosis of SS. In contrast, parotid flow rates are decreased in SS and Non-SS sicca patients. Sialochemistry of collected glandular saliva samples may show several characteristic changes in electrolytes and proteins (enzymes) in SS (Van der Reijden Kwaak et al., 1996). The Na^+ concentration level in the parotid glandular saliva is six fold higher in SS patients as compared to non-SS and healthy volunteers (Kalk et al., 2001).

4.2 Sialography

Sialography consists in the radiography of the salivary glands and its associated ducts following the injection of a contrast radiopaque substance. This technique enables the assessment of the anatomical changes occurring in the salivary gland ductal system. The procedure of sialography is indeed invasive in that it necessitates the cannulation of the salivary gland and ductal system being evaluated. Two types of radiocontrast substance can be utilized: fat soluble and water-soluble compounds. Water-soluble contrast media are usually preferred in that they induce less localized inflammation in contrast to fat-soluble compounds, which provide better radiographic imaging and contrast but can entail chronic inflammatory changes if leakage of the product occurs.

The changes observed in SS consist of salivary glands duct dilatations, duct strictures, sialectasis and occasionally peripheral duct narrowing. The sensitivity of parotid sialography ranges from 48%to 86% and specificity values stretching from 61% to 100%.

4.3 Salivary gland scintigraphy

Salivary scintigraphy is a valid and non-invasive procedure to assess the involvement of salivary glands in patients with xerostomia. After intravenous ^{99m}Tc-sodium pertechnetate administration, sequential images of the head, on anterior projection, are acquired during a variable time interval, usually between 20 and 40 minutes. The images are then stored and glandular regions of interest (ROI) and a background ROI, usually in the skull, are manually drawn. Computer software generates time-activity curves for each major salivary gland. Time-activity curves are divided in two phases: the uptake phase, corresponding to the accumulation of the tracer by the glandular parenchyma, the duration of which depends on the protocol; and the excretion phase, initiated by the administration of a salivary stimulus, usually lemon juice, which corresponds to the tracer elimination through the oral cavity, providing information on the patency of salivary ducts and the overall functional integrity of the system (Vinagre et al., 2009). Abnormal salivary scintigraphy findings include delayed uptake, reduced concentration and/or delayed uptake of the tracer, according to the method proposed by Schall (Schall et al., 1971). According to the Schall classification, salivary gland functional impairment is classified into four grades, following the intensity of uptake and activity present at the mouth after administration of the salivary stimulus; grade 1 classified as normal tracer uptake and grade 4 as complete absence of uptake and mouth activity. This widely diffused classification is considered the standard method for salivary scintigram interpretation but is observer dependent. The overall sensitivity and specificity of salivary scintigraphy is 54% and 98% respectively (Kohn et al., 1992). The most common and early scintigraphic abnormality observed in SS is the impairment of excretion, followed by a decrease in tracer accumulation, reflecting glandular parenchyma destruction. The preferential involvement of the submandibular glands in SS and the decrease of non-stimulated salivary secretion by these glands are correlated to the degree of xerostomia. Recently, quantitative evaluation of salivary gland dysfunction has been developed and there is data supporting the fact that quantitative salivary scintigraphy can detect minimal salivary glands abnormalities, detecting as low as 25% of glandular destruction and is therefore important to identify glandular dysfunction in early SS (Bohuslavizki et al., 1995).

4.4 Tear function tests

4.4.1 Schirmer's test

The Schirmer's test consists in assessing the function of the lachrymal gland. The Schirmer's I test consists in measuring the amount of wetting on a strip of filter paper placed in the lower eyelid over 5 minutes. In the normal non-anesthetized eye, at least 15mm of wetting is expected in patients younger than 40 years old, and at least 10mm of wetting is expected in elderly patients. If no anesthetic is placed onto the eye, the expected wetting of the filter strip sums up to at least 10 mm in a healthy patient younger than 40 years and at least 5 mm in a patient older than 40years. The schirmer's I test is considered to be anormal if it results in less than 5 mm of wetting confirms the clinical diagnosis of dry eye syndrome. A result of 6–10 mm of wetting suggests a dry eye problem (Lemp, 2000). The Schirmer's II test is quite similar to the I test, the difference being that a cotton swab is used to trigger the tear reflex inside the nose.

The phenol red thread test has been developed to obviate the disadvantages of Schirmer's test by eliminating the need for anesthesia. Three millimeters of a fine dye-impregnated 75 mm cotton thread is placed under the lateral one fifth of the inferior palpebral lid margin for 15 seconds; alkalinity changes its color to bright orange from tear contact. Direct stimulation of the nasociliary nerve through irritation of the nasopharynx confirms the presence or absence of reflex tearing. More recently the combination of the phenol red thread test with the Schirmer's test was found to be highly predictive of severe ocular sicca syndrome (De Monchy et al., 2011).

Hyperosmolarity is a common endpoint for all dry eye syndromes and its measurement is a sensitive, but not specific, test since it does not distinguish between tear-deficient and tear-sufficient dry eye. Other rarely performed tests for reduced tear function include fluorophotometry for decreased protein content, lysozyme levels, ocular ferning, impression cytology, and lactoferrin assays.

4.4.2 Diagnostic dye evaluation

Fluorescein is a large molecule unable to traverse normal corneal epithelial tight junctions. In advanced dry eye syndrome, these junctions are disrupted, allowing characteristic diffuse subepithelial or punctate staining. Rose Bengal, a derivative of fluorescein, in a 1% solution or impregnated strips stains devitalized epithelial cells. Alternatively, lissamine green stains for cell death or degeneration, as well as cell-to-cell junction disruption, but does not irritate the eye. Van Bijsterveld created a grading scale for rose Bengal dye that divides the ocular surface into three zones: nasal bulbar conjunctiva, cornea, and temporal bulbar conjunctiva, each graded 0-3 (0, none; 3, confluent staining) (Van Bijsterveld, 1969). A maximum of nine can be obtained and a score ≥ 4 is considered as positive test. The Van Bijsterveld score is the most specific ocular test for evaluation of SS (Kalk et al., 2002).

4.4.3 Tear film stability

Tear film instability can be due to either tear deficiency or evaporative dry eye syndrome. In tear breakup time, fluorescein dye is instilled and the time interval is measured between a complete blink to the first appearance of a dry spot in the precorneal tear film. As such, tear breakup time shorter than the blink interval of 5 seconds could imply ocular surface damage while very short tear breakup time (less than 2 seconds) is suggestive of KCS.

4.5 Salivary gland biopsy

The histopathology of labial salivary glands is a key feature in the diagnosis of SS. A widely accepted criterion for histopathological confirmation of SS is focal lymphocytic sialadenitis of the labial salivary glands. Minor labial salivary glands biopsy is performed by midline incision (of about 1.5-2.0 cm) of lower lip under local anesthesia. Four to six lobules of minor salivary glands are harvested because of prominent variation in the degree of inflammatory and destructive involvement of salivary glands and lobes (Greenspan et al., 1974)

Assessment of inflammatory infiltrates in the salivary gland is based on the number of foci present in the glands, classified as the focus score (FS) (Greenspan et al., 1974). The FS is the number of foci per $4mm^2$ of salivary gland section. The FS represents an extension of the grade 4 classification of labial salivary gland biopsies of Chisholm and Masson (Table 1). The FS is graded from 0 to 12, with a FS of 0 representing the absence of one focus, while a FS of 12 represent those specimens where the foci are so numerous that they have become confluent. A FS ≥ 1 is considered as positive for the diagnosis of SS. It has to be underlined that a FS ≥ 1 can also be observed in other systemic autoimmune diseases such as RA, SLE and in 5-10% of healthy subjects thereby reducing its specificity for SS (Bodeutsch et al., 1992, Lindahl & Hedfors, 1989; Lindahl et al., 1989). Moreover, the sensitivity of FS is reduced in smokers and in patients taking corticosteroids ((Manthorpe et al., 2000), (Zandbelt et al., 2001). The combination of FS ≥ 1 and immunological staining for IgA has been shown to increase the diagnostic specificity for SS (Zandbelt et al., 2002). Indeed, the presence of a Fs ≥ 1 and quantitative immunohistogical staining of IgA < 70%, had greater sensitivity and specificity than the FS alone.

Grade	**Lymphocytes and plasma cells per $4mm^2$ of gland tissue**
0	Absent
1	Slight infiltrate
2	Moderate infiltrate or less than 50 lymphocytes/$4mm^2$
3	One focus per $4mm^2$
4	More than one focus per 4 mm^2

Table 1. represents the grading of labial salivary gland biopsies according to the classification by Chisholm and Mason (Chisholm & Mason, 1968).

Parotid gland biopsy can also be an adjunct diagnostic tool for the diagnosis of SS. Previous prospective studies have shown that the performance of minor salivary gland biopsy is comparable to parotid gland biopsy, which explains why parotid gland biopsy is less often performed (Pijpe et al. 2007,Wise et al., 1988). As such, incisional parotid biopsy is not performed because of the fear of facial nerve injury, sialoceles and fistulae. One of the advantages of parotid gland biopsy over labial salivary gland biopsy is that lymphoepithelial islands or lymphoepithelial lesions (LELs) are often observed in parotid gland tissue of SS patients. These LELs, a characteristic histological feature of the major salivary glands in SS develop as a result of hyperplasia of ductal basal cells within a lymphocytic infiltrate. In addition, well-formed lymphoid follicles or germinal centers, often adjacent to ductal epithelium, can be found in the major salivary glands (Jordan & Speight, 1996).

4.6 New diagnostic tools in SS

Ultrasonography is an inexpensive, noninvasive technique that is used to detect several abnormalities in the major salivary glands. The normal parotid gland appears homogeneous, with increased echogenicity relative to adjacent muscle on ultrasonography. Ultrasonography of salivary gland is a useful tool to detect anatomical changes in the parotid and submandibular glands, with similar diagnostic ability to sialography. Hypoechoic or anechoic areas are believed to represent lymphocytic infiltration, damaged salivary parenchyma, and dilated ducts. As the disease progresses, numerous cystic spaces appear, which most likely reflect progressive glandular destruction and prominent intra-glandular sialectasis (Madani & Beale, 2006). Moreover, submandibular glands of patients with SS have a lower volume and increased parenchymal heterogenicity compared with normal individuals. Receiver operating characteristic (ROC) curve analyses showed that these findings could reliably discriminate patients from healthy individuals (specificity >90%), but could detect only one-half of patients with SS (sensitivity 48–64%). Detection of hypoechoic areas, echogenic streaks, cysts and irregular gland margins are highly suggestive of SS (Takagi et al., 2010).

Similarly, parotid MRI can also prove to be an adjunct diagnostic tool to detect heterogeneity in the salivary glands and specific cystic lésions (Roberts et al., 2008). Niemela *et al.* recently showed that magnetic resonance sialography was the most sensitive method for detecting glandular changes (96%), followed by MRI (81%) and ultrasonography (78%)(Niemela et al., 2001). However, the changes detected did not correlate with saliva secretion, whereas the focus scores the intensity of lymphocytic infiltration in salivary gland biopsy specimens were related only to parotid MRI findings (Niemela et al., 2004).

The involvement of epigenetic mechanisms in disease processes were established when DNA methylation was first identified as an important factor in tumor biology. Nevertheless, impaired epigenetic control has been linked to various autoimmune diseases including rheumatoid arthritis, systemic lupus erythematosus, systemic sclerosis and SS ((Pan & Sawalha, 2009; Richardson, 2007). In salivary glands from SS patients undergoing extracellular matrix remodelling, mechanotransduction may affect epigenetic control of gene expression (Gonzalez et al., 2011a). Global DNA methylation of salivary glands from SS patients appears to be decreased, while specific genes appear to be hypermethylated (i.e: BP230) (Gonzalez et al., 2011b). Over-expression of 2 miRNAs (miR-574 and miR-768-3p) also contributes to the epigenetic control of gene expression in salivary glands from SS patients (Alevizos et al., 2011). These two micro-RNAs were associated with high degree inflammation and correlated with the histological focus score. Moreover, the distinctive signatures of these micro-RNA's could also distinguish SS patients from normal healthy controls (Alevizos & Illei, 2010). As such, they could represent future diagnostic and prognostic biomarkers of inflammation in SS patients.

4.7 Diagnosis and classification criteria for SS

SS is a complex autoimmune disease with protean nonspecific features, thereby hampering the diagnostic process.

Because of this, many patients often remain either under diagnosed or diagnosis is made after a long lapse of time when full-fledged symptoms are obvious. The seminal importance of making an early diagnosis relies on the fact that appropriate treatment can be tailored and proper management of patients set down. Actually, there are no definite diagnostic criteria for SS and diagnosis is essentially based on the clinical insights of the experienced physician in the light of a set of biological and clinical manifestations. Even if classification criteria have been established for SS, they do not have a sensitivity and specificity of 100%, and therefore cannot be used as diagnostic criteria. As a general rule, classification criteria are used as diagnostic criteria in clinical studies in order to standardize diagnosis for patients participating in multicenter clinical studies and therefore enable analysis of data in an unbiased fashion, or for teaching purposes. The stumbling block for devising diagnostic criteria for SS as in other autoimmune diseases is the temporal progression of the clinical manifestations. In very early disease, the clinical manifestations are not overt, thereby fostering further hurdles in the adequate diagnosis.

In 2002, an American–European consensus group was created and a new set of classification criteria for SS has been proposed (Table 2) (Vitali et al., 2002). These criteria comprise subjective criteria: ocular symptoms and oral symptoms, and objective criteria: ocular signs, histopathological signs (focus score ≥ 1), oral signs, and serological signs (presence of antinuclear antibodies: anti-SSA or anti-SSB). Patients are classified as SS if 4 of the 6 mentioned criteria are present, as long as histopathology or serology is positive, or if 3 of any 4 objective criteria are present.

1. Ocular symptoms
   Ocular symptoms are present if there is a positive answer to at least one of the following questions:
   - Have you had daily persistent, troublesome dry eyes for >3 months?
   - Do you have recurrent sensation of sand or gravel in the eyes?
   - Do you use tear substitutes > 3times daily?

2. Oral symptoms
   Oral symptoms are present if there is a positive response to at least one of the following questions:
   - Do you have a daily feeling of dry mouth > 3 months?
   - Have you had recurrent or persistent swollen salivary glands as an adult?
   - Do you drink frequently liquids to help in swallowing dry food?

3. Objective evidence of ocular involvement as defined by a positive result for at least one of the following tests:
   - Positive Schirmer's test without anesthesia ("5mm)
   - Rose Bengal or other ocular dye staining score (≥4 according to Van Bijsterveld's scoring system)
4. Histopathology
   - Focal lymphocyte sialoadenitis in minor salivary glands, evaluated by an expert histopathologist, with a focus score ≥ 1 (defined as a number of lymphocytic foci that are adjacent to normal appearing mucous acini and contain more than 50 lymphocytes per $4mm^2$ of glandular tissue
5. Objective evidence of salivary gland involvement defined as positive result of at least one of the following diagnostic tests:
   - Parotid sialography showing the presence of diffuse sialectasis (punctuate, cavitary or destructive pattern) without evidence of obstruction of major salivary ducts
   - Salivary scintigraphy showing delayed uptake, reduced concentration and/or delayed excretion of tracer
6. Presence of autoantibodies to Ro/SSA or La/SSB, or both, in the serum.

Exclusion Criteria

- Past head and neck radiation treatment
- Hepatitis C or HIV infection
- Pre-existing lymphoma
- Sarcoidosis
- Graft versus host disease
- Use of anticholinergic drugs

Classification of Primary and secondary Sjögren's syndrome

In the absence of any underlying disease, primary Sjögren's syndrome is defined as the presence of any four diagnostic criteria as long as either item4 (histopathology) or 6(serologic autoantibody) is positive or as the presence of any 3 of the 4 objective criteria items (items 3,4,5,6).

In the presence of any potentially associated disease (such as another autoimmune disease; systemic lupus erythematosus for example)), the presence of item 1or 2 plus any other 2 items 3,4 and 5 might be suggestive of secondary Sjögren's disease.

Table 2. American-European classification criteria for SS

4.8 Differential diagnosis of SS

The differential diagnosis of SS includes diseases that present with sicca symptoms and parotid gland enlargement. Sarcoidosis can mimic SS, but salivary gland biopsy usually depicts non-caseating granuloma and autoantibodies are absent and clinical features such as hilar lymphadenopathy, uveitis or hypercalcemia are more suggestive of sarcoidosis (Ramos-Casals et al., 2004). Other medical conditions masquerading as SS include lipoproteinemias (types II, IV and V), chronic graft-versus-host disease, amyloidosis, and infection with viruses such as human immunodeficiency virus (HIV), human T-lymphocytic virus-I (HTLV-I) and HCV. Patients with HIV infection may present with sicca manifestations, parotid gland enlargement, pulmonary involvement, and lymphadenopathy.

These patients have an increased prevalence of HLA-DR5 alloantigen (Itescu et al., 1990). The two diseases can easily be distinguished, as patients with HIV infection are usually young males, have no autoantibodies to Ro (SS-A) and La (SS-B), and the lymphocytic infiltrates of the salivary glands consist of CD8+ T cells. HCV can produce a chronic lymphocytic sialadenitis that ressembles SS (Haddad et al., 1992). These patients have a higher mean age, a lower prevalence of parotid gland enlargement and a higher prevalence of liver involvement than patients with pSS. However, patients with SS do not possess an increased frequency of antibodies to HCV in their sera. In cases with isolated dry mouth or dry eyes, other potential causes including deficiency disorders (vitamin A deficiency for example), drugs, infections, endocrinopathies, or degenerative diseases should be excluded.

4.9 Measuring disease activity in SS

In an attempt to provide tools to assess pSS patients in clinical practice as well as in therapeutic trials, several disease activity indices have been designed. These include the SSDAI (SS Disease Activity Index), SCAI (Sjögren's Systemic Clinical Activity Index) and ESSDAI (EULAR SS Disease Activity Index). SSDAI and ESSDAI are global scores. SCAI is a composite score. Validity is a limitation for SSDAI and SCAI (Campar & Isenberg, 2010). ESSDAI is complemented by ESSPRI for the assessment of subjective features. It is more accurate in detecting changes in activity. Comparing the three disease activity indices, it was observed that for patients with improved activity, the 3 disease activity indices showed similar, large sensitivity to change. However, the ESSDAI seemed to detect changes in activity more accurately than other disease activity indexes. Notably, for patients with stable activity, the ESSDAI did not show erroneous improvement (Seror et al., 2010). The ESSDAI consists of 12 organ-specific domains, which are predominantly clinical; only 2 of them include haematological (cytopenias) or biological (clonal component, serum complement levels, serum IgG and cryoglobulins) findings (Seror et al., 2010). For each domain, features of disease activity were classified in 3 or 4 levels according to their severity (Table 3).

Domain	Activity level	Description
Constitutional	0-2	0=no symptoms; 1=mild fever and 5-10% weight loss; 2=severe fever and >10% weight loss
Lymphadenopathy	0-3	0= absence of the following features; 1=Lymphadenopathy ≥ 1 cm in any nodal region or ≥ 2 cm in inguinal region; 2=Lymphadenopathy ≥ 2 cm in any nodal region or ≥ 3 cm in inguinal region, and/or splenomegaly (clinically palpable or assessed by imaging); 3=Current malignant B-cell proliferative disorder
Glandular	0-2	0=no glandular swelling; 1=Small glandular swelling with enlarged parotid (≤ 3 cm), or limited submandibular or lachrymal swelling; 2=Major glandular swelling with enlarged parotid (> 3 cm), or important submandibular or lachrymal swelling

Domain	Activity level	Description
Articular	0-3	0= no articular symptoms; 1=Arthralgias in hands, wrists, ankles and feet accompanied by morning stiffness (>30 min); 2=1 to 5 (of 28 total count) synovitis; 3=≥ 6 (of 28 total count) synovitis.
Cutaneous	0-3	0=absence of active cutaneous involvement; 1=Erythema multiforma; 2=Limited cutaneous vasculitis, including urticarial vasculitis, or purpura limited to feet and ankle, or subacute cutaneous lupus; 3=Diffuse cutaneous vasculitis, including urticarial vasculitis, or diffuse purpura, or ulcers related to vasculitis
Pulmonary	0-3	0=absence of active pulmonary involvement; 1= Persistent cough or bronchial involvement with no radiographic abnormalities on radiography Or radiological or HRCT evidence of interstitial lung disease with: No breathlessness and normal lung function test; 2=Moderately active pulmonary involvement, such as interstitial lung disease shown by HRCT with shortness of breath on exercise (NHYA II) or abnormal lung function tests restricted to: 70% >DL_{CO}≥ 40% or 80%>FVC≥60%; 3=Highly active pulmonary involvement, such as interstitial lung disease shown by HRCT with shortness of breath at rest (NHYA III, IV) or with abnormal lung function tests: DL_{CO}< 40% or FVC< 60%.
Renal	0-3	0=Absence of currently active renal involvement with proteinuria< 0.5 g/d, no hematuria, no leucocyturia, no acidosis, or long-lasting stable proteinuria due to damage; 1=Evidence of mild active renal involvement, limited to tubular acidosis without renal failure or glomerular involvement with proteinuria (between 0.5 and 1 g/d) and without hematuria or renal failure (GFR ≥60 ml/min); **2**=Moderately active renal involvement, such as tubular acidosis with renal failure (GFR <60 ml/min) or glomerular involvement with proteinuria between 1 and 1.5 g/d and without hematuria or renal failure (GFR ≥60 ml/min) or histological evidence of extra-membranous glomerulonephritis or important interstitial lymphoid infiltrate; **3**=Highly active renal involvement, such as glomerular involvement with proteinuria >1.5 g/d or hematuria or renal failure (GFR <60 ml/min), or histological evidence of proliferative glomerulonephritis or cryoglobulinemia related renal involvement

Domain	Activity level	Description
Muscular	0-3	0= absence of muscular involvement; 1=Mild active myositis shown by abnormal EMG or biopsy with no weakness and creatine kinase ($N < CK \leq 2N$); 2=Moderately active myositis proven by abnormal EMG or biopsy with weakness (maximal deficit of 4/5), or elevated creatine kinase ($2N < CK \leq 4N$); 3=Highly active myositis shown by abnormal EMG or biopsy with weakness (deficit ≤ 3/5) or elevated creatine kinase ($>4N$)
PNS	0-3	0 = absence of PNS involvement; 1=Mild active peripheral nervous system involvement, such as pure sensory axonal polyneuropathy shown by NCS or trigeminal (V) neuralgia; 2= Moderately active peripheral nervous system involvement shown by NCS, such as axonal sensory-motor neuropathy with maximal motor deficit of 4/5, pure sensory neuropathy with presence of cryoglobulinemic vasculitis, ganglionopathy with symptoms restricted to mild/moderate ataxia, inflammatory demyelinating polyneuropathy (CIDP) with mild functional impairment (maximal motor deficit of 4/5or mild ataxia),Or cranial nerve involvement of peripheral origin (except trigeminal (V) neuralgia) ;3=Highly active PNS involvement shown by NCS, such as axonal sensory-motor neuropathy with motor deficit ≤3/5, peripheral nerve involvement due to vasculitis (mononeuritis multiplex etc.), severe ataxia due to ganglionopathy, inflammatory demyelinating polyneuropathy (CIDP) with severe functional impairment: motor deficit ≤3/5 or severe ataxia
CNS	0-3	0= absence of CNS involvement; 1=Moderately active CNS features, such as cranial nerve involvement of central origin, optic neuritis or multiple sclerosis-like syndrome with symptoms restricted to pure sensory impairment or proven cognitive impairment; 3=Highly active CNS features, such as cerebral vasculitis with cerebrovascular accident or transient ischemic attack, seizures, transverse myelitis, lymphocytic meningitis, multiple sclerosis-like syndrome with motor deficit.

Domain	Activity level	Description
Hematological	0-3	0=absence of autoimmune cytopenia; 1=Cytopenia of auto-immune origin with neutropenia (1000 < neutrophils < 1500/mm3), and/or anemia (10 < hemoglobin < 12 g/dl), and/or thrombocytopenia (100,000 < platelets < 150,000/mm3) Or lymphopenia (500 < lymphocytes < 1000/mm3); 2= Cytopenia of auto-immune origin with neutropenia (500 ≤ neutrophils ≤ 1000/mm3), and/or anemia (8 ≤ hemoglobin ≤ 10 g/dl), and/or thrombocytopenia (50,000 ≤ platelets ≤ 100,000/mm3) Or lymphopenia (≤500/mm3) ;3=Cytopenia of auto-immune origin with neutropenia (neutrophils < 500/mm3), and/or or anemia (hemoglobin < 8 g/dl) and/or thrombocytopenia (platelets <50,000/mm3
Biological	0-2	0=absence of any of the following biological feature; 1=Clonal component and/or hypocomplementemia (low C4 or C3 or CH50) and/or hypergammaglobulinemia or high IgG level between 16 and 20 g/L; 2=Presence of cryoglobulinemia and/or hypergammaglobulinemia or high IgG level > 20 g/L, and/or recent onset hypogammaglobulinemia or recent decrease of IgG level (<5 g/L)

Table 3. ESSDAI index for measuring disease activity in SS (modified according to Seror et al., 2010)

4.10 Biological markers of disease activity in SS

Biological biomarkers are of pivotal importance in determining which patients are at risks of developing systemic complications of SS and those who could benefit from therapeutic immunomodulation. Classical markers of inflammation such as C-reactive protein and erythrocyte sedimentation rate are of limited value to assess disease activity in SS. These past ten years, significant progress has been made in deciphering the molecular mechanisms underscoring the pathogenesis of SS. As such, the pivotal role of B-cell in pathophysiology of SS has been unearthed (Groom et al., 2002, Gottenberg et al., 2006, Mackay et al., 2007). The B-cell activating factor (BAFF) is significantly increased in the sera and in the salivary glands of pSS patients (Mariette et al., 2003, Lavie et al., 2004). BAFF levels in the sera of pSS patients correlate with the presence of anti-SSA autoantibodies and with the ESSDAI index. Serum beta macroglobulin, another marker of B lymphocyte activation, has been shown to be useful marker of disease activity in pSS, in that it correlated with the presence of disease flare as well as with the occurrence of extraglandular manifestations (Gottenberg et al., 2005). More recently, the levels of serum beta-microglobulin have been observed to correlate with the ESSDAI index (Pertovaara & Korpela, 2011). Serum free light chains have also been detected to be increased in pSS patients and shown to correlate with disease activity (Gottenberg et al., 2007). Several studies are ongoing to evaluate other biomarkers of disease activity of pSS such as chemokines induced by interferon pathway and IL-21, and also other markers of B-cell activation are being currently investigated.

5. Prognostic features of SS

Much knowledge has been gathered these last ten years about the outcome of patients with SS. Although not a benign disease, primary SS has a slow insidious progression with no rapid deterioration in salivary gland function, systemic markers or dramatic changes in clinical manifestations (Gannot et al., 2000). Primary SS, as such is a relatively chronic stable condition, with only mild deterioration of main disease characteristics (Theander et al., 2005). Significant loss of glandular function and quality of life are highlighted during the first years of disease (median of 6 years) and remain stable afterwards. The presence of immunological abnormalities such as the presence of anti-SSA autoantibodies, hypocomplemententemia, increased levels of IgG, high focus scores and low unstimulated whole saliva, is associated with more severe glandular dysfunction (Haldorsen et al., 2008), Theander et al., 2005, Pijpe et al. 2007). It has to be underlined that even if the clinical course of the disease is usually stable, similarly to other autoimmune diseases, individual patients might present some flares and remissions. However, there are two exceptions to this classical benign course, which include a high incidence of lymphoma and the development of systemic manifestations, pertaining to a worsened prognostic significance. The presence of autoantibodies is correlated with the number of systemic manifestations and more specifically anti-SSA autoantibodies are the strongest predictors of extra-glandular manifestations (Ter Borg et al., 2011). Furthermore, serum free light chains and serum β2 microglobulin are increased and correlate with extra-glandular involvement in pSS (Gottenberg et al., 2007; Gottenberg et al., 2005). These findings reflect that enhanced disturbance of the immune system portrayed by B-cell hyperactivity with hypergammaglobulinemia and autoantibody formation, is associated with systemic manifestations in primary SS. A steady clinical course is usually observed in patients with peri-epithelial lesions (tubulointerstitial nephritis, lung and liver involvement), while those presenting with extra-epithelial lesions such as polyneuropathy, vasculitis, glomerulonephritis, purpura and vasculitis, have increased morbidity and mortality (Skopouli et al., 2000, Ioannidis et al., 2002). The cardinal role of cryoglobulinemia has been underlined in this latter group of patients as being the harbinger of the extraepithelial manifestations. These extraepithelial characteristics are associated with a high risk of developing life-threatening conditions and require tailoring treatment with higher doses of corticosteroids and immunosuppressive agents. On the other hand, in patients presenting with peri-epithelial lesions, treatment requires less use of steroids and immunosuppressive drugs and a less frequent clinical monitoring is recommended.

Several reports have noted an increased incidence of malignant non-Hodgkin lymphomas (NHL) in SS patients, with an estimated risk of up to 44 times greater as compared to general population (Kassan et al., 1978). This risk increases with disease duration, is maintained with time and is not related to the patient age at time of diagnosis of pSS (Solans-Laque et al., 2011). Several predictors of lymphoma development have been detailed and include anemia, lymphadenopathy, lymphopenia, hypocomplementemia, peripheral neuropathy, cutaneous vasculitis, bilateral parotid gland swelling, severe involvement in parotid scintigraphy, and cryoglobulinemia (Voulgarelis, Dafni, Isenberg, & Moutsopoulos,

1999), (Brito-Zeron et al., 2007). It has been observed that patients with two of three following factors (parotid scintigraphy, vasculitis, hypocomplementemia) were associated with a lower survival as compared to patients with no factor. More recently, hypocomplementemia and lymphocytopenia were independent risk factors for developing lymphoma but only hypocomplementemia was related to earlier development of NHL and higher mortality ((Brito-Zeron et al., 2007; Solans-Laque et al., 2011). Furthermore, it has been also observed that the detection of germinal center-like lesions in pSS diagnostic salivary biopsies is a highly predictive marker of NHL (Theander et al., 2011). Patients with high-to-intermediated grade lymphoma have significantly worse survival while large tumor diameters and the presence of B symptoms are additional risk factors for increased mortality (Voulgarelis et al., 1999).

6. Conclusions

SS is a chronic autoimmune disease characterized by glandular and systemic manifestations. Because of the increased risk of developing lymphoma in pSS patients, making the diagnosis of SS is of pivotal importance. The herald of newer diagnostic tools could help clinicians and thereby provide significant relief to patients through earlier treatments. Deciphering mechanistic processes inherent to the pathophysiology of SS should in the future provide more sophisticated means for early diagnosis of SS.

7. References

Aasarod, K., Haga, H. J., Berg, K. J., Hammerstrom, J., & Jorstad, S. (2000). Renal involvement in primary Sjogren's syndrome. *QJM: monthly journal of the Association of Physicians, 93*(5), 297-304.

Alevizos, I., Alexander, S., Turner, R. J., & Illei, G. G. (2011). MicroRNA expression profiles as biomarkers of minor salivary gland inflammation and dysfunction in Sjogren's syndrome. *Arthritis and rheumatism, 63*(2), 535-544.

Alevizos, I., & Illei, G. G. (2010). MicroRNAs as biomarkers in rheumatic diseases. [Review]. *Nature reviews. Rheumatology, 6*(7), 391-398.

Bodeutsch, C., de Wilde, P. C., Kater, L., van Houwelingen, J. C., van den Hoogen, F. H., Kruize, A. A., et al. (1992). Quantitative immunohistologic criteria are superior to the lymphocytic focus score criterion for the diagnosis of Sjogren's syndrome. . *Arthritis and rheumatism, 35*(9), 1075-1087.

Bohuslavizki, K. H., Brenner, W., Wolf, H., Sippel, C., Tonshoff, G., Tinnemeyer, S., et al. (1995). Value of quantitative salivary gland scintigraphy in the early stage of Sjogren's syndrome. *Nuclear medicine communications, 16*(11), 917-922.

Bossini, N., Savoldi, S., Franceschini, F., Mombelloni, S., Baronio, M., Cavazzana, I., et al. (2001). Clinical and morphological features of kidney involvement in primary Sjogren's syndrome. *Nephrology, dialysis, transplantation: official publication of the European Dialysis and Transplant Association - European Renal Association, 16*(12), 2328-2336.

Brito-Zeron, P., Ramos-Casals, M., Bove, A., Sentis, J., & Font, J. (2007). Predicting adverse outcomes in primary Sjogren's syndrome: identification of prognostic factors. *Rheumatology, 46*(8), 1359-1362.

Campar, A., & Isenberg, D. A. (2010). Primary Sjogren's syndrome activity and damage indices comparison. *European journal of clinical investigation, 40*(7), 636-644.

Chisholm, D. M., & Mason, D. K. (1968). Labial salivary gland biopsy in Sjogren's disease. *Journal of clinical pathology, 21*(5), 656-660.

Delaleu, N., Jonsson, M. V., Appel, S., & Jonsson, R. (2008). New concepts in the pathogenesis of Sjogren's syndrome. *Rheumatic diseases clinics of North America, 34*(4), 833-845, vii.

De Monchy, I., Gendron, G., Miceli, C., Pogorzalek, N., Mariette, X., & Labetoulle, M. (2011). Combination between Schirmer I test and Phenol Red Thread as a rescue strategy for diagnosis of ocular dryness associated with Sjogren's syndrome. *Investigative ophthalmology & visual science.*

Fauchais, A. L., Ouattara, B., Gondran, G., Lalloue, F., Petit, D., Ly, K., et al. (2010). Articular manifestations in primary Sjogren's syndrome: clinical significance and prognosis of 188 patients. *Rheumatology, 49*(6), 1164-1172.

Feist, E., Kuckelkorn, U., Dorner, T., Donitz, H., Scheffler, S., Hiepe, F., et al. (1999). Autoantibodies in primary Sjogren's syndrome are directed against proteasomal subunits of the alpha and beta type. . *Arthritis and rheumatism, 42*(4), 697-702.

Fox, R. I. (2005). Sjogren's syndrome. [Review]. *Lancet, 366*(9482), 321-331.

Gannot, G., Lancaster, H. E., & Fox, P. C. (2000). Clinical course of primary Sjogren's syndrome: salivary, oral, and serologic aspects. *The Journal of rheumatology, 27*(8), 1905-1909.

Gonzalez, S., Aguilera, S., Alliende, C., Urzua, U., Quest, A. F., Herrera, L., et al. (2011). Alterations in type I hemidesmosome components suggestive of epigenetic control in the salivary glands of patients with Sjogren's syndrome. [Research Support, Non-U.S. Gov't]. *Arthritis and rheumatism, 63*(4), 1106-1115.

Gonzalez, S., Aguilera, S., Urzua, U., Quest, A. F., Molina, C., Alliende, C., et al. (2011). Mechanotransduction and epigenetic control in autoimmune diseases. *Autoimmunity reviews, 10*(3), 175-179.

Goransson, L. G., Haldorsen, K., Brun, J. G., Harboe, E., Jonsson, M. V., Skarstein, K., et al. (2011). The point prevalence of clinically relevant primary Sjogren's syndrome in two Norwegian counties. *Scandinavian journal of rheumatology, 40*(3), 221-224.

Gottenberg, J. E., Busson, M., Cohen-Solal, J., Lavie, F., Abbed, K., Kimberly, R. P., et al. (2005). Correlation of serum B lymphocyte stimulator and beta2 microglobulin with autoantibody secretion and systemic involvement in primary Sjogren's syndrome. *Annals of the rheumatic diseases, 64*(7), 1050-1055.

Gottenberg, J. E., Cagnard, N., Lucchesi, C., Letourneur, F., Mistou, S., Lazure, T., et al. (2006). Activation of IFN pathways and plasmacytoid dendritic cell recruitment in target organs of primary Sjogren's syndrome. *Proceedings of the National Academy of Sciences of the United States of America, 103*(8), 2770-2775.

Gottenberg, J. E., Aucouturier, F., Goetz, J., Sordet, C., Jahn, I., Busson, M., et al. (2007). Serum immunoglobulin free light chain assessment in rheumatoid arthritis and primary Sjogren's syndrome. *Annals of the rheumatic diseases, 66*(1), 23-27.

Greenspan, J. S., Daniels, T. E., Talal, N., & Sylvester, R. A. (1974). The histopathology of Sjogren's syndrome in labial salivary gland biopsies. [Review]. *Oral surgery, oral medicine, and oral pathology, 37*(2), 217-229.

Groom, J., Kalled, S. L., Cutler, A. H., Olson, C., Woodcock, S. A., Schneider, P., et al. (2002). Association of BAFF/BLyS overexpression and altered B cell differentiation with Sjogren's syndrome. [Comparative Study.*The Journal of clinical investigation, 109*(1), 59-68

Haddad, J., Deny, P., Munz-Gotheil, C., Ambrosini, J. C., Trinchet, J. C., Pateron, D., et al. (1992). Lymphocytic sialadenitis of Sjogren's syndrome associated with chronic hepatitis C virus liver disease. *Lancet, 339*(8789), 321-323.

Haldorsen, K., Moen, K., Jacobsen, H., Jonsson, R., & Brun, J. G. (2008). Exocrine function in primary Sjogren syndrome: natural course and prognostic factors. *Annals of the rheumatic diseases, 67*(7), 949-954.

He, J., Guo, J. P., Ding, Y., Li, Y. N., Pan, S. S., Liu, Y., et al. (2011). Diagnostic significance of measuring antibodies to cyclic type 3 muscarinic acetylcholine receptor peptides in primary Sjogren's syndrome. *Rheumatology, 50*(5), 879-884.

Iagnocco, A., Modesti, M., Priori, R., Alessandri, C., Perella, C., Takanen, S., et al. (2010). Subclinical synovitis in primary Sjogren's syndrome: an ultrasonographic study. *Rheumatology, 49*(6), 1153-1157.

Itescu, S., Brancato, L. J., Buxbaum, J., Gregersen, P. K., Rizk, C. C., Croxson, T. S., et al. (1990). A diffuse infiltrative CD8 lymphocytosis syndrome in human immunodeficiency virus (HIV) infection: a host immune response associated with HLA-DR5. *Annals of internal medicine, 112*(1), 3-10.

Jordan, R. C., & Speight, P. M. (1996). Lymphoma in Sjogren's syndrome. From histopathology to molecular pathology. *Oral surgery, oral medicine, oral pathology, oral radiology, and endodontics, 81*(3), 308-320.

Kalk, W. W., Mansour, K., Vissink, A., Spijkervet, F. K., Bootsma, H., Kallenberg, C. G., et al. (2002). Oral and ocular manifestations in Sjogren's syndrome. *The Journal of rheumatology, 29*(5), 924-930.

Kalk, W. W., Vissink, A., Spijkervet, F. K., Bootsma, H., Kallenberg, C. G., & Nieuw Amerongen, A. V. (2001). Sialometry and sialochemistry: diagnostic tools for Sjogren's syndrome. *Annals of the rheumatic diseases, 60*(12), 1110-1116.

Kassan, S. S., Thomas, T. L., Moutsopoulos, H. M., Hoover, R., Kimberly, R. P., Budman, D. R., et al. (1978). Increased risk of lymphoma in sicca syndrome. *Annals of internal medicine, 89*(6), 888-892.

Kittridge, A., Routhouska, S. B., & Korman, N. J. (2011). Dermatologic manifestations of Sjogren syndrome. [Review]. *Journal of cutaneous medicine and surgery, 15*(1), 8-14.

Kohn, W. G., Ship, J. A., Atkinson, J. C., Patton, L. L., & Fox, P. C. (1992). Salivary gland 99mTc-scintigraphy: a grading scale and correlation with major salivary gland flow rates. *Journal of oral pathology & medicine : official publication of the International Association of Oral Pathologists and the American Academy of Oral Pathology, 21*(2), 70-74.

Lafitte, C., Amoura, Z., Cacoub, P., Pradat-Diehl, P., Picq, C., Salachas, F., et al. (2001). Neurological complications of primary Sjogren's syndrome. *Journal of neurology, 248*(7), 577-584.

Launay, D., Hachulla, E., Hatron, P. Y., Jais, X., Simonneau, G., & Humbert, M. (2007). Pulmonary arterial hypertension: a rare complication of primary Sjogren syndrome: report of 9 new cases and review of the literature. *Medicine, 86*(5), 299-315.

Lavie, F., Miceli-Richard, C., Quillard, J., Roux, S., Leclerc, P., & Mariette, X. (2004). Expression of BAFF (BLyS) in T cells infiltrating labial salivary glands from patients with Sjogren's syndrome. *The Journal of pathology, 202*(4), 496-502.

Lemp, M. A. (2000). Evaluation and differential diagnosis of keratoconjunctivitis sicca. *The Journal of rheumatology. Supplement, 61*, 11-14.

Lindahl, G., & Hedfors, E. (1989). Lymphocytic infiltrates and epithelial HLA-DR expression in lip salivary glands in connective tissue disease patients lacking sicca: a prospective study. *British journal of rheumatology, 28*(4), 293-298.

Lindahl, G., Lonnquist, B., & Hedfors, E. (1989). Lymphocytic infiltrations of lip salivary glands in bone marrow recipients. A model for the development of the histopathological changes in Sjogren's syndrome? *Journal of autoimmunity, 2*(4), 579-583.

Mackay, F., Groom, J. R., & Tangye, S. G. (2007). An important role for B-cell activation factor and B cells in the pathogenesis of Sjogren's syndrome. [Review]. *Current opinion in rheumatology, 19*(5), 406-413.

Madani, G., & Beale, T. (2006). Inflammatory conditions of the salivary glands. *Seminars in ultrasound, CT, and MR, 27*(6), 440-451.

Manoussakis, M. N., & Kapsogeorgou, E. K. (2010). The role of intrinsic epithelial activation in the pathogenesis of Sjogren's syndrome. [Review]. *Journal of autoimmunity, 35*(3), 219-224.

Manthorpe, R., Benoni, C., Jacobsson, L., Kirtava, Z., Larsson, A., Liedholm, R., et al. (2000). Lower frequency of focal lip sialadenitis (focus score) in smoking patients. Can tobacco diminish the salivary gland involvement as judged by histological examination and anti-SSA/Ro and anti-SSB/La antibodies in Sjogren's syndrome? *Annals of the rheumatic diseases, 59*(1), 54-60.

Mariette, X., Roux, S., Zhang, J., Bengoufa, D., Lavie, F., Zhou, T., et al. (2003). The level of BLyS (BAFF) correlates with the titre of autoantibodies in human Sjogren's syndrome. *Annals of the rheumatic diseases, 62*(2), 168-171.

Mariette, X., & Gottenberg, J. E. (2010). Pathogenesis of Sjogren's syndrome and therapeutic consequences. *Current opinion in rheumatology, 22*(5), 471-477.

Mavragani, C. P., & Moutsopoulos, H. M. (2010). The geoepidemiology of Sjogren's syndrome. [Review]. *Autoimmunity reviews, 9*(5), A305-310.

Niemela, R. K., Paakko, E., Suramo, I., Takalo, R., & Hakala, M. (2001). Magnetic resonance imaging and magnetic resonance sialography of parotid glands in primary Sjogren's syndrome. *Arthritis and rheumatism, 45*(6), 512-518.

Niemela, R. K., Takalo, R., Paakko, E., Suramo, I., Paivansalo, M., Salo, T., et al. (2004). Ultrasonography of salivary glands in primary Sjogren's syndrome. A comparison with magnetic resonance imaging and magnetic resonance sialography of parotid glands. *Rheumatology, 43*(7), 875-879.

Pan, Y., & Sawalha, A. H. (2009). Epigenetic regulation and the pathogenesis of systemic lupus erythematosus. *Translational research : the journal of laboratory and clinical medicine, 153*(1), 4-10.

Parambil, J. G., Myers, J. L., & Ryu, J. H. (2006). Diffuse alveolar damage: uncommon manifestation of pulmonary involvement in patients with connective tissue diseases. *Chest, 130*(2), 553-558.

Parke, A. L. (2008). Pulmonary manifestations of primary Sjogren's syndrome. *Rheumatic diseases clinics of North America, 34*(4), 907-920, viii.

Pelstring, R. J., Essell, J. H., Kurtin, P. J., Cohen, A. R., & Banks, P. M. (1991). Diversity of organ site involvement among malignant lymphomas of mucosa-associated tissues. *American journal of clinical pathology, 96*(6), 738-745.

Pertovaara, M., & Korpela, M. (2011). Serum {beta}2 microglobulin correlates with the new ESSDAI in patients with Sjogren's syndrome. *Annals of the rheumatic diseases.*

Pijpe, J., Kalk, W. W., Bootsma, H., Spijkervet, F. K., Kallenberg, C. G., & Vissink, A. (2007). Progression of salivary gland dysfunction in patients with Sjogren's syndrome. *Annals of the rheumatic diseases, 66*(1), 107-112.

Pijpe, J., Kalk, W. W., van der Wal, J. E., Vissink, A., Kluin, P. M., Roodenburg, J. L., et al. (2007). Parotid gland biopsy compared with labial biopsy in the diagnosis of patients with primary Sjogren's syndrome. *Rheumatology, 46*(2), 335-341.

Ramos-Casals, M., Anaya, J. M., Garcia-Carrasco, M., Rosas, J., Bove, A., Claver, G., et al. (2004). Cutaneous vasculitis in primary Sjogren syndrome: classification and clinical significance of 52 patients. *Medicine, 83*(2), 96-106.

Ramos-Casals, M., Brito-Zeron, P., Garcia-Carrasco, M., & Font, J. (2004). Sarcoidosis or Sjogren syndrome? Clues to defining mimicry or coexistence in 59 cases. *Medicine, 83*(2), 85-95.

Ramos-Casals, M., Cervera, R., Yague, J., Garcia-Carrasco, M., Trejo, O., Jimenez, S., et al. (1998). Cryoglobulinemia in primary Sjogren's syndrome: prevalence and clinical characteristics in a series of 115 patients. *Seminars in arthritis and rheumatism, 28*(3), 200-205.

Ramos-Casals, M., Garcia-Carrasco, M., Cervera, R., Gaya, J., Halperin, I., Ubieto, I., et al. (2000). Thyroid disease in primary Sjogren syndrome. Study in a series of 160 patients. . *Medicine, 79*(2), 103-108.

Richardson, B. (2007). Primer: epigenetics of autoimmunity. . *Nature clinical practice. Rheumatology, 3*(9), 521-527.

Roberts, C., Parker, G. J., Rose, C. J., Watson, Y., O'Connor, J. P., Stivaros, S. M., et al. (2008). Glandular function in Sjogren syndrome: assessment with dynamic contrast-enhanced MR imaging and tracer kinetic modeling--initial experience. *Radiology, 246*(3), 845-853.

Royer, B., Cazals-Hatem, D., Sibilia, J., Agbalika, F., Cayuela, J. M., Soussi, T., et al. (1997). Lymphomas in patients with Sjogren's syndrome are marginal zone B-cell neoplasms, arise in diverse extranodal and nodal sites, and are not associated with viruses. *Blood, 90*(2), 766-775.

Schall, G. L., Anderson, L. G., Wolf, R. O., Herdt, J. R., Tarpley, T. M., Jr., Cummings, N. A., et al. (1971). Xerostomia in Sjogren's syndrome. Evaluation by sequential salivary scintigraphy. *JAMA : the journal of the American Medical Association, 216*(13), 2109-2116.

Segal, B., Carpenter, A., & Walk, D. (2008). Involvement of nervous system pathways in primary Sjogren's syndrome. [Review]. *Rheumatic diseases clinics of North America, 34*(4), 885-906, viii.

Seror, R., Mariette, X., Bowman, S., Baron, G., Gottenberg, J. E., Boostma, H., et al. (2010). Accurate detection of changes in disease activity in primary Sjogren's syndrome by the European League Against Rheumatism Sjogren's Syndrome Disease Activity Index. *Arthritis care & research, 62*(4), 551-558.

Seror, R., Ravaud, P., Bowman, S. J., Baron, G., Tzioufas, A., Theander, E., et al. (2010). EULAR Sjogren's syndrome disease activity index: development of a consensus systemic disease activity index for primary Sjogren's syndrome. *Annals of the rheumatic diseases, 69*(6), 1103-1109.

Skopouli, F. N., Dafni, U., Ioannidis, J. P., & Moutsopoulos, H. M. (2000). Clinical evolution, and morbidity and mortality of primary Sjogren's syndrome. *Seminars in arthritis and rheumatism, 29*(5), 296-304.

Solans-Laque, R., Lopez-Hernandez, A., Angel Bosch-Gil, J., Palacios, A., Campillo, M., & Vilardell-Tarres, M. (2011). Risk, Predictors, and Clinical Characteristics of Lymphoma Development in Primary Sjogren's Syndrome. *Seminars in arthritis and rheumatism.*

Takagi, Y., Kimura, Y., Nakamura, H., Sasaki, M., Eguchi, K., & Nakamura, T. (2010). Salivary gland ultrasonography: can it be an alternative to sialography as an imaging modality for Sjogren's syndrome? *Annals of the rheumatic diseases, 69*(7), 1321-1324.

Ter Borg, E. J., Risselada, A. P., & Kelder, J. C. (2011). Relation of Systemic Autoantibodies to the Number of Extraglandular Manifestations in Primary Sjogren's Syndrome: A Retrospective Analysis of 65 Patients in the Netherlands. *Seminars in arthritis and rheumatism, 40*(6), 547-551.

Theander, E., Andersson, S. I., Manthorpe, R., & Jacobsson, L. T. (2005). Proposed core set of outcome measures in patients with primary Sjogren's syndrome: 5 year follow up. *The Journal of rheumatology, 32*(8), 1495-1502.

Theander, E., Henriksson, G., Ljungberg, O., Mandl, T., Manthorpe, R., & Jacobsson, L. T. (2006). Lymphoma and other malignancies in primary Sjogren's syndrome: a cohort study on cancer incidence and lymphoma predictors. *Annals of the rheumatic diseases, 65*(6), 796-803.

Theander, E., Vasaitis, L., Baecklund, E., Nordmark, G., Warfvinge, G., Liedholm, R., et al. (2011). Lymphoid organisation in labial salivary gland biopsies is a possible predictor for the development of malignant lymphoma in primary Sjogren's syndrome. *Annals of the rheumatic diseases, 70*(8), 1363-1368.

Trontzas, P. I., & Andrianakos, A. A. (2005). Sjogren's syndrome: a population based study of prevalence in Greece. The ESORDIG study. [Letter]. *Annals of the rheumatic diseases, 64*(8), 1240-1241.

Tzioufas, A. G., & Voulgarelis, M. (2007). Update on Sjogren's syndrome autoimmune epithelitis: from classification to increased neoplasias. [Review]. *Best practice & research. Clinical rheumatology, 21*(6), 989-1010.

Van Bijsterveld OP. Diagnostic tests in the Sicca syndrome. Arch Ophthalmol 1969; 82:10-14.

Van der Reijden, W. A., van der Kwaak, J. S., Veerman, E. C., & Nieuw Amerongen, A. V. (1996). Analysis of the concentration and output of whole salivary constituents in patients with Sjogren's syndrome. *European journal of oral sciences, 104*(4 (Pt 1)), 335-340.

Vinagre, F., Santos, M. J., Prata, A., da Silva, J. C., & Santos, A. I. (2009). Assessment of salivary gland function in Sjogren's syndrome: the role of salivary gland scintigraphy. [Review]. *Autoimmunity reviews, 8*(8), 672-676.

Voulgarelis, M., Dafni, U. G., Isenberg, D. A., & Moutsopoulos, H. M. (1999). Malignant lymphoma in primary Sjogren's syndrome: a multicenter, retrospective, clinical study by the European Concerted Action on Sjogren's Syndrome. *Arthritis and rheumatism, 42*(8), 1765-1772.

Voulgarelis M & Moutsopoulos HM (2008). Mucosa-associated lymphoid tissue lymphoma in Sjögren's syndrome: risks, management, and prognosis Rheum Dis Clin North Am; 34:921-933.

Willeke P, Gaubitz M, Schotte H, Becker H, Mickholz E, Domschke W & Schlüter B (2007). Clinical and immunological characteristics of patients with Sjögren's syndrome in relation to alpha-fodrin antibodies. Rheumatology; 46:479-483.

Wise, C. M., Agudelo, C. A., Semble, E. L., Stump, T. E., & Woodruff, R. D. (1988). Comparison of parotid and minor salivary gland biopsy specimens in the diagnosis of Sjogren's syndrome. *Arthritis and rheumatism, 31*(5), 662-666.

Witte, T. (2005). Antifodrin antibodies in Sjogren's syndrome: a review. [Review]. *Annals of the New York Academy of Sciences, 1051*, 235-239.

Zandbelt, M. M., van den Hoogen, F. H., de Wilde, P. C., van den Berg, P. J., Schneider, H. G., & van de Putte, L. B. (2001). Reversibility of histological and immunohistological abnormalities in sublabial salivary gland biopsy specimens following treatment with corticosteroids in Sjogren's syndrome. [Case Reports]. *Annals of the rheumatic diseases, 60*(5), 511-513.

Zandbelt, M. M., Wentink, J. R., de Wilde, P. C., van Damme, P. A., van de Putte, L. B., & van den Hoogen, F. H. (2002). The synergistic value of focus score and IgA% score of sublabial salivary gland biopsy for the accuracy of the diagnosis of Sjogren's syndrome: a 10-year comparison. *Rheumatology, 41*(7), 819-823.

9

Oral Aspects of Sjögren's Syndrome

Sertan Ergun
Istanbul University, Faculty of Dentistry, Department of Oral Surgery, Istanbul, Turkey

1. Introduction

1.1 General aspects of Sjögren's syndrome

1.1.1 Definition

Sjögren's syndrome (SS) is a chronic autoimmune disease associated with the production of autoantibodies and characterized by a progressive lymphocytic and plasma cell infiltration of the salivary and lacrimal glands leading to xerostomia and keratoconjunctivitis sicca (1). A Danish ophthalmologist named Henrik Sjögren in 1932 was the first one, who reported the triad of keratoconjunctivitis sicca, xerostomia, and rheumatoid arthritis and then Sjögren introduced the term keratoconjunctivitis sicca for this syndrome, to distinguish it from dry eyes caused by lack of vitamin A (2). It is characterized by lymphocytic infiltration and subsequent destruction of the exocrine glands (3–5) including those found in the nose, ears, skin, vagina, respiratory and gastrointestinal systems (6).

1.2 Diagnosis

1.2.1 Differential diagnosis

The diagnosis of SS is not straightforward as many of the symptoms are subjective (Figure 1) (5).

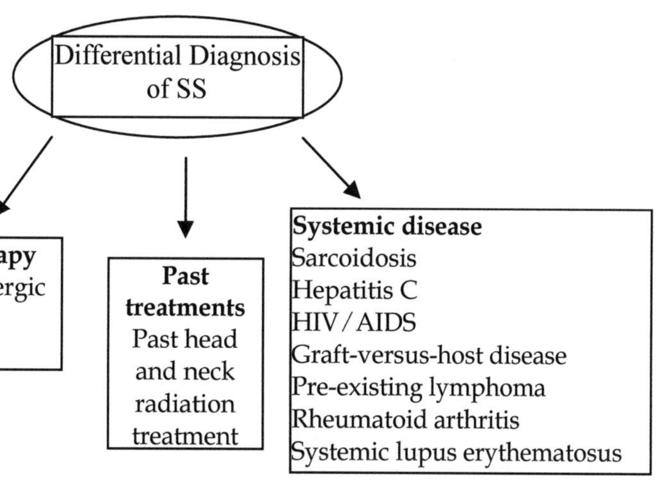

Fig. 1. Differential Diagnosis of SS (5)

1.2.2 Diagnostic criteria

The criteria for diagnosis of SS remain controversial, and different diagnostic criteria have been proposed. The syndrome can present primary or secondary. Generally, SS is classified as secondary (SS-2) when it is associated with other autoimmune diseases such as rheumatoid arthritis (RA), systemic lupus erythematosus (SLE), systemic sclerosis and polymyositis and as primary (SS-1) when there is no other connective tissue disease (7, 8). There are at least 6 international diagnostic criteria, such as Fox criteria, San Diego criteria, San Francisco criteria, European criteria (EEC), American-European Consensus Group (AECG) criteria, and Copenhagen criteria. San Diego criteria requires evidence for an autoimmune process associated with destruction of salivary and lacrimal gland tissues while the Copenhagen and EEC study group have based their diagnostic criteria on clinical findings of dry eyes and mouth with no absolute requirement for gland biopsy or presence of autoantibodies.

On the other hand, Sjögren's Syndome Foundation (SSF) stressed that the classification criteria for Sjögren's syndrome currently used by clinicians and researchers around the world is the American-European Consensus Classification Criteria (Table 1). Because many different criteria previously were used both within the U.S. and in other countries, the Sjögren's Syndrome Foundation and members of the European Study Group on Classification Criteria brought international leaders in Sjögren's together to develop consensus on one set of guidelines (9). SSF mentioned that that classification criteria is the strictest criteria available to prove a definitive diagnosis of Sjögren's for research purposes. Physicians usually diagnose SS for clinical purposes on a more individual, medically intuitive and broader basis. However, none of them was approved by the World Health Organization, which suggested better diagnostic criteria should be established.

1.3 Prevalance

Sjögren's syndrome occurs worldwide and in all ages. The peak incidence is in the fourth and fifth decades of life, with a female : male ratio of 9:1 (13). A number of studies have shown great variation in the frequency of Sjögren's syndrome (14). Prevalence studies have demonstrated that sicca symptoms and primary Sjögren's syndrome affects a considerable percentage of the population, with precise numbers dependent on the age group studied and on the criteria used (15). A cautious but realistic estimate from the studies presented thus far is that primary Sjögren's syndrome is a disease with a prevalence not exceeding 0.6% of the general population (15).

1.4 Aetiology and pathogenesis

The etiology of Sjogren's syndrome remains unidentified (16). Interactions between environmental contributors such as viruses or stress in conjunction with genetic susceptibility factors and hormonal effects are currently believed to result in disease development (16, 17). Intrinsic activation of epithelium in various target organs was demonstrated (18), based on inappropriate expression of MHC molecules, overexpression of costimulatory molecules and capacity for cytokine production, and the term "autoimmune epithelitis" was proposed (19). In the context of SS, Epstein Barr, HTLV-1, Hepatitis-C and enteroviruses have been previously proposed as potential initiating factors of the SS

I. Ocular Symptoms (at least one) - Dry eyes >3 months? - Foreign body sensation in the eyes? - Use of artificial tears >3x per day?
II. Oral Symptoms (at least one) - Dry mouth >3 months? - Recurrent or persistently swollen salivary glands? - Need liquids to swallow dry foods?
III. Ocular Signs (at least one) - Schirmer's test, (without anesthesia) $\leq$5 mm/5 minutes - Positive vital dye staining (van Bijsterveld $\geq$4)
IV. Histopathology Lip biopsy showing focal lymphocytic sialoadenitis - focus score $\geq$1 per 4 mm^2)[2]
V. Oral Signs (at least one) - Unstimulated whole salivary flow ($\leq$1.5 mL in 15 minutes) - Abnormal parotid sialography[3] - Abnormal salivary scintigraphy[4]
VI. Autoantibodies (at least one) - Anti-SSA (Ro) or Anti-SSB (La)
For a primary Sjögren's syndrome diagnosis: a. Any 4 of the 6 criteria, must include either item IV (Histopathology) or VI (Autoantibodies) b. Any 3 of the 4 objective criteria (III, IV, V, VI)
For a secondary Sjögren's syndrome diagnosis: In patients with another well-defined major connective tissue disease, the presence of one symptom (I or II) plus 2 of the 3 objective criteria (III, IV and V) is indicative of secondary SS.
Exclusion Criteria Past head and neck radiation treatment Hepatitis C infection Acquired immunodeficiency syndrome (AIDS) Pre-existing lymphoma Sarcoidosis Graft versus host disease Current use of anticholinergic drugs

Table 1. American-European Consensus Classification Criteria accepted by Sjögren's Syndome Foundation (9-12)

(16, 20) However, the mechanisms that account for the epithelial activation remain stil unclear (16). Recent data suggest the central role of the type I interferon (IFN) system in the pathogenesis of many autoimmune disorders including SS (16).

A genetic predisposition to SS has been suggested because of multiple reports of two or more members of the same family developing the syndrome (21). A family history of the disease puts people at an increased risk of developing SS compared to the general population (22). This is also supported by the development of SS in twins (22). A genetic susceptibility may be required for the development of autoantibodies which are found in SS (22) and this may be associated with a link between polymorphic major histocompatibility complex (MHC) genes and the development of autoimmune diseases (21).

High cDNAlevels in patients with SS may result with a disease at worst prognosis which should the clinician let to follow-up the patients with SS both, clinically and serologicallly (23). The study of Alevizos *et al.* revealed that microRNA are promising candidate biomarkers of inflammation and salivary gland dysfunction in patients with SS (24). Further exploration of the predicted pathways associated with decreased salivary flow in this study will provide insight into the pathophysiology of SS and may identify novel therapeutic targets (24-25).

1.5 Complications

SS systemic disease may affect many other body systems. The most serious complication of SS could be accepted as the increased incidence of malignant lymphoma (26). This fhenemenon was first reported in patients with SS in 1963 (26) and has been shown to be 44 times higher than the general population in some studies (27). Additionally, multiple case reports supported the association of lymphoma with Sjögren syndrome and stressed lymphoma as the major complication in the progression of the disease (28, 29). When it occurs, patients with SS are accepted as they are in stage 3 who consist of %5 of the general SS population.

Severeal studies have shown different involvements in patients with SS such as hematological system, respiratory system, cardiac, liver, pancreatic, renal, thyroid and finally exocrine glands involvements. Bayetto and Logan have summerized extraglandular manifestations of SS in a table perfectly (Table 2) (27, 57).

Malaise Peripheral neuropathy Primary biliary cirrhosis
Fatigue Autoimmune thyroiditis GI symptoms
Fibromyalgia Renal tubular acidosis Respiratory diseases
Fever Myositis Psychosis
Arthralgia Chronic hepatitis Lymphadenopathy
Synovitis Purpura Splenomegaly
Raynaud's phenomenon Vasculitis Lymphoma

Table 2. Symptoms associated with extraglandular manifestations of Sjögren's syndrome by (27, 57)

Briefly, leucopenia (approximately 45% of all SS cases), thromboycytopenia (approximately 25% of all SS cases), hemolytic anemia (approximately 5% of all SS cases) and lower thrombopoietin levels (approximately 20% of all SS cases) are accepted as hematological system involvement of the disease. Respiratory system involvement of the disease reveals interstitial lung disease (approximately 20% of all SS cases), pulmonary hypertension (approximately 12% of all SS cases) and multiple nodules (approximately 5% of all SS cases). pericardial effusion (approximately 15% of all SS cases) and atrioventricular conduction block (approximately 5% of all SS cases) are the cardiac complications of the disease. The liver damage could be seen almost one third of the patients with SS. Likewise approximately one third of the patients with SS revealed hepatosplenomegaly. Elevated gamma-glutamyl transpeptidase, alaine transferase and alkaline phosphatase levels are seen approximately in one fifth of the patients with SS. Renal involvement in SS are relatively common. Proteinuria (approximately 20% of all SS cases), Renal tubular acidosis (approximately 15% of all SS cases) and kidney stones and/or renal calcification (approximately 10% of all SS cases) are the most important renal complications of the disease. Thyroid disorders are also common among the patients with SS (33% of all cases). Abnormal thyroid function was seen in one forfth of the whole SS population (30).

1.6 Pediatric cases

SS is very rare in childhood and is frequently undiagnosed (31). Literature search revealed 200 pediatric cases of SS. The most important clinical manifestations in children with SS is the recurrent parotid swelling (31). Pathologic and laboratory findings are similar to those found in adults, with characteristic lymphocytic infiltration of exocrine glands, the presence of hypergammaglobulinemia, elevated erythrocyte sedimentation rate, and positive anti-SS antigen A, anti-SS antigen B, antinuclear antibody, and rheumatoid factor (32-34). Inflammation characterized by recurrent episodes of painful unilateral or bilateral parotid enlargement associated with swelling, fever, redness, and reduction in salivary flow (35-39).

1.7 Management

Sicca symptoms of the disease could be treated by using topical agents wheras extraglandular features are managed with glucocorticoids and immunosuppressive drugs (40). But, literature search revealed no evidence based therapeutic guidelines for the management of primary Sjögren syndrome which is also universally accepted (41). The results of one excellent systematic review about the treatment of SS shows that B cell targeted agents seem to be the most promising future therapy, especially rituximab, which has been used in more than 100 reported cases. Agents that block B cell-activating factor of the tumor necrosis factor family may also be a promising therapy (41, 42). Advances in knowledge of the molecular mechanisms involved in the etiopathogenesis of Sjögren's syndrome may allow the development of more effective, highly selective therapies without the adverse effects often associated with standard, less-selective drugs (41). Today, current treatment options are decided upon a mix of personal experience, expert opinion, and reported studies (41).

2. Oral aspects of Sjögren's syndrome

2.1 Saliva, glandular involvement, xerostomia and treatment

2.1.1 Saliva

Saliva is secreted from three major paired glands which are parotid, submandibular and sublingual glands and from hundreds of minor salivary glands which are localized over most parts of the oral mucosa (43). About 90% of mixed saliva is derived from three pairs of major salivary glands (parotid, submandibular and sublingual) and the remaining 10% is from numerous minor salivary glands distributed in the oral mucosa (43). In healthy humans, the daily production of whole saliva (mixed saliva) normally ranges from 0Æ5 to 1Æ5 L (43).

The salivary secretion is mainly induced during eating (43). Stimulated saliva which is also called as reflex salivation helps the chewing of food, formation and swallowing of a food bolus and digestion of starch and lipids (43). Saliva takes also part in the detection of food taste through the diffusion of taste substances to taste receptors, chemical interaction with taste substances and changes in the sensitivity of taste receptors (43). On the other hand, resting saliva, which is a lesser amount of saliva, covers the surface of the oral and pharyngeal cavities (43). When compared to the stimulated saliva resting saliva is accapted as more important in the maintenance of oral health (43). Protection properties against bacteria / - viruses / fungi are based on the salivary anti-microbial action [such as lysozyme, peroxidase, secretory immunoglobulin A (IgA) and histatins] and also on adhesion (mucins) and rinsing properties (43). Saliva is also responsible by taking part in speech, denture holding, anticaries activity, controlling breath odour and maintaining the integrity of oral and gastrointestinal mucosa (43).

Acinar cells produce saliva at first (43). Two types of these cells have been detected: serous and mucous cells (43). The parotid gland has serous acinar cells and secretes a thin, watery and amylase-rich saliva through its main excretory duct which is called as Stenson ductus; it opens onto the buccal mucosa near the upper molar teeth (43). The submandibular gland produces a more viscous and mucin-rich saliva and it consists of serous and mucous acinar cells whereas the sublingual gland has mucous acinar cells and also produces a viscous mucin rich saliva (43).

The sympathetic and parasympathetic autonomic nervous systems control mainly the salivary secretion (44). The sympathetic nerve is mainly responsible for the secretion of proteins accompanied by exocytosis in acinar cells, while the parasympathetic nerve is mainly responsible for the secretion of water and electrolytes (44). These are adequate stimuli for salivation, and secreted saliva is called stimulated saliva (43). Saliva secreted in the absence of apparent sensory stimuli related to eating refers to resting or unstimulated saliva (43). This saliva may have two components; one is spontaneous secretion, which is the continuous production of small amounts of saliva without any extraneous stimuli (43). There are prominent differences between stimulated and resting salivary secretions in their flow rate and viscosity (43). The flow rate of resting whole saliva is far less than that of stimulated whole saliva, whereas the viscosity of resting whole saliva is 2–3 times that of stimulated whole saliva in healthy adults which implies that resting whole saliva is rich in mucins mainly secreted by sublingual, submandibular and palatal glands (45). Resting whole saliva contains a higher concentration of high-molecular-weight mucin (MG1) than stimulated whole saliva, whereas low-molecular weight mucin (MG2) shows similar concentrations under resting and stimulated conditions (46).

One of two main roles of saliva in taste perception is the relatively short-term effect of saliva seen in the initial processes of taste perception (47). Taste substances should be dissolved in the salivary fluid layer to reach and stimulate taste receptors (43). The solubilization of taste substances in saliva, the chemical interaction between taste substances and salivary compositions, and the diffusion and dilution of taste substances in saliva are the ones which are responsible (43). Additionally, some components which can also stimulate taste receptors and / or change taste sensitivity by chemical interaction with the receptor are contained in the saliva (43). One other long-term effect of saliva is maintaining the health and function of the taste receptor site (43).

2.1.2 Glandular involvement

Garcio-Carrasco *et al.* summarized the mechanism of gland-induced dysfunction in primary SS in their excellent review article (Figure 2) (58).

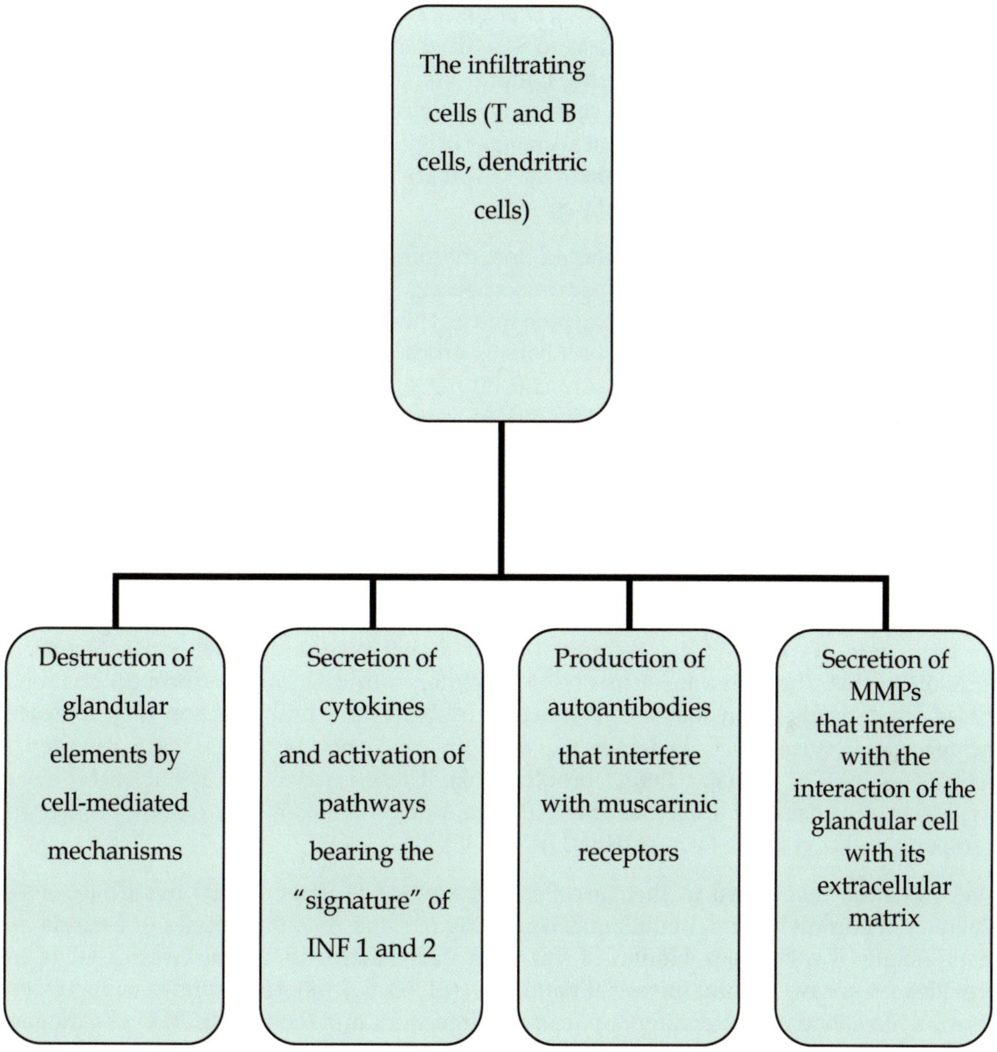

Fig. 2. Main mechanisms of gland-induced dysfunction in pSS. INF, interferon; MMP, metalloproteinase (58).

2.1.3 Xerostomia & treatment

Xerostomia is defined as a subjective complaint of dry mouth that may result from deficient production of saliva (48). Xerostomic patients complain mostly about burning mouth, loss of taste, difficulty in swallowing, unpleasant taste and odor, oral dryness, increased thirst, chewing, speaking, gastroesophageal reflux, oral breathing, malfunction of removable prosthesis and sensitive teeth (49-54). Allec *et al.* concluded in their prospective cross-sectional descriptive observational study that patients with SS have voice, speech and swallowing abnormalities, not only associated with to xerosis but perhaps also to neurological abnormalities, probably secondary to the syndrome (55). On the other hand, subjective xerostomia has been reported in higher percentages (75.18% to 91.84%) in patients with SS (56). In addition to that, Skopouli *et al.* showed that the rate of dry mouth increased from 41% of patients at initial diagnosis to 84% 10 years after diagnosis (57). Salivary gland dysfunction appears due to progressing lymphocytic infiltration in salivary acini, which in turn leads to inflammatory reaction causing acinar atrophy and proliferation of connective tissue (58). Sometimes such pathological changes originate in the minor salivary glands and may result in early symptoms of xerostomia, which are less intense than those in cases when the major salivary glands are affected (48).

Alcohol and smoking should be avoided and thorough oral hygiene is essential (40, 59). Saliva replacement products and sugarfree chewing gums may be effective for mild to moderate dry mouth (41). Oral pilocarpine and cevimeline are the treatment of choice for patients with SS (41). The doses that best balance efficacy and adverse effects are reported to be 5 mg every 6 hours for pilocarpine and 30 mg every 8 hours for cevimeline (41). In patients with contraindications or intolerance to muscarinic agonists, N-acetylcysteine may be an alternative (41).

2.2 Risk of dental caries and erosions & treatment

2.2.1 Risk of dental caries and erosions

The reduced salivary flow and its altered composition influence the bacterial clearance in the oral cavity as well as the accumulation of dental plaque on teeth surfaces (60). In addition to that, the saliva loses its ability to buffer, lubricate, and perform antimicrobial duties which leads to an increase in mucosal friability and oral infection (61). Increased incidence of cervical, incisal, decays in cusps tips and root caries has been reported in patients with SS as a major dental problem (62). These types of decays are accepted as atypical or unusual dental decays. This is constant demineralization, a rapidly progressing (rampant) and aggressive form of dental decay (43).

Mathews *et al.* mentioned in their excellent review article named ‘Oral manifestations of Sjögren's syndrome’ that dental plaque, consisting of more than 500 species of bacteria in a mature state, is a complex biofilm of microbes that adheres to the surfaces of teeth and provides a reservoir for oral microbial pathogens (61, 63, 64). Sjögren's syndrome increases a person's likelihood of contracting opportunistic infections and the proliferation of cariogenic micro-organisms (61, 65). Pederson *et al.* have reported that persons with primary Sjögren's syndrome have lower numbers of periopathogenic microorganisms and higher numbers of cariogenic and acidophilic micro-organisms in comparison with those found in control individuals (61, 66). Pederson *et al.* concluded in another study that patients with a labial salivary gland biopsy focus score of one or more (as per the American-European Classification Criteria) or the presence of Ro/SSA and La / SSB antibodies in serum, had a significantly higher DMFT/DMFS score than patients without these two factors (67).

Boutsi *et al.* mentioned in their study investigating dental and periodontal status of patients with SS that the number of cervical decay lesions correlated negatively with the salivary flow (56). It is known that because of reduced salivary flow, bacterial plaque accumulates more rapidly on the tooth surface and especially at the marginal gingiva and crevicular areas which results in a higher prevalence of cervical caries (56). In patients with SS, an increased number of decayed and filled teeth surfaces have been referred previously by several investigators (62, 68). The very low salivary secretion rates, the decreased buffering effect and neutralization of bacterial acids as well as the high counts of lactobacilli and streptococci found in patients with SS, may be responsible for this effect (69). It is interesting that in their study, the number of cervical decay lesions correlated negatively with the salivary flow, while the number of distal or mesial decay lesions correlated negatively with age (56). It seems that the lack of salivary flow affects more extensively the cervical surfaces of the teeth, and predisposes them to a more rapid development of caries (56).

2.2.2 Treatment

Mese and Matsua stressed that patients should be advised to maintain impeccable hygiene, schedule frequent examinations and use topical fluoride regimens (43). The choice of the fluoride-delivery system varies with the clinical need and patient compliance (43). Common sources of fluoride in toothpaste are sodium monofluorophosphate and sodium fluoride (70-72). But Mathews *et al* reported that even with excellent oral hygiene, individuals with Sjögren's syndrome have elevated levels of dental caries, along with the loss of many teeth early in the disease (61). Pedersen *et al.* reported that persons who brushed their teeth with toothpaste containing fluoride and visited their dentist more frequently still had higher numbers of missing, filled, and decayed teeth, along with a higher gingival index (66).

2.3 Periodontal status & treatment

2.3.1 Periodontal status

The reduced salivary flow and its altered composition influence the bacterial clearance in the oral cavity, as well as the increased accumulation of dental plaque on tooth surfaces. Studies have demonstrated a higher gingival bleeding and plaque index in subjects with hyposalivation but without shown a correlation between salivary flow rate and gingival bleeding index or plaque index (73, 74).

Few studies have managed to report an increased risk of periodontal disease in Sjögren's syndrome (75-77). Ergun *et al.* had summarised the studies that evaluated the periodontal status of the patients with Sjögren's syndrome (78) (Table 3).

Number of the teeth (NT), bleeding on probing (BOP) (expressed as the % of sites which bled upon gentle probing), approximal plaque index (API) (expressed as the % of sites which presented plaque), probing pocket depth (PPD) were used in studies evaluating the periodontal status of patients with SS since they are easy to perform and produced adequate results for this kind of evaluation (78). Ergun *et al.* found out a significant difference between patients with SS and healthy controls in regard to API and BOP (78). This result is in agreement with the studies which have found that the API, PPD and BOP are significantly higher in SS patients than healthy subjects (75-77, 79). Other studies, however, have shown that SS patients are not at higher risk of having periodontitis (56, 79-83).

It is well known that BOP is strongly corralated to API and both are correlated with tooth brushing efficiency (84). Ergun *et al* concluded that as there was no statistically significant

Author	*Study group(s)*	*Control group(s)*	*Difference inapproximal plaque index (API)*	*Difference in bleeding on probing (BOP)*	*Difference in periodontal probing depth (PPD)*	*Difference in attachment loss*	*Difference in supragingival calculus*	*Difference in subgingival calculus*	*Difference in alveolar bone loss*	*Difference in GCF volume*	*Difference in DMF-T*	*Conclusion: Higher risk of having periodontitis ?*
Tseng *(1991)*	SS (n=14)	HS (n=14)	NS	NS	NS	NS	NS	NS	-	-	S	No
Celenligil *et al (1994)*	SS (n=17)	HS (n=14)	S	S	S	-	-	-	-	-	S (missing)	Yes
Najera *et al (1997)*	SS-1 (n=23) SS-2 (n=2)	HS (n=24)	S	NS	NS	S	-	-	S	-	S	Yes
Ravald and List *(1998)*	SS-1 (n=22)	HS (n=21)	NS	NS	NS	NS	-	-	-	-	S (decay)	No
Pedersen *et al (1999)*	SS-1 (n=16)	HS (n=13)	NS	NS	NS	-	-	-	-	-	S	No
Boutsi *et al (1999)*	SS-1 (n=8) SS-2 (n=16)	Patients with other autoimmune diseases (n=27) HS (n=29)	NS	NS	NS	NS	-	-	-	-	NS	No
Schiodt *et al (2001)*	SS-1 (n=57)	HS (n=75)	-	NS	NS	-	S	NS	-	-	-	No
Kuru *et al (2002)*	SS-1 (n=8) SS-2 (n=10)	HS (n=11)	NS	NS	NS	NS	-	-	-	-	-	No
Jorkjend *et al (2003)*	SS-2 (n=33)	HS (n=33)	-	-	-	S (mandibular teeth)	-	-	-	-	S (teeth) NS (fillings)	No
Leung *et al (2004)*	SS-1 (n=26) SS-2 (n=25)	HS (n=29)	-	-	-	-	-	-	-	-	S	-
Rhodus *et al (2005)*	SS-1 (n=10)	HS (n=10)	S	NS	NS	S	-	-	-	S	-	No (but more gingival recession)
Pers *et al (2005)*	SS-1 (n=9)	Patients with xerostomia (n=15) and with periodontal disease (n=10)	NS	NS	NS	-	-	-	-	-	NS	-
Marton *et al (2006)*	SS-1 (n=38)	HS (n=34)	-	S	S	-	-	-	-	-	S	Yes

Table 3. Studies which evaluated the periodontal status of the patients with Sjögren's syndrome (*GCF*: gingival creviculer fluid, *DMF-T*: decayed, missing, and filled permanent teeth, *HS*: healthy subjects, *S*: statistical significant; *NS*: not statistical significant) (78).

difference between patients with SS and healthy controls regarding to their tooth brushing habits (p>0.05) it can be concluded that the significant difference in terms of API could have been occurred due to the low SFR levels of the subjects participated in the study group which is in agreement with Marton *et al.* (75, 78). Their results indicate that patients with SS carry a higher risk of having periodontitis.

There is a limited number of the studies regarding evaluation of the periodontal status of the subgroups of SS patients in terms of plaque accumulation, gingival inflammation and pocket depth. Most of these studies did not find a statistically significant difference between primary and secondary SS patients in terms of their periodontal status (56, 75, 82, 83, 85, 86). Najera *et al.* (77) found a significant difference in plaque index, but they did not find a statistically significant difference in gingival bleeding and periodontal pocket depth between SS-1 and SS-2 patients. The lack of difference in periodontal status between SS-1 and SS-2 subjects may indicate that both types of SS do not play significant role in periodontal status (66, 78, 80).

2.3.2 Treatment

As mentioned before, the treatment of SS is palliative and turns to the xerostomia related complications. One of these is the increased periodontal damage seen in patients with SS as accepted as some authors who found out possible correlations between the disease and the periodontal status of this type of patients. The aim is to maintain impeccable hygiene by having regular follow-ups, teaching oral hygiene instructions and some topical applications. The treatment should be conservative aiming to reduce the bacterial clearance in the oral cavity, as well as the accumulation of dental plaque on tooth surfaces.

2.4 Oral mucosal lesions

Oral health status of patients with SS has been investigated in many studies, previously (56, 75, 87-91). Subjective xerostomia has been reported in higher percentages (75.18% to 91.84%) in the patients with SS (56, 75, 88, 91). Additional dryness-related signs in patients with SS are angular chelitis, redness of the tongue, atrophy of filiform papilae (Figure 3 and 4), erythematous buccal mucosa (Figure 5), hardpalate and softpalate, difficulties and pain on swallowing, burning syndrome, sensitivity to acid and/or spicy food, dysgeusia and bitter taste (8, 87-93). Most of the subjective symptoms such as dry mouth feeling and dysphagia have been reported to be in direct correlation with the decreased salivary flow rate which could also affect the sensory process of swallowing that leads to pain and difficulties on swallowing (73, 94).

Ergun *et al* have shown that oral objective and subjective signs on oral clinical examination are very common among patients with SS regardless its type. Similarly, a recent study demonstrated that oral health related quality of life was poor in patients with SS (95). The reason why dysgeusia was a common subjective symptom of SS-2 when compared with that of SS-1, could be related to the use of D-penicillamine which has found as common drug-therapy for patients with RA. Dysgeusia was reported to be seen as a frequent problem of patients using D-penicillamine (96).

Ergun *et al* have shown that oral examination of the patients with SS revealed no statistically significant difference between SS-1 and SS-2 patients in regard to presence of angular stomatitis, oral ulcerations, atrophic, reddened and dry mucosa, dysgeusia and atrophy of filiform papilla (78). Similar percentage of the two subgroups of SS complained about

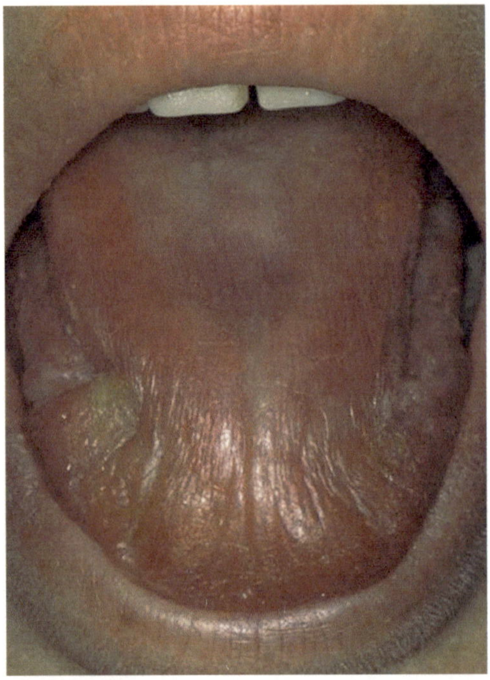

Fig. 3. Atrophy of filiform papillae

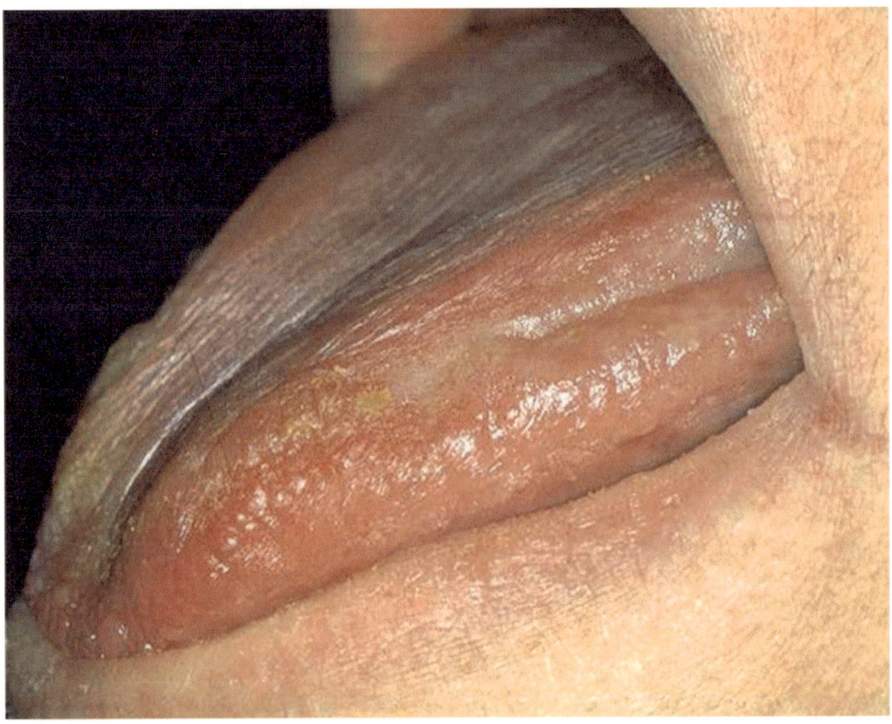

Fig. 4. Redness of the tongue

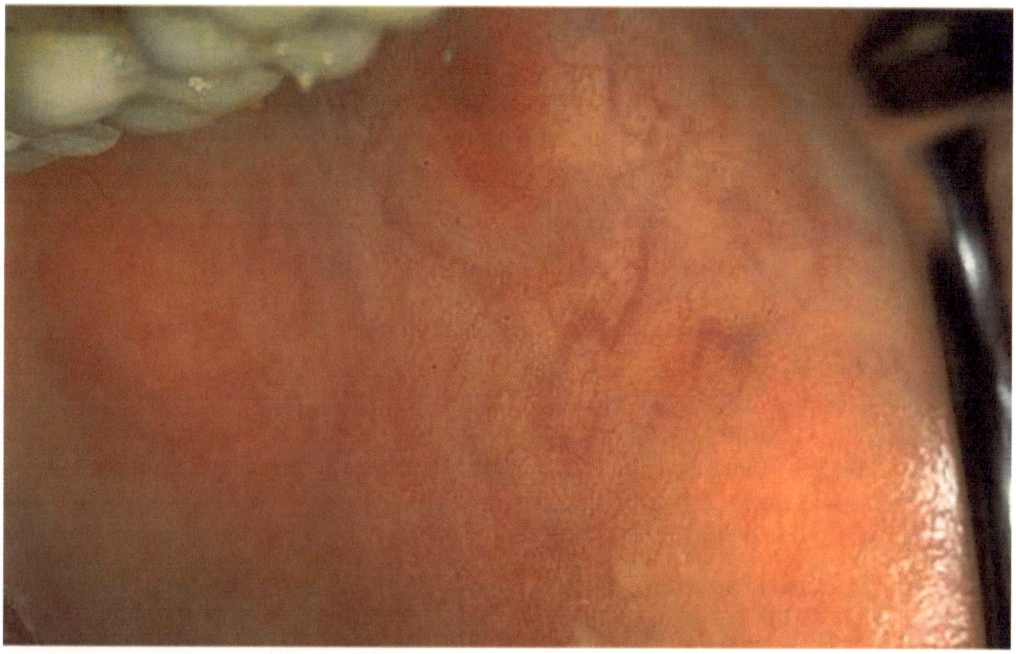

Fig. 5. Erythematous buccal mucosa

subjective xerostomia, burning sensation, pain on swallowing and hypersensitivity. They observed significant differences between patients with SS and healthy subjects in terms of the clinical oral findings associated with SS (Table 4).

	SS *(n=37)* N, %,	*HS* *(n=37)* N, %,	*p*
Angular Chelitis	8 (21.62%)	0 (0%)	0.005 *(S)*
Oral Ulcerations	13 (35.13%)	0 (0%)	0.0001 *(S)*
Atrophic Mucosa	28 (75.67%)	3 (8.10%)	0.0001 *(S)*
Dry Mucosa	23 (62.16%)	1 (2.70%)	0.0001 *(S)*
Reddened Mucosa	23 (62.16%)	5 (13.51%)	0.0001 *(S)*
Atrophy of Filiform Papilla	18 (48.65%)	4 (10.81%)	0.001 *(S)*
Xerostomia	32 (86.49%)	5 (13.51%)	0.0001 (S)
Burning Sensation	29 (78.38%)	5 (13.51%)	0.0001 (S)
Pain on Swallowing	23 (62.16%)	4 (10.81%)	0.0001 (S)
Dysgeusia	30 (81.08%)	3 (8.10%)	0.0001 (S)
Hypersensitivity	22 (59.46%)	0 (0%)	0.0001 (S)

Table 4. Positive objective and subjective signs on oral clinical examination of the patients with SS (78)

2.5 Oral flora & treatment

2.5.1 Oral flora

A continuous flow of saliva is important in preventing oral colonization by *Candida*, as the constant flushing action of saliva may remove the unattached or loosely attached *Candida* from the oral cavity (86). It has been shown that high *Candida albicans* counts in saliva are associated with clinical signs of candidiasis (97). Also there has also been shown an inverse association between salivary flow rate and *C. albicans* counts in saliva (98-100). Various investigators have reported a high prevalence of oral *Candida* species in patients with SS when compared with those of healthy controls (90, 101-104), while others have found that there is no significant difference between patients with SS and healthy controls in terms of presence of candidiasis (86, 101). Most reports indicate that *C. albicans* is the predominant yeast isolated in gingival crevicular fluid and in periodontal pockets of the periodontal patients as well as in healthy subjects, although *Candida glabrata* and *Candida tropicalis* have also been found, albeit infrequently (33, 86, 100, 102, 104). Additionally, one study showed that *C. albicans* was detected in gingival crevicular fluid at one measurement site in one of the SS-1 subjects but not in the control group (79).

Saliva has antibacterial, remineralizing, digestive, soft tissue reparative, lubricative, buffering, and cleansing properties. Therefore, decreased saliva production, which occurs in SS, can directly contribute to the oral and dental complications experienced by these patients. An inverse relationship between salivary flow rates and the level of *Candida* infection has been described, previously (86). Additionally, infection by *C. albicans* has been reported more frequently in individuals with SS than in the general population (87). While an even higher proportion of the total population (up to 60%) carry *C. albicans* in their mouths without clinical symptoms. The amount of the candidal load is important for development of candidiasis (105). As the quantification is essential for candidal assessment, we have detected the salivary *Candida* levels of the study population. Ergun *et al* have found out that *Candida* counts in saliva were statistically higher either in SS-1 or SS-2 patients as compared with that of the healthy control, which is in agreement with the results of other similar studies (78, 89, 99).

For successful colonization and infection, adhesion to oral surfaces is necessity. *C. albicans* can adhere to epithelial cells of buccal mucosa, the tongue, tooth surfaces, various oral prostheses such as dentures, and other oral micro-organisms that have already colonized these surfaces. Clinically, *C. albicans* can be cultured from swabs of the buccal mucosa, tongue, teeth, denture surfaces, and dental plaque samples. The flushing effect of saliva and anti-candidal salivary components such as lysozyme, histatins, lactoferrin, and calprotectin are the innate host defenses which act to remove or kill invading yeasts (106). The decreased salivary flow means the decreased host defense. Ergun *et al.* showed that candidal colonization on the buccal epithelial and the dorsal tongue was found to be in higher in SS patients than in healthy controls. In colonized individuals with no clinical symptoms of candidiasis, *C. albicans* is most frequently found on the dorsum of the tongue. Although Almståhl & Wikström (107) did not find an increase of frequency of *Candida* in subjects with hyposalivation, those authors did not analyse *Candida* colonization on the tongue's dorsal surface, which is the main ecological niche for *Candida* in the oral cavity.

Denture wearing is one of the major predisposing factor in humans for oral candidiasis. In denture wearers, the fitting surface of the denture is the main reservoir of the yeasts (108). Angular chelitis is commonly associated with denture-induced stomatitis. Ergun *et al.* stressed that no statistically significant difference was found between SS and healthy subjects on the prevalence of *C. albicans* colonization on dentures, palatinal and angular areas who use dentures with similar cleaning habits. Absence of normal salivary flow results with candidal colonization on the denture surfaces, palatinal mucosa and angular area in denture wearers even with normal or decreased salivary flow rate.

As there is limited findings in healthy subjects, yeasts especially *C. albicans* have been recovered from periodontal pockets of patients with chronic periodontitis in different rates (7.1-19.6%) (104, 109-112). Brill considered gigngival crevicular fluid a transudate, a passage of fluid from bloodstream (113). But it's also known that amount of gigngival crevicular fluid increases with periodontal disease and decreases during health (114). According to Cimasoni, gigngival crevicular fluid flow rate in slightly inflamed gingiva is about 0.1mg in 3 minutes, which leads us to think that gigngival crevicular fluid renews itself continuously (115). Ergun *et al* concluded that population it is found that the subjects showed slight to moderate signs of inflammation (78). Finding only one subject (2.70%) in each group who has *C. albicans* colonization in the gigngival crevicular fluid, might be because of this continuous flow despite high scores of positive *candida* albicans colonization in different areas of the mouth. Rhodus and Michalowicz (25) found almost the same result in their pilot study, in which they compared the periodontal status and prevalence of sulcular *C. albicans* between subjects with SS-1 and healthy control subjects.

Ergun *et al* have found out that there were direct correlations between positive *candida* albicans colonization on buccal area and dry mucosa, hypersensitivity and pain on swallowing with no spesific reason (78). Additionally, they have shown a weak correlation between *Candida* carriage in saliva and pain on swallowing (78). Volter *et al.* and Logemann *et al.* reported that xerestomia affects the sensory process of swallowing (94, 116). It is well known that positive *Candida* carriage in saliva is mostly the result of the lower levels of salivary flow rate. From this available evidence, it can be assumed that difficulties and pain on swallowing could occur due to positive *Candida* carriage in saliva. But more studies with higher number of patients with SS are needed to confirm or refute this association.

2.5.2 Treatment

Reduced saliva predisposes patients to an overgrowth of *Candida* albicans (43). This may be augmented by the use of dentures, smoking and diabetes (43, 51). Recurrent oral candidiasis can be treated with topical anti-fungal medications. Oral rinses with anti-fungal medications such as nystatin and fluconazole are effective in the treatment of oral candidiasis and for relieving oraldiscomfort (43, 117, 118). Management of chronic erythematous candidiasis and angle cheilitis can be based on the prescription of nystatin in tablets or solution (100,000 IU 4-6 times a day), or miconazole gel 4 times a day (119). Removable dental prostheses should be treated separated by soaking in anti-fungal medication. Angular cheilitis can be treated with nystatin ointment or clotrimazole cream. Milillo *et al.* recently reported that 5% amorolfine anti-fungal varnish was effective for *Candida*-related denture stomatitis (120).

As mentioned before dentures may not be suitable for patients SS; however, dentures could be the only restorative choice (43). The tongue adheres to and dislodges the denture, causing decreased retention of partial and totally removable prosthesis and resulting in abrasions, sore spots, ulceration and irritation, all unpleasant and painful experiences for the patient (4, 43). Despite this, an implant-supported denture may be successful; however, the high cost of this denture could represent a problem for patients. If dryness is a continuous problem, the manufacture of dentures with reservoirs or chambers for artificial saliva is suggested for continuous delivery of saliva, although these dentures should not be worn during eating (43, 121-123).

3. References

[1] Fox RI, Howell FV, Bone RC, *et al.* (1984) Primary Sjögren syndrome: clinical and immunopathologic features. *Semin Arthritis Rheum.*;14:77–105.

[2] Bloch KJ, Buchanan WW, Wohl MJ, Bunim JJ. (1965) Sjögren's syndrome: a clinical, pathological and serological study of 62 cases. *Medicine (Baltimore)* 1965;44:187e231.

[3] Kasper D, Braunwald E, Fauci A, Hauser S, Longo D, Jameson L, eds. (2006) *Harrison's Rheumatology*. New York: McGraw-Hill,.

[4] Al-Hashimi I. (2001) The management of Sjögren's syndrome in dental practice. *J Am Dent Assoc*;132:1409–1417.3.

[5] von Bultzinglowen I, Sollecito T, Fox P, *et al.* (2007) Salivary dysfunctionassociated with systemic diseases: systematic review and clinical management recommendations. *Oral Surg Oral Med Oral Pathol Oral Radiol Endod*;103:S57.e1–15.

[6] Al-Hashimi I. (2005) Xerostomia secondary to Sjo¨ gren's syndrome in the elderly: recognition and management. *Drugs Aging* ;22:887–899.

[7] Yamamoto K: (2003) Pathogenesis of Sjögren's syndrome. *Autoimmun Rev*;1:13-8.

[8] Soto-Rojas AE, Kraus A: The oral side of Sjögren syndrome. Diagnosis and treatment. A review. *Arch Med Res* 2002;2:95-106.

[9] Vitali C, Bombardieri S, Jonsson R, Moutsopoulos HM, Alexander EL, Carsons SE, Daniels TE, Fox PC, Fox RI, Kassan SS, Pillemer SR, Talal N, Weisman MH, (2002)European Study Group on Classification Criteria for Sjögren's Syndrome. Classification criteria for Sjögren's syndrome: a revised version of the European criteria proposed by the American-European Consensus Group. *Ann Rheum Dis.* Jun;61(6):554-8.

[10] Daniels TE, Whitcher JP. (1994) Association of patterns of labial salivary gland inflammation with keratoconjunctivitis sicca. Analysis of 618 patients with suspected Sjögren's syndrome. *Arthritis Rheum.* ;37:869-877.

[11] Rubin H, Holt M. (1957) Secretory sialography in diseases of the major salivary glands. *AJR Am J Roentgenol.* 77:575-598.

[12] Shall GL, Anderson LG, Wolf RO, Herdt JR, Tarpley TM Jr, Cummings NA, *et al.* (1971) Xerostomia in Sjögren's syndrome: evaluation by sequential scintigraphy. *JAMA.*;216:2109-2116.

[13] Bolstad AI, Jonsson R. (2002) Genetic aspects of Sjögren's syndrome. *Arthritis Res.* 4(6):353-9.

[14] Jonsson R, Haga H-J, Gordon T. (2001) Sjögren´s syndrome. In: Arthritis and Allied Contitions: *a Textbook of Rheumatology*, 14th ed. Edited by Koopman WJ. Philadelphia: Lippincott, Williams & Wilkins,:1736-1759.

[15] Silman AJ, Rooney BK: (1999) Epidemiology of Sjögren's syndrome. In: *The 100-year Anniversary of Henrik Sjögren.* Edited by ErikssonE, Jonsson R. Jönköping: Hygiea,:53-57.

[16] Mavragani CP, Crow MK. (2010) Activation of the type I interferon pathway in primary Sjogren's syndrome. *J Autoimmun.* Nov;35(3):225-31.

[17] Mavragani CP, Moutsopoulos HM. (2010) The geoepidemiology of Sjogren's syndrome. *Autoimmun Rev*;9(5):A305e10.

[18] Manoussakis MN, Kapsogeorgou EK. (2007) The role of epithelial cells in the pathogenesis of Sjogren's syndrome. *Clin Rev Allergy Immunol*;32:225e30.

[19] Skopouli FN, Moutsopoulos HM. (1994) Autoimmune epitheliitis: Sjogren's syndrome. *Clin Exp Rheumatol*;12(Suppl. 11):S9e11.

[20] Triantafyllopoulou A, Moutsopoulos H. (2007) Persistent viral infection in primary Sjogren's syndrome: review and perspectives. *Clin Rev Allergy* Immunol; 32:210e4.

[21] Jonsson R, Moen K, Vesterheim D, Szodoray P. (2002) Current issues in Sjögren's syndrome. *Oral Dis*;8:130–140.

[22] Al-Hashimi I. (2005) Xerostomia secondary to Sjögren's syndrome in theelderly: recognition and management. *Drugs Aging*;22:887–899.

[23] Bartoloni E, Ludovini V, Alunno A, Pistola L, Bistoni O, Crinò L, Gerli R. (2011) Increased levels of circulating DNA in patients with systemic autoimmune diseases: a possible marker of disease activity in Sjogren's syndrome. *Lupus.* May 25. [Epub ahead of print)

[24] Alevizos I, Alexander S, Turner RJ, Illei GG. (2011) MicroRNA expression profiles as biomarkers of minor salivary gland inflammation and dysfunction in Sjögren's syndrome. *Arthritis Rheum.* Feb;63(2):535-44.

[25] Fox RI, Stern M, Michelson P. (2000) Update in Sjögren syndrome. *Curr Opin Rheumatol*;12:391e398.

[26] Bunim JJ, Talal N. (1963) Development of malignant lymphoma in the course of Sjögren's syndrome. *Trans Assoc Am Physicians.*;76:45–56.

[27] Bayetto K, Logan RM. (2010) Sjögren's syndrome: a review of aetiology, pathogenesis, diagnosis and management. *Aust Dent J.* Jun;55 Suppl 1:39-47.

[28] Kassan SS, Thomas TL, Moutsopoulos HM, *et al.* (1978) Increased risk of lymphoma in sicca syndrome. Ann Intern Med.;89:888–892.

[29] Talal N, Sokoloff L, Barth WF. (1967) Extrasalivary lymphoid abnormalities in Sjögren's syndrome (reticulum-cell sarcoma, "pseudolymphoma" macroglobulinemia). *Am J Med.*;43:50–65.

[30] LIN Dong-fang, YAN Shu-min, ZHAO Yan, ZHANG Wen, LI Meng-tao, ZENG Xiao-feng, ZHANG Feng-chun and DONG Yi. (2010) Clinical and prognostic characteristics of 573 cases of primary Sjögren's syndrome. *Chin Med J*;123(22):3252-3257

[31] Civilibal M, Canpolat N, Yurt A, Kurugoglu S, Erdamar S, Bagci O, Sever L, Kasapcopur O, Caliskan S, Arisoy N. (2007) A child with primary Sjögren syndrome and a review of the literature. *Clin Pediatr* (Phila). Oct;46(8):738-42

[32] Nikitakis NG, Rivera H, Lariccia C, Papadimitriou JC, Sauk JJ. (2003) Primary Sjögren syndrome in childhood: report of a case and review of the literature. *Oral Surg Oral Med Oral Pathol Oral Radiol Endod.*;96:42-47.

[33] Fox R. (2005) Sjögren's syndrome. Lancet.;366:321-331.

[34] Houghton KM, Cabral DA, Petty RE, Tucker LB. (2005) Primary Sjögren syndrome in dizygotic adolescent twins: one case with lymphocytic interstitial pneumonia. *J Rheumatol.*;32:1603-1606.

[35] Sardenberg F, Goursand D, Polletto LT, Vale MP, Zarzar PM, Paiva SM. (2010) Oral manifestations and treatment of a child with Sjögren's syndrome. *J Dent Child* (Chic). May-Aug;77(2):102-5.

[36] Hara T, Nagata M, Mizuno Y, Ura Y, Matsuo M, Ueda K. (1992) Recurrent parotid swelling in children: Clinical features useful for differential diagnosis of Sjögren's syndrome. *Acta Paediatr*;81:547-9.

[37] Mizuno Y, Hara T, Hatae K, *et al.* (1989) Recurrent parotid gland enlargement as an initial manifestation of Sjögren's syndrome in children. *Eur J Pediatr*;148:414-6.

[38] Anaya JM, Ogawa N, Talal N. (1995) Sjögren's syndrome in childhood. *J Rheumatol*;22:1152-8.

[39] Isaacs D. (2002) Recurrent parotitis. *J Paediatr Child Health*;38:92-4.

[40] Ramos-Casals M, Font J. (2007) Primary Sjögren syndrome. In: Imboden J, Hellman D, Stone JH, eds. *Current Diagnosis and Treatment in Rheumatology*. New York,NY: McGraw-Hill;:237-245.

[41] Ramos-Casals M, Tzioufas AG, Stone JH, Sisó A, Bosch X. (2010) Treatment of primary Sjögren syndrome: a systematic review. *JAMA*. Jul 28;304(4):452-60.

[42] Pers JO, Devauchelle V, Daridon C, *et al.* (2007) BAFFmodulated repopulation of B lymphocytes in the blood and salivary glands of rituximab-treated patients with Sjögren's syndrome. *Arthritis Rheum.*;56 (5):1464-1477

[43] Mese H, Matsuo R. (2007) Salivary secretion, taste and hyposalivation. *J Oral Rehabil.* Oct;34(10):711-23.

[44] Garrett JR, Suleiman AM, Anderson LC, Proctor GB. (1991) Secretory responses in granular ducts and acini of submandibular glands in vivo to parasympathetic or sympathetic nevre stimulation in rats. *Cell Tissue Res*;264:117–126.

[45] Rantonen PJF, Meurman JH. (1998) Viscosity of whole saliva. *Acta Odont Scand.*;56:210–214.

[46] Rayment SA, Liu B, Soares RV, Offner GD, Oppenheim FG, Troxler RF. (2001) The effects of duration and intensity of stimulation on total protein and mucin concentrations in resting and stimulated whole saliva. *J Dent Res*;80:1584–1587.

[47] Matsuo R. (2000) Role of saliva in the maintenance of taste sensitivity. *Crt Rev Oral Biol Med.*;11:216–229.

[48] Guobis Z, Baseviciene N, Paipaliene P, Niedzelskiene I, Januseviciūte G. (2008) Aspects of xerostomia prevalence and treatment among rheumatic inpatients. *Medicina* (Kaunas).;44(12):960-8.

[49] Atkinson JC, Wu AJ. (1994) Salivary gland dysfunction: causes,symptoms, treatment. J *Am Dent Assoc*;125(4):409-16.

[50] Aguirre A. (1997) Recognizing and managing the oral clues that point to Sjögren's syndrome. *Medscape Womens Health*;2(9):2.

[51] Guggenheimer J, Moore PA. (2003) Xerostomia: etiology, recognitionand treatment. *J Am Dent Assoc*;134(1):61-9.

[52] Patinen P, Aine L, Collin P, Hietanen J, Korpela M, EnckellG, *et al.* (2004) Oral findings in coeliac disease and Sjögren's syndrome. *Oral Dis*;10(6):330-4

[53] Humprey SP, Williamson RT. (2001) A review of saliva: normal composition, flow and function. *J Prosthet Dent*;85: 162-9.
[54] Tenovuo J. (1998) Invited review: antimicrobial function of human saliva - how important is it for oral health. *Acta Odontol Scand*;56(5):250-6.
[55] Ruiz Allec LD, Hernández López X, Arreguín Porras JB, Velasco Ramos R, Pacheco Del Valle JC, Pérez García AI. (2011) Alterations in voice, speech and swallowing in patients with Sjögren's syndrome. *Acta Otorrinolaringol Esp*. Feb 21.
[56] Boutsi EA, Paikos S, Dafni UG, Moutsopoulos HM, Skopouli FN. (2000) Dental and periodontal status of Sjögren's syndrome. *J Clin Periodontol*. Apr;27(4):231-5.
[57] Skopouli F, Dafni U, Ioannidis J, Moutsopoulos H. Clinical evolution, and morbidity and mortality of primary Sjögren'ssyndrome. Semin Arthritis Rheum 2000;29:296–304.
[58] García-Carrasco M, Fuentes-Alexandro S, Escárcega RO, Salgado G, Riebeling C, Cervera R. (2006) Pathophysiology of Sjögren's syndrome. *Arch Med Res*. Nov;37(8):921-32.
[59] Kassan SS, Moutsopoulos HM. (2004) Clinical manifestations and early diagnosis of Sjögren syndrome. *Arch Intern Med.*;164(12):1275-1284.
[60] Melvin, J. E. (1991) Saliva and dental diseases. *Curr. Opin. Dent.* 1, 795–801.
[61] Mathews SA, Kurien BT, Scofield RH. (2008) Oral manifestations of Sjögren's syndrome. *J Dent Res*. Apr;87(4):308-18.
[62] Atkinson, J. C. & Fox, P. C. (1993) Sjogren's syndrome: oral and dental considerations. *J. Am. Dent. Assoc.* 91, 838–845.
[63] Paster BJ, Boches SK, Galvin JL, Ericson RE, Lau CN, Levanos VA, *et al.* (2001). Bacterial diversity in human subgingival plaque. *J Bacteriol* 183:3770-3783.
[64] Matsumoto N, Salam MA, Watanabe H, Amagasa T, Senpuku H (2004). Role of gene E2f1 in susceptibility to bacterial adherence of oral streptococci to tooth surfaces in mice. *Oral Microbiol Immunol* 19:270- 276.
[65] Astor FC, Hanft KL, Ciocon JO (1999). Xerostomia: a prevalent condition in the elderly. *Ear Nose Throat J* 78:476-479.
[66] Pedersen AM, Bardow A, Nauntofte B (2005). Salivary changes and dental caries as potential oral markers of autoimmune salivary gland dysfunction in primary Sjögren's syndrome. *BMC Clin Pathol* 5:4.
[67] Pederson A, Reibel J, Bergem H, Jensen J, Nauntofte B. (1999) Primary Sjögren's syndrome: salivary gland function and clinical oral findings. *Oral Dis*;5:128–138.
[68] MacFarlane, T. W. & Mason, D. K. (1974) Changes in the oral flora in Sjo¨gren's syndrome. *J. Clin. Pathol.* 27, 416–419.
[69] Lundstrom, I. M. C. & Lindstrom, F. D. (1995) Subjective and clinical oral symptoms in patients with primary Sjo¨gren's syndrome. *Clin. Experiment. Rheumatol.* 13, 725–731.
[70] Pardo GI, Sreebny LM. (1992) Management for the highly cariessusceptible patient. *J Prosthet Dent*;67:637–644.
[71] Mandel ID. (1996) Current strategies, new directions. *J Am Dent Assoc*;127:1477–1488.
[72] Anusavice KJ. (1995) Treatment regimens in preventive and restorative dentistry. *J Am Dent Assoc*;126:727–743.

[73] Márton K, Madléna M, Bánóczy J, Varga G, Fejérdy P, Sreebny LM, Nagy G: (2008) Unstimulated whole saliva flow rate in relation to sicca symptoms in Hungary. *Oral Dis.*;14:472-7.

[74] Crow HC, Ship JA: (1995) Are gingival and periodontal conditions related to salivary gland flow rates in healthy individuals? *J Am Dent Assoc.*;126:1514-20.

[75] Márton K, Boros I, Varga G, Zelles T, Fejérdy P, Zeher M *et al.* (2006) Evaluation of palatal saliva flow rate and oral manifestations in patients with Sjögren's syndrome. *Oral Dis*;5:480-6.

[76] Celenligil H, Eratalay K, Kansu E, Ebersole JL: (1998) Periodontal status and serum antibody responses to oral microorganisms in Sjögren's syndrome. *J Periodontol*;5:571-7.

[77] Najera MP, al-Hashimi I, Plemons JM, Rivera-Hidalgo F, Rees TD, Haghighat N, Wright JM: (1997) Prevalence of periodontal disease in patients with Sjögren's syndrome. *Oral Surg Oral Med Oral Pathol Oral Radiol Endod*;4:453-7.

[78] Ergun, S., A. Çekici, N. Topcuoglu, D.A. Migliari, G. Külekçi, H. Tanyeri ve G. Isık, (2010) "Oral status and *Candida* colonization in patients with Sjögren syndrome", *Medicina Oral, Patologia Oral y Cirurgia Bucal,* 1;15 (2):e310-5

[79] Rhodus NL, Michalowicz BS: (2005) Periodontal status and sulcular *Candida* albicans colonization in patients with primary Sjögren's Syndrome. *Quintessence Int*;3:228-33.

[80] Kuru B, McCullough MJ, Yilmaz S, Porter SR: (2002) Clinical and microbiological studies of periodontal disease in Sjögren syndrome patients. *J Clin Periodontol*;2:92 102.

[81] Pers JO, d'Arbonneau F, Devauchelle-Pensec V, Saraux A, Pennec YL, Youinou P: (2005) Is periodontal disease mediated by salivary BAFF in Sjögren's syndrome? *Arthritis Rheum*;8:2411-4.

[82] Schiødt M, Christensen LB, Petersen PE, Thorn JJ: (2001) Periodontal disease in primary Sjögren's syndrome. *Oral Dis*;2:106-8.

[83] Tseng CC: (1991) Periodontal status of patients with Sjögren's syndrome: a cross-sectional study. *J Formos Med Assoc*;1:109-11.

[84] Keene HJ, Horton IM, Handler SF: (1981) Streptococcus mutans approximal plaque index as a new epidemiologic tool for defining the parameters of Streptococcus mutans infection in human populations.*Arch Oral Biol*;26:345-5.

[85] Kamagata-Kiyoura Y, Abe S, Yamaguchi H, Nitta T: (2004) Protective effects of human saliva on experimental murine oral candidiasis. *J Infect Chemother*;4:253-5.

[86] Kindelan SA, Yeoman CM, Douglas CW, Franklin C: (1998) A comparison of intraoral *Candida* carriage *in Sjögren's syndrome patients with healthy xerostomic controls. Oral Surg Oral Med Oral Pathol Oral Radiol Endod*;2:162-7.

[87] Alves MB, Motta AC, Messina WC, Migliari DA: (2004) Saliva substitute in xerostomic patients with primary Sjögren's syndrome: a single-blind trial. *Quintessence Int*;5:392-6.

[88] Koseki M, Maki Y, Matsukubo T, Ohashi Y, Tsubota K: (2004) Salivary flow and its relationship to oral signs and symptoms in patients with dry eyes. *Oral Dis*;2:75-80.

[89] Leung KC, McMillan AS, Leung WK, Wong MC, Lau CS, Mok TM: (2004) Oral health condition and saliva flow in southern Chinese with Sjögren's syndrome. *Int Dent J*;3:159-65.

[90] Soto-Rojas AE, Villa AR, Sifuentes-Osornio J, Alarcón-Segovia D, Kraus A: (1998) Oral candidiasis and Sjögren's syndrome. *J Rheumatol*;5:911-5.

[91] Soto-Rojas AE, Villa AR, Sifuentes-Osornio J, Alarcón-Segovia D, Kraus (1998) A: Oral manifestations in patients with Sjögren's syndrome. *J Rheumatol*;5:906-10.

[92] Porter SR, Scully C, Hegarty AM: (2004) An update of the etiology and management of xerostomia. *Oral Surg Oral Med Oral Pathol Oral Radiol Endod*,1:28-46.

[93] Scully C: (1989) Oral parameters in the diagnosis of Sjögren's syndrome. *Clin Exp Rheumatol*;2:113-7.

[94] Volter F, Fain O, Mathieu E, Thomas M: (2004) Esophageal function and Sjögren's syndrome. *Dig Dis Sci.*;49:248-53.

[95] Stewart CM, Berg KM, Cha S, Reeves WH: (2008) Salivary dysfunction and quality of life in Sjögren syndrome: a critical oral-systemic connection. *J Am Dent Assoc*;3:291-9;

[96] Taggart AJ, Hill J, Astbury C, Dixon JS, Bird HA, Wright V: (1987) Sulphasalazine alone or in combination with D-penicillamine in rheumatoid arthritis. *Br J Rheumatol*;1:32-6.

[97] Epstein JB, Pearsall NN, Truelove EL: (1980) Quantitative relationships between *Candida* albicans in saliva and the clinical status of human subjects. *J Clin Microbiol*;3:475-6.

[98] Navazesh M, Wood GJ, Brightman VJ: (1995) Relationship between salivary flow rates and *Candida* albicans counts. *Oral Surg Oral Med Oral Pathol Oral Radiol Endod*;3:284-8.

[99] Radfar L, Shea Y, Fischer SH, Sankar V, Leakan RA, Baum BJ *et al.* (2003) Fungal load and candidiasis in Sjögren's syndrome. *Oral Surg Oral Med Oral Pathol Oral Radiol Endod*;3:283-7.

[100] Torres SR, Peixoto CB, Caldas DM, Silva EB, Akiti T, Nucci M *et al.* (2002) Relationship between salivary flow rates and *Candida* counts in subjects with xerostomia. *Oral Surg Oral Med Oral Pathol Oral Radiol Endod.*;2:149-54.

[101] Abraham CM, al-Hashimi I, Haghighat N: (1998) Evaluation of the levels of oral *Candida* in patients with Sjögren's syndrome. *Oral Surg Oral Med Oral Pathol Oral Radiol Endod*;1:65-8.

[102] Leung KC, McMillan AS, Cheung BP, Leung WK: (2008) Sjögren's syndrome sufferers have increased oral yeast levels despite regular dental care. *Oral Dis*;2:163-73.

[103] Tawara Y, Honma K, Naito Y: (1996) Methicillin-resistant Staphylococcus aureus and *Candida* albicans on denture surfaces. *Bull Tokyo Dent Coll*;3:119-28.

[104] Reynaud AH, Nygaard-Østby B, Bøygard GK, Eribe ER, Olsen I, Gjermo P: (2001) Yeasts in periodontal pockets. *J Clin Periodontol.*;9:860-4.

[105] Cannon RD, Chaffin WL: (1999) Oral colonization by *Candida* albicans. *Crit Rev Oral Biol Med*;10:359-83.

[106] Cannon RD, Chaffin WL: (2001) Colonization is crucial factor in oral candidiasis. *Journal of Dental Education*;65:785-787.

[107] Almståhl A, Wikström M: (1999) Oral microflora in subjects with reduced salivary secretion. *J Dent Res*;8:1410-6.

[108] Scully C, El-Kabir M, Samaranayake LP: (1994) *Candida* and oral candidosis: a review. *Crit Rev Oral Biol Med*;5:125-157.

[109] Slots J, Rams TE, Listgarten MA: (1988) Yeasts, enteric rods and pseudomonads in the subgingival .ora of severe adult periodontitis. *Oral Microbiol Immunol*;3:47–52.

[110] Dahlen G, Wikstrom M: (1995) Occurrence of enteric rods, staphylococci and *Candida* in subgingival samples. *Oral Microbiol Immunol*;10:42–46.
[111] Rams TE, Flynn MJ, Slots J: (1997) Subgingival microbial associations in severe human periodontitis. *Clin Inf Dis*;25:224–226.
[112] A Jarvensivu, J Hietanen, R Rautemaa, T Sorsa, M Richardson: (2004) *Candida* yeasts in chronic periodontitis tissues and subgingival microbial biofilms in vivo. *Oral Diseases*;10:106-112.
[113] Brill N: (1969) The gingival pocket fluid.Studies of its occurrence, composition and effect. *Acta Odontol Scand*;2:159.
[114] Löe H, Holm-Pedersen P: (1965) Absence and presence of fluid from normal and inflamed gingiva. *Periodontics*; 3:171.
[115] Cimasoni G: (1983) Crevicular fluid updated. In myers H (ed): *Monographs in Oral Science*, vol 12 Basel, S Krager,.
[116] Logemann JA, Pauloski BR, Rademaker AW, Lazarus CL, Mittal B, Gaziano J, Stachowiak L, MacCracken E, Newman LA: (2003) Xerostomia: 12-month changes in saliva production and its relationship to perception and performance of swallow function, oral intake, and diet after chemoradiation. *Head Neck.*;25:432-7.
[117] Johnson JT, Ferretti GA, Nethery WJ, Valdez IH, Fox PC, Ng D, Muscoplat CC, Gallagher SC. (1993) Oral pilocarpine for post-irradiation irradiation xerostomia in patients with head and neck cancer. *Nengl J Med*;329:390–395.
[118] Epstein JB, Gorsky M, Caldwell J. (2002) Fluconazole mouth rinses for oral candidiasis in postirradiation, transplant and other patients. *Oral Surg Oral Med Oral Pathol Oral Radiol Endod*;93:671–675.
[119] Gallud D, Delgado W. Micosis. (2006) In: Bagán-Sebastián JV, Scully C. Medicina y patología oral. Valencia: *Medicia Oral* S.L;. p. 47-54.
[120] Milillo L, Lo Muzio L, Carlino P. (2005) *Candida*-related denture stomatitis: a pilot study of the efficacy of an amorolfine antifungal varnish. *Int J Prosthodont.*;18:55–59.
[121] Binon PP, Fowler CN. (1993) Implant-supported fixed prosthesis treatment of a patient with Sjogren's syndrome: a clinical report. *Int J Oral Maxillofac Implants*;8:54–58.
[122] Frost PM. (1997) A preliminary assessment of intra-oral lubricating systems for dry mouth patients. *Gerodontology*;14:54–58.
[123] Gravenmade EJ, Vissink A. (19929 Management of oral features of Sjogren's syndrome. *Neth J Med*;40:117–124.

10

Mechanisms of Salivary Gland Secretory Dysfunction in Sjögren's Syndrome

Kaleb M. Pauley, Byung Ha Lee, Adrienne E. Gauna and Seunghee Cha
University of Florida
USA

1. Introduction

Sjögren's syndrome (SS) is a systemic chronic autoimmune disorder affecting exocrine organs such as the salivary and lacrimal glands. SS is characterized by severe dryness of the mouth and eyes due to inflammatory reactions against salivary and lacrimal glands, respectively. Dryness of other mucosal surfaces such as skin, gastrointestinal tract, lungs, and vagina, has also been observed. SS patients also exhibit systemic symptoms such as Raynaud's phenomenon, arthritis, fatigue, peripheral neuropathies, and cognitive impairment. SS exists in two forms: primary SS, unassociated with other autoimmune disesases; and secondary SS, accompanied by another autoimmune disease such as scleroderma, rheumatoid arthritis, or systemic lupus erythematosus (Fox and Kang 1992). SS is the second most common autoimmune rheumatic disease, with a prevalence in the United States estimated at 2-4 million people (Kassan and Moutsopoulos 2004), with a female to male ratio of 9:1. Although SS affects men and children as well, it is most commonly seen if peri- or postmenopausal women.

Diagnostic criteria for SS have been defined most recently by the modified American-European Consensus Group (Vitali et al. 2002). These criteria include histological evaluation of a minor salivary gland for lymphocytic infiltration, serological presence of autoantibodies against SSA or SSB antigens, and assessment of ocular and oral symptoms. Oral involvement is assessed by the patient's subjective symptoms of oral dryness, parotid sialography showing the presence of diffuse sialectasis, salivary scintigraphy showing delayed uptake, reduced concentration, and/or delayed excretion of tracer, and/or the evaluation of unstimulated saliva production. Ocular involvement is assessed by the patient's subjective symptoms of ocular dryness, a Schirmer's test to measure tear secretion or a Rose Bengal test to measure the ocular surface abrasion in patients.

Originally, it was thought that loss of secretory function, a clinical hallmark of SS, was due to apoptotic destruction of acinar cells mediated by $CD8^+$ T lymphocytes in the lymphocytic infiltration in the salivary and lacrimal glands. However, research has demonstrated that transfer of human SS patient IgG to the B-cell deficient SS-prone NOD mouse resulted in altered saliva production in the absence of immune cell infiltration in the glands, indicating a role for autoantibodies in the functional impairment of secretory processes in SS (Robinson, Brayer et al. 1998). This resulted in a paradigm shift in the field, leading to the belief that lymphocytic infiltration was not the only contributing factor to secretory dysfunction in SS. In addition to autoantibodies targeting muscarinic receptors, pro-inflammatory cytokines have been shown to play a role in SS pathogenesis by contributing to damage of glandular tissue and secretory dysfunction. Nitric oxide production has also been implicated as a potential cause of loss of secretion, as loss of nitric oxide synthase activity in salivary glands paralleled the decline in salivary secretion. A role for apoptotic cell death of acinar cells still remains in SS pathogenesis, however; our group has demonstrated that increased apoptosis is detectable in the salivary glands of SS-prone mice prior to disease onset or lymphocytic infiltration (Bulosan et al. 2008). In this review, these mechanisms and other possibilities that can contribute to loss of secretory function in SS will be discussed in detail.

2. Mechanisms

The clinical hallmark of SS is dryness due to loss of secretory function in the salivary and lacrimal glands. However, the etiology of SS is still not understood. There are numerous underlying mechanisms thought to contribute to this loss of secretory function in salivary glands, though no single mechanism has been identified as the primary cause. Lymphocytic infiltration, autoantibodies targeting muscarinic receptors, pro-inflammatory cytokines, nitric oxide, and apoptotic cell death of acinar cells have all been implicated as potential causes of secretory dysfunction in the salivary glands.

2.1 Lymphocytic infiltration and proinflammatory cytokines in the salivary glands

SS is characterized by lymphocytic infiltration and aberrant activation of epithelial tissues, which appear in salivary and lacrimal glands. It has been reported that this lymphocytic infiltration within the salivary and lacrimal glands consists mostly of CD4+ T cells, B cells, and lesser numbers of CD8+ T cells (Robinson, Cornelius et al. 1998, ; Tapinos et al. 1998). Balance between T and B cells in the lymphocyte infiltrates varies according to disease progression in the mouse model of SS (Robinson, Cornelius et al. 1998, ; Tapinos et al. 1998). It has been shown that leukocytes expressing pro-inflammatory cytokines infiltrate the exocrine glands, and T cells are recruited first to the site of infiltration followed by B cells, establishing lymphocytic infiltrates (Kong et al. 1998). CD8+ T cells, which have been shown to have increased expression of adhesion molecules and Fas/FasL, can also directly kill acinar cells in the salivary glands. Salivary gland dryness and/or formation of lymphocytic infiltration may be the result of glandular destruction mediated by effector cytokines/chemokines from T and B cells, as well as cytotoxic effects of CD8+ T cells.

2.1.1 Cytokines contributing to salivary gland dysfunction

Tumor necrosis factor- α (TNF-α) is one of the proinflammatory cytokines produced in response to infection, tissue damage, and environmental challenges and also known as an Interferon-γ (IFNγ)-inducing cytokine along with IL-12 and IL-18 (Locksley 1993, ; Billiau 1996). TNF-α production has been implicated in many human diseases including autoimmune diseases such as inflammatory bowel disease (IBD), rheumatoid arthritis (RA), systemic lupus erythematosus (SLE). TNF-α activated the extrinsic apoptotic pathway and induced upregulation of intercellular adhesion molecule-1 (ICAM-1) and CCL20 in human salivary gland (HSG) cells *in vitro* (Wang et al. 2009). In addition, TNF-α can disrupt tight junction structure in salivary glands from SS patients, potentially resulting in secretory dysfunction (Ewert et al. 2010, ; Baker 2010).

IL-18 and its inducer IL-12 are cytokines that play an important role in T_H1 driven autoimmune responses and inflammatory tissue disease by activating IFNγ secretion. The elevation of these cytokines triggered the inflammatory response in SLE and RA patients (Mosaad et al. 2003). Increased circulating levels and salivary gland expression of IL-18 was observed in SS patients, and IL-18 was detected in periductal inflammatory foci and saliva as well (Bombardieri et al. 2004, ; Bulosan et al. 2009). In addition, increased labial salivary gland IL-18 levels in primary SS patients correlated with increased disease activity parameters (Bikker et al. 2010, ; Bombardieri et al. 2004). Moreover, salivary gland infiltration by macrophages and dendritic cells (DCs), along with the expression of IL-18 and IL-12, appear to play active roles in the expansion and organization of infiltrative injuries and have a correlation with the lymphoma development in the patients with primary SS (Manoussakis et al. 2007). IL-12 transgenic mice showed decreased stimulated salivary flow by pilocarpine than in wild type controls. Also, IL-12 transgenic mice exhibited increased number and size of lymphocytic foci with increased anti-SSB/La antibodies, compared to glands from age-matched controls (Vosters et al. 2009).

IFNγ is the major cytokine which is released from T_H1 cells and regulates cell-mediated immune responses through activation of natural killer (NK) cells, macrophages, and CD8+ T cells. IFN-γ or receptor knockout mouse models (NOD. $IFN\gamma^{-/-}$ and NOD. $IFN\gamma R^{-/-}$) showed normal development of salivary glands, maintained secretory function, and failed to develop any SS-like phenotypes (Cha et al. 2004). However, its parental strain NOD and a recently developed SS mouse model C57BL/6.NOD-*Aec1Aec2* showed retarded salivary gland growth and acinar cell apoptosis prior to disease onset and proceed to developing full-blown disease phenotype including loss of secretory function (Lee, Tudares, and Nguyen 2009). This indicates that IFN-γ plays an important role in loss of secretory function in SS. In addition, it has been found that IFNγ-induced T cells can produce chemokines (IFN-inducible protein 10 (IP-10)/CXCL9, CXCL10), which can attract NK cell and T cells in SS ductal epithelial cells (Ogawa et al. 2002, ; Ogawa et al. 2004).

There are also cytokines released from T_H2 cells that can play an important role in SS. Elevated levels of IL-4 were found in the serum of primary SS patients who have lymphocytic infiltration and ectopic germinal center formation in their minor salivary glands (Reksten et al. 2009). Studies using the NOD.$IL4^{-/-}$ and NOD.B10-H2b.$IL4^{-/-}$ mice indicated that IL-4 gene knockout mice have pathophysiological abnormalities and leukocyte infiltration in the salivary glands but salivary gland secretion was normal in the absence of IL-4 (Gao et al. 2006). Considering that IL-4 knockout mice fail to produce IgG1 isotypic autoantibodies against cell surface receptor muscarinic type 3 receptor (M3R), isotypic anti-M3R autoantibody is critical in the development of secretory dysfunction (Gao et al. 2004). Moreover, purified IgG fractions isolated from the sera of Stat6 (downstream signal transduction factor of IL-4) knockout mice, which are unable to produce IgG1, were not able to inhibit saliva flow rates when infused to wild type control mice (C57BL/6) (Nguyen et al. 2007). Therefore, IL-4 can affect saliva secretion via antibody production and its isotype switching.

Recently, not only T_H1 and T_H2 effector cells but also T_H17 cells, which mainly release pro-inflammatory cytokine IL-17, are being investigated for their role in disease pathogenesis of many autoimmune diseases including SS. The presence of T_H17 cells and T_H17-associated cytokines, IL-6, IL-23, IL-17, and IL-1β were reported in the serum and minor salivary glands of primary SS patients (Nguyen et al. 2008, ; Sakai et al. 2008, ; Reksten et al. 2009, ; Katsifis et al. 2009). It is also known that IL-18 synergizes with IL-17 to induce secretion of pro-inflammatory cytokines IL-6 and IL-8 in human parotid gland cells (Sakai et al. 2008). Serum levels of IL-17, IL-6, and IL-23 were significantly elevated in primary SS. A recent study in which an adenovirus vector expressing IL-17 was infused into the salivary glands of wild type mice (C57BL/6J) demonstrated the appearance of lymphocytic infiltrates, increased proinflammatory cytokine levels, changes in antinuclear antibody profiles, and temporal loss of saliva flow after infusion (Nguyen et al. 2010). In the reverse approach, infusion of IL-17R:Fc-blocking factor into the SS mouse model to block IL-17 binding to IL-17 receptor showed decreased lymphocytic infiltration in salivary glands, normalization of the antinuclear antibody repertoire, and increased saliva secretion (Nguyen et al. 2011). Therefore, these studies indicate that IL-17 is critical in inducing SS-phenotype in wild type mice. However, the mechanism by which IL-17 functions in altering secretory function in SS needs to be defined.

2.1.2 B cell involvement in SS

In addition to pathogenic T cells and cytokines, loss of B cell tolerance is critical in autoimmune diseases including SS. Levels of the B cell activating factor belonging to the TNF family (BAFF) in serum were higher in patients with SLE, RA and pSS than in normal individuals (Cheema et al. 2001, ; Groom et al. 2002, ; Zhang et al. 2001). BAFF overexpression caused self-reactive B cells at the transitional B cell stage and is responsible for B cell hyperactivity. It is known that over-expressing BAFF in BAFF-transgenic mice resulted in SLE-like disease with increased number of marginal-zone (MZ) like B cells, and at 16-18 months of age, these mice exhibited a SS-like disease with MZ like B cells in the salivary glands (Mackay et al. 1999, ; Groom et al. 2002). However, recent findings indicated that BAFF expression alone is not correlated with disease activity (Cheema et al. 2001, ; Zhang et al. 2001, ; Stohl et al. 2003). Nonetheless, BAFF influences the survival, proliferation, and differentiation of B cells in combination with IL-17 in patients with SLE and its combination can promote the persistence of self-reactive B cells (Doreau et al. 2009).

As described above, T cells and B cells clearly contribute to SS onset and progression. However, activation of T cells and B cells are required for normal immune function, and the trigger for autoimmune reactivity in SS has yet to be identified. Also, studies using immune-deficient mice revealed that secretory dysfunction and other salivary gland abnormalities can still occur in the absence of infiltrating immune cells and their cytokines.

2.2 Autoantibodies targeting muscarinic receptors

The assumption that secretory dysfunction in SS was a direct consequence of acinar tissue loss after lymphocytic infiltration was deeply ingrained in the SS research community for more than 60 years. However, more recently, our understanding of the pathogenesis of secretory dysfunction in SS has undergone a dramatic change. Questions arose concerning

SS patients with viable acinar tissue in their salivary glands but who still suffer from xerostomia. These observations suggest that the salivary gland secretory dysfunction in many SS patients is the result of a disruption of acinar cell function rather than acinar tissue destruction.

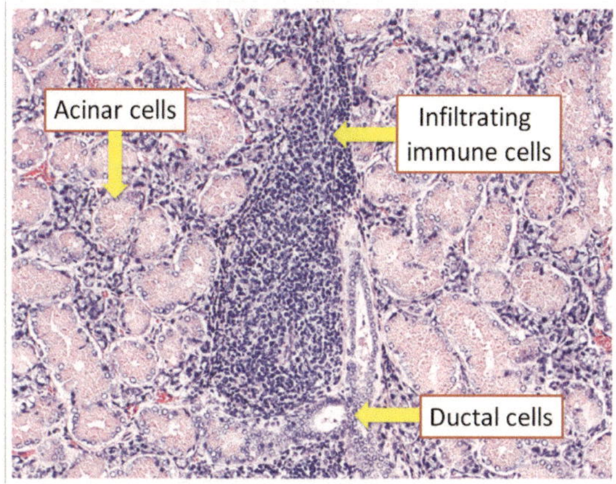

Fig. 1. Immune cell infiltration in the salivary gland of 34 week old SS-prone C57BL/6.NOD-*Aec1Aec2* male mouse.

In addition to salivary gland lymphocytic infiltration, SS patients exhibit hypergammaglobulinemia with a range of autoanitbodies targeting cell surface, cytoplasmic, and nuclear proteins of exocrine tissue (Chan et al. 1991, ; Fox and Kang 1992, ; Haneji et al. 1997). Approximately 90% of patients are positive for antinuclear antibodies (ANA), the most common of which are directed against two ribonucleoprotein antigens known as Ro or SSA and La or SSB. These autoantibodies are included in the modified European-American Diagnostic Criteria for Sjögren's Syndrome (Vitali et al. 2002), but are also found in other autoimmune diseases, particularly systemic lupus erythematosus (SLE). Autoantibodies to other immunoglobulins (known as rheumatoid factors) are also frequently found in SS. Primary SS (pSS) sera can also contain many different autoantibodies against organ or tissue specific autoantigens, including acetylcholine receptors, the carbonic anhydrase and thyroid peroxidase. Finally, autoantibodies directed against the cytoskeletal protein β-fodrin, and the muscarinic receptors M3, have also been described in primary SS, the latter of which we will focus on here.

2.2.1 Muscarinic receptor function in salivary glands

Acetylcholine (ACh) control of fluid secretion in salivary acinar cells is mediated through the G protien-linked muscarinic M3 receptor (M3R). ACh binds to M3R, which causes phospholipase C to generate inositol 1,4,5-trisphosphate (IP3). IP3 binds to and opens the IP3 receptor on the endoplasmic reticulum, which releases Ca^{2+}. The increased concentration of intracellular Ca^{2+} activates the apical membrane Cl^- channel and the basolateral K^+ channel. Efflux of Cl^- into the acinar lumen draws Na^+ across the cells, and the osmotic gradient generates fluid secretion (Tobin, Giglio, and Lundgren 2009). Therefore, blocking or desensitizing muscarinic receptors is detrimental to this signaling pathway and ultimately results in loss of secretory function.

2.2.2 Initial characterization of anti-muscarinic antibodies

In 1994, it was observed that in the NOD mouse model, which exhibits an autoimmune-associated lymphocytic attack on the salivary glands and loss of secretory function, decreased response to beta-adrenergic receptor stimulation was related to a decrease in receptor density and changes in the level of intracellular second messenger signalling (Hu et al. 1994). It was hypothesized that these changes could be due to an autoantibody targeting the β1-adrenergic receptor present in the sera of NOD mice.

In 1996, futher study of the NOD mouse model revealed a reduction in muscarinic receptor density on the salivary glands of prediabetic and diabetic NOD mice compared to BALB/c mice corresponding to reduced secretory function in the NOD (Yamamoto et al. 1996). Additionally, sera from the diabetic NOD but not the BALB/c immunoprecipitated radiolabeled muscarinic receptor, indicating the presence of autoantibody to the receptor in NOD mice (Yamamoto et al. 1996).

Autoantibodies against M3R were first described in human SS patients in 1996 (Bacman et al. 1996). It was demonstrated that IgG present in the sera of primary SS patients could bind and activate muscarinic receptors of rat parotid glands (Bacman et al. 1996). They also demonstrated that the IgG fraction from the sera of pSS patients mimicked the biological effects of muscarinic cholingergic agonists by modifying intracellular events associated with specific receptor activation, such as decreasing cAMP and increasing phosphoinositide turnover (Bacman et al. 1996). These findings suggested that autoantibodies targeting M3R could potentially play a role in SS pathogenesis.

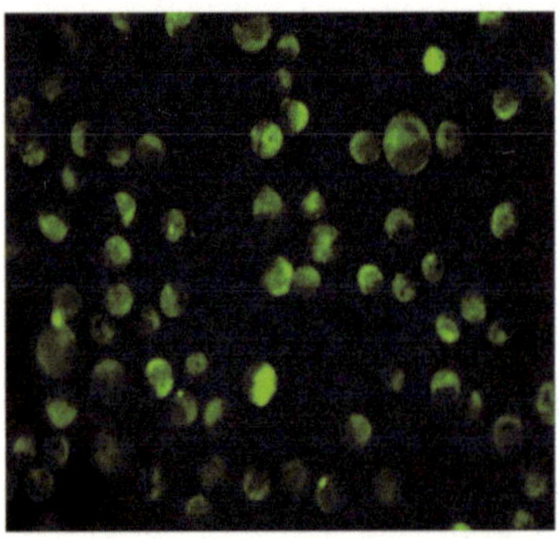

Fig. 2. pSS IgG staining of hM3R-transfected Flp-In CHO cells. Flp-In CHO cells were transfected with hM3R and then incubated with pSS sera (1:50 dilution) containing anti-M3R autoantibodies. Fluorescein isothiocyanate (FITC)-conjugated goat anti-mouse antibody at 1:250 dilution was used for detection.

2.2.3 Roles for anti-muscarinic receptor antibodies in SS

In 1998, Robinson, et al. were the first to demonstrate that transferring human SS patient IgG to NOD.Igμ^{null} mice resulted in secretory gland dysfunction (Robinson, Brayer et al. 1998). NOD.Igμ^{null} mice lack functional B lymphocytes, and therefore lack the IgG autoantibodies that are produced by their NOD counterparts and human SS patients. NOD.Igμ^{null} mice do exhibit lymphocytic infiltration of the salivary and lacrimal glands, but fail to lose secretory function. However, when treated with IgG from SS patient sera, a 54% reduction in saliva production was observed, while treatment with IgG from healthy control mice and healthy humans had no significant effect on secretory function (Robinson, Brayer et al. 1998). Furthermore, after prolonged treatment with SS IgG fractions, there was an increase in apoptotic cell death of salivary acinar cells (Robinson, Brayer et al. 1998). These data indicate that anti-M3R autoantibodies play a critical role in the clinical presentation of dryness in SS.

Further evidence for anti-M3R autoantibody-mediated secretory dysfunction in NOD mice was presented in 2000. Infusion of monoclonal antibodies to mouse M3R into NOD-*scid* mice resulted in significantly reduced saliva secretion within 72 hours, while infusion with antibodies to Ro (SSA), La (SSB), or parotid secretory protein (PSP) had no effect on secretory function (Nguyen et al. 2000). Mechanistic studies revealed that translocation of aquaporin-5 to the plasma membrane was inhibited by anti-M3R antibodies, but not the other antibodies again showing a role for anti-M3R autoantibodies in SS pathogenesis (Nguyen et al. 2000).

In 2004, Li, et al. demonstrated the inhibitory effects of autoantibodies from SS patients on muscarinic receptors by showing that carbachol-induced intracellular calcium release was inhibited by SS IgG treatment of HSG cells (Li et al. 2004). Aquaporin-5 trafficking to the apical membrane of rat parotid acinar cells was also inhibited by SS IgG (Li et al. 2004). Additionally, other groups found abnormal translocation of aquaporin-5 in the NOD mouse model of SS and in salivary glands of SS patients (Konttinen et al. 2005, ; Steinfeld et al. 2001). However, these findings are somewhat controversial since others have shown no differences in the subcellular distribution of aquaporin-5 in salivary glands of primary SS patients (Beroukas et al. 2001, ; Tsubota et al. 2001). Our unpublished findings show a definite alteration in GFP-tagged aquaporin-5 trafficking in human salivary gland cells that were pre-treated with SS plasma compared to healthy control plasma. Taken together, these data further support a role for anti-muscarinic receptor autoantibodies in loss of secretory function in SS.

The chronic effects of anti-M3R autoantibodies were examined in 2006 by analyzing the contraction of bladder smooth muscle strips from diseased NOD mice (Cha et al. 2006). The results indicated that the presence of anti-M3R autoantibodies in NOD mice resulted in a desensitization of M3R as measured by direct carbachol-induced responses and an accelerated loss of responses to repeated pilocarpine injections (Cha et al. 2006). This data supports the hypothesis that frequent use of pilocarpine by SS patients who have already progressed to M3R desensitization induced by anti-M3R autoantibodies will be less effective due to a desensitizing synergy between pilocarpine and anti-M3R autoantibodies.

Anti-muscarinic receptor antibodies have also been shown to affect the autonomic nervous system. In 2000, it was demonstrated that sera from primary and secondary SS patients inhibited parasympathetic neurotransmission as measured by carbachol-stimulated bladder contraction using bladder and colon smooth muscle strips in vitro, while sera from healthy controls or SLE patients had no effect (Waterman, Gordon, and Rischmueller 2000). These findings suggest that autoantibodies targeting M3R may contribute to sicca symptoms as well as autonomic dysfunction such as bladder symptoms in some patients (Waterman, Gordon, and Rischmueller 2000).

In vivo evidence was presented in 2004, when passive transfer of SS IgG with anti-M3R activity to BALB/c mice resulted in an increased response to cholinergic stimulation of bladder smooth muscle (Wang et al. 2004). This cholinergic hyperresponsiveness was found to be specifically induced by anti-M3R antibodies following passive transfer (Wang et al. 2004). These findings are consistent with the overactive bladder symptoms experienced by many SS patients, indicating that overactive bladder in SS is an autoantibody-mediated disorder of the autonomic nervous system that could also account for a broad range of cholinergic hyperresponsiveness.

Most recently, it has been demonstrated that primary SS IgG with anti-M3R activity inhibited contraction of the smooth muscle of the GI tract and disrupted contractile motility in the colon (Park et al. 2011). These data may explain the widespread impairment of the GI tract in SS patients including delayed gastric emptying and abnormalities in colonic motility (Cai et al. 2008, ; Kovacs et al. 2003).

2.2.4 Conclusions

Overall, these findings strongly support a role for anti-M3R autoantibodies in the pathogenesis of SS. The data suggest that a number of primary and secondary SS patients have serum IgG capable of binding to and inhibiting muscarinic receptors on salivary acinar cells in vitro. However, due to the lack of a reliable screening assay, relatively few subjects have been tested, and the percentage of SS patients estimated to be positive for anti-muscarinic antibodies varies wildly from 0 to almost 100%. Future studies in this field should focus on the development of a screening assay for anti-muscarinic antibodies to confirm the number of SS patients positive for these autoantibodies and establish or rule-out anti-M3R antibodies as a diagnostic marker for SS.

2.3 Nitric oxide and nitric oxide synthase

In 1986 nitric oxide (NO) was first described as endothelially derived relaxing factor (EDRF) (Palmer, Ferrige, and Moncada 1987). Subsequently, it has been shown to be involved in a multitude of diverse physiological and pathophsiological processes, including potential functions in the regulation of salivary gland secretion and in the development of secretory hypofunction. *In vivo*, NO is found to be synthesized in a wide variety of cell types by the enzyme NO synthase (NOS). There are three known isoforms of NOS, each produced from a distinct set of genes. The two constitutive isoforms are neuronal NOS (nNOS, NOS-1) and endothelial NOS (eNOS, NOS-3), whereby their names reflect the original tissues from which they were discovered. The functional activity of these two isoforms is dependent on a rise in Ca^{2+} and therefore generate low, transient, concentrations of NO. The other isoform, inducible NOS (iNOS, NOS-2), is mainly found in inflammatory cell types including: macrophages, neutrophils, and fibroblasts (Knowles and Moncada 1994). Expression of iNOS can be induced by bacterial lipopolysaccharides (LPS) and inflammatory cytokines. The concentrations of NO produced by iNOS are much greater than either eNOS or nNOS, and at levels that are typically cytotoxic and bactericidal (Kimura-Shimmyo et al. 2002).

2.3.1 Sources of NO in human salivary glands

The increased presence of nitrite (NO_2^-, the oxygenation product of NO) in the saliva of healthy individuals in response to stimulated secretion (Bodis and Haregewoin 1993) implies a system by which endogenous, constitutively expressed, NO may be produced in glandular cells and in turn alter saliva secretion. Surprisingly, immunohistochemical analyses of human minor and major salivary glands revealed that nNOS is strongly restricted to the non-neuronal duct epithelium and only a minority of the major salivary gland nerve fibers (surrounding acini, tubuli, ducts and blood vessels) expressed nNOS (Soinila, Nuorva, and Soinila 2006). In addition, salivary gland acinar cells have been demonstrated to express NOS (Looms et al. 2002, ; Looms et al. 2000, ; Soinila, Nuorva, and Soinila 2006). Human labial salivary gland acinar cells possess NOS activity and exhibit a very low level of NO production without stimulation *in vitro* (Looms et al. 2000). Stimulation of NO production, with a concomitant rise in Ca^{2+}, in human labial acinar cells was shown to be directly mediated through activation of β-adreneric receptors, which could not be mimicked by a rise in Ca^{2+} alone (Looms et al. 2000). As expected, the expression of eNOS in human minor and major salivary glands is restricted mostly to the vascular endothelium (Soinila, Nuorva, and Soinila 2006). The constitutive expression of NOS and NO in human salivary gland acini and ducts suggests a potential contribution to secretion. However, their exact roles in healthy salivary glands are still undetermined.

2.3.2 Potential function of NO in secretion

Saliva secretion signaling pathways and mechanisms have been studied closely, where the involvement of NO in these pathways is still of great interest. The classical signaling pathway involves autonomic receptor stimulation of acinar cells, which leads to increased IP3-mediated intracellular Ca^{2+} release from the endoplasmic reticulum and cAMP activation of protein phosphorylation. An additional receptor/channel involved in the release of Ca^{2+} from intracellular stores is the ryanodine receptor (RyR), of which, cyclic ADP-ribose (cADPR) has been suggested as an endogenous ligand (Galione, Lee, and Busa 1991, ; Looms et al. 2001). One potential means by which endogenous NO exerts an effect in the salivary gland acinar cells is by binding to the heme moiety of soluble guanylyl cyclases (Denninger and Marletta 1999) thus activating the synthesis of cyclic guanosine monophosphate (cGMP), which can promote the synthesis of the Ca^{2+}-mobilizing cADPR (Galione et al. 1993, ; Looms et al. 2001, ; Willmott et al. 1996). This NO-induced intracellular Ca^{2+} release is proposed to coordinate cellular activation and to have a role in determining the magnitude and time course of the secretory response (Caulfield et al. 2009, ; Harmer, Gallacher, and Smith 2001). Alterations in this response could play a role in salivary gland hypofunction via a disruption in the normal Ca^{2+} signaling pathways.

2.3.3 Potential roles of NO and iNOS in exocrine hypofunction

Evidence suggests that the loss of secretory function associated with SS may occur due to factors which alter Ca^{2+} signaling and not only through direct tissue destruction by infiltrating lymphocytes. One hypothesis for salivary gland exocrine hypofunction is based from the observation that the sera from NOD mice, prone to developing SS, were found to contain autoantibodies against β-adrenergic and muscarinic receptors (Hu et al. 1994, ; Yamamoto et al. 1996). The blockage of the β-adrenergic agonist binding down-regulated receptor density due to the chronic stimulation (Hu et al. 1994). Therefore, according to the previously described model for NO-induced Ca^{2+} release, saliva secretion could be diminished due to blockage of these receptors (Looms et al. 2002).

On the contrary, elevated nitrite is present at increased concentrations in SS patient saliva and serum compared to healthy controls (Konttinen et al. 1997, ; Wanchu et al. 2000). The effects of this possible elevation in NO concentration has been explored in recent experiments where the acute exposure of NO to human submandibular gland acinar cells were able to transiently (20-30 minutes) enhance Ca^{2+} signaling, but a more chronic exposure to NO eventually desensitized these cells to stimulation (Caulfield et al. 2009). The mechanism by which NO exerts its inhibitory effects on the stimulation of secretion is still not understood, but it is most likely not mediated through cGMP nor due to a depletion of the Ca^{2+} stores. It is hypothesized that the inhibition of activity could be due to the NO-mediated nitrosylation of receptors or other proteins involved in the secretion signal transduction pathways (Caulfield et al. 2009). However, this relationship between increased nitrite concentrations and salivary gland hypofunction is more complicated, since other oral inflammatory disorders exhibit increased nitrite concentrations in saliva as well (Kendall et al. 2000, ; Kendall, Marshall, and Bartold 2001, ; Ohashi, Iwase, and Nagumo 1999).

The role of iNOS in the loss of secretory function has also been investigated due to the pro-inflammatory environment present in the salivary glands of SjS patients. As expected, iNOS expression is increased in resident cells of the labial salivary glands of patients with SS when compared to healthy controls (Konttinen et al. 1997). Cytokines (for example: IFN-γ, IL-18, IL-1β and TNF-α) or LPS induction of iNOS leads to a significant increase in NO production (Dinarello 1997, ; Kimura-Shimmyo et al. 2002, ; Liew 1994). NO production from iNOS is long-lasting and at relatively high concentrations when compared to the other two Ca^{2+}-dependent isotypes (Nathan and Xie 1994). This increased NO has been hypothesized to directly nitrosylate functional proteins and thus could induce cell death by potentially disrupting essential cellular processes (Kimura-Shimmyo et al. 2002, ; Sarih, Souvannavong, and Adam 1993). In another course of altering cellular functioning, the product of the reaction of NO with superoxide, peroxynitrite, has also been suggested to promote modulations of cell signaling and even produce oxidative injury (Pacher, Beckman, and Liaudet 2007). It has been shown in several cases how the upregulation of iNOS expression may ultimately lead to secretory hypofunction due to the accumulated damage from NO (Dawson, Fox, and Smith 2006, ; Kimura-Shimmyo et al. 2002, ; Konttinen et al. 1997, ; Takeda et al. 2003).

2.4 Altered glandular homeostasis

In addition to the immune cell-mediated mechanisms that contribute to secretory gland dysfunction, there is also evidence for altered glandular homeostasis in SS glands that appears even prior to disease onset. Specifically, aberrant expression and proteolytic cleavage of PSP, increased serine and cysteine protease enzyme activity, elevated numbers of apoptotic cells, enhanced matrix metalloproteinase activities in salivary gland lysates and decreased amylase activity and epidermal growth factor gene expression are all observed irrespective of the presence of lymphocytic infiltration or detectable autoimmune phenotype. Additionally, submandibular glands of NOD neonates revealed some genetically programmed glandular defects such as retarded salivary gland development. How these early defects influence the onset and development of SS is still under active investigation.

2.4.1 Defects in salivary glands of NOD mouse models after disease onset

NOD mice develop chronic lymphocytic infiltration in the salivary glands that correlate with decreased saliva production concurrently with infiltration in the pancreas that results in phenotypes similar to insulin-dependent diabetes mellitus and SS. To differentiate between immune cell-mediated and non-immune cell-mediated mechanisms in the SS phenotype, salivary glands were characterized in NOD-*scid* mice and other NOD derivatives.

In the absence of a functional immune system, the salivary flow rate of >20 week old NOD-*scid* is similar to 10-12 week old mice (Robinson et al. 1996). However, saliva analysis revealed that epidermal growth factor (EGF, a product of submandibular gland ductal cells) and amylase (a product of salivary acinar cells) were significantly decreased in the saliva of >20 week old NOD-*scid* compared to 10-12 week old mice (Robinson et al. 1996). Additionally, PSP was detected in submandibular gland lysates of 10 week old NOD-*scid* and increased in quantity by 20 weeks of age, while PSP was not detected in control BALB/c glands, and (Robinson et al. 1996). Histological examination of NOD-*scid* submandibular glands revealed a progressive loss of acinar tissue and a decline in the acinar to ductal cell ratio in the absence of lymphocytic infiltrates (Robinson et al. 1996). These differences in salivary protein composition and glandular histology in the absence of lymphocytic infiltration indicate that glandular defects in the NOD genetic background may contribute to the onset of the autoimmune reaction in the salivary glands.

Further analysis of these findings revealed increased cysteine protease activity in the saliva and gland lysates of 20 week old NOD and NOD-*scid* mice compared to age matched BALB/c or 8 week old NOD mice (Robinson et al. 1997). This increased activity was highest in the NOD-*scid* mice indicating that infiltrating immune cells are not responsible for these changes. Additional protease activity in the saliva and gland lysates of older NOD and NOD-*scid* mice generated an enzymatically cleaved PSP (Robinson et al. 1997). These findings suggest that proteolytic enzyme activity contributes to loss of exocrine gland tolerance by generating abnormally processed protein constituents.

2.4.2 Defects in salivary glands of NOD mice prior to disease onset

The changes in the protein composition of saliva, PSP expression, and protease activity in the absence of lymphocytic infiltration or functional immune cells indicate that innate genetic differences in the NOD salivary glands exist and may contribute to the SS phenotype. To further support this theory, salivary gland organogenesis was examined in neonatal NOD mice and compared to wild type mice (Cha et al. 2001). Histomorphological analyses of submandibular glands at 1 day postpartum revealed delayed morphological differentiation during organogenesis in NOD mice compared to wild type mice, acinar cell proliferation was reduced, and expression of Fas, FasL and bcl-2 were increased (Cha et al. 2001). Prior to weaning (up to 21 days) the NOD strains showed increased matrix metalloprotease (MMP)-2 and MMP-9 activity (Cha et al. 2001). This altered glandular development may contribute to an environment capable of triggering autoimmunity.

As mentioned previously, a role for interferon-γ (IFN-γ) in these pre-disease aberrations was discovered when neither NOD.IFNγ $^{-/-}$ and NOD.IFNγR$^{-/-}$ mice exhibited increased acinar cell apoptosis or abnormal salivary protein expression prior to disease (Cha et al. 2004). Strikingly, without these abnormalities, the NOD.IFNγ $^{-/-}$ and NOD.IFNγR$^{-/-}$ mice showed no autoimmune attack of the salivary glands at 20 weeks old (Cha et al. 2004). Also, NOD-*scid.IFNγ* $^{-/-}$ mice, unlike NOD-*scid* and NOD, showed normal glandular morphogenesis at birth (Cha et al. 2004). These data suggest that IFN-γ has a critical role during the pre-immune phase disease independent of effector functions of immune cells.

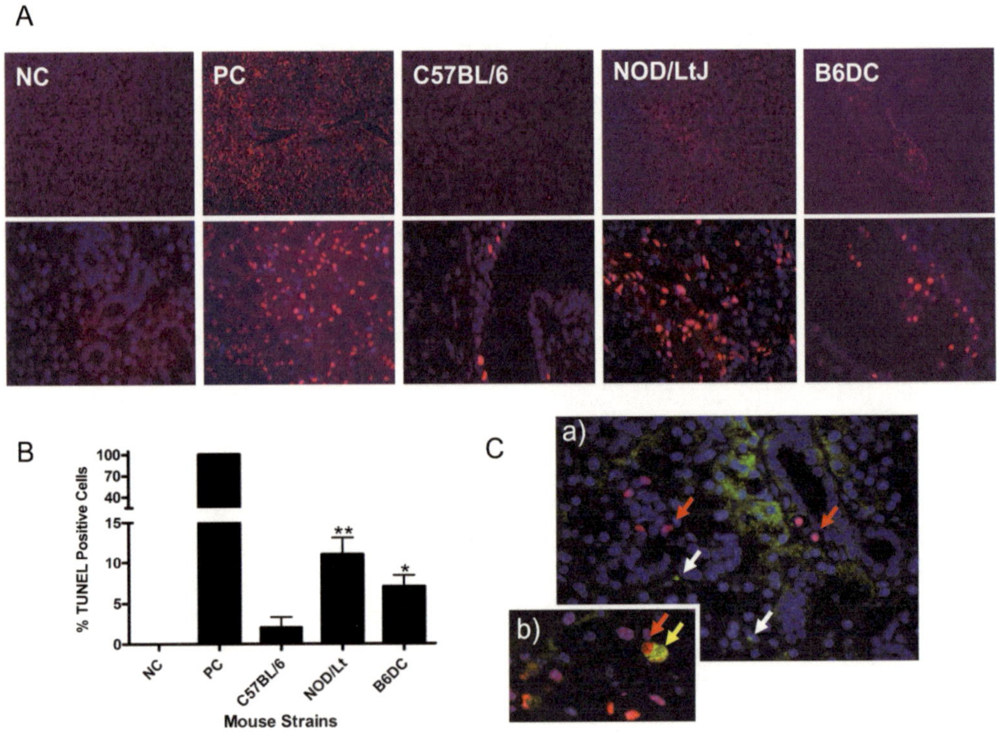

Fig. 3. Increased epithelial cell death in the glands of disease-prone mice at 8 weeks and lack of direct colocalization of caspase-11 with TUNEL-positive cells. (**A**) TUNEL staining was performed on the prediseased salivary glands; upper panel at × 10 and lower panel at × 40 magnifications. (**B**) Percentages of TUNEL-positive cells are shown as a bar graph. For each mouse, three slides were evaluated for TUNEL-positive cells, which were counted using a cell counter. (**C**) Caspase-3-positive cells (yellow arrows in **b**) were colocalized with TUNEL-positive cells (red arrows). White arrows indicate caspase-11-positive cell. Magnification, × 40. NC, negative control; PC, positive control treated with nuclease; TUNEL, transferase-mediated dUTP-biotin nick end labeling. Figure previously published in (Bulosan et al. 2009).

The NOD mouse model was/is used extensively to study SS pathogenesis; however, this model is genetically predisposed to develop at least three autoimmune diseases. To create a primary SS mouse model that only exhibits SS-like phenotype, two chromosomal intervals from the NOD mouse that conferred sialadenitis were bred to non-autoimmune C57BL/6 mice (Cha et al. 2002). These mice, designated C57BL/6.NOD-*Aec1Aec2*, enabled the study of disease-associated genes alone, and were used to characterize early pathogenic events associated with SS-like disease through microarray analysis of gene expression in the salivary glands during the pre-disease stage (Killedar et al. 2006). Interestingly, C57BL/6.NOD-*Aec1Aec2* exhibited upregulated genes encoding proteins associated with IFN-γ signal transduction pathway (*Jak/Stat*), TLR-3 (*Irf3 and Traf6*), and apoptosis (*casp11 and casp3*) compared to C57BL/6 (Killedar et al. 2006).

The upregulation of caspase-11 in 8 week old C57BL/6.NOD-*Aec1Aec2* mice was detected in our study. Concomitantly, apoptotic cells were more readily detected in this mouse model compared to wild type mice. Further studies were then conducted to determine whether upregulated caspase-11 is responsible for this phenomenon. In these studies it was shown that the upregulated caspase-11 expression from the salivary glands activated caspase-1, but not caspase-3. In effect, apoptotic cells were not positive for caspase-11 staining, suggesting that caspase-11 plays an indirect role in increased apoptotic acinar cell death in the salivary glands before disease onset (Bulosan et al. 2009). This finding led to the hypothesis that inflammatory caspases, such as caspase-11 indirectly functions in apoptosis by activating caspase-1 and resulting in the subsequent release of proinflammatory cytokines into the glandular environment. This hypothesis was tested by co-culturing human salivary gland cells with a human monocyte cell line, THP-1, stimulated with LPS in the presence or absence of IFN-γ. In the presence of IFN-γ, there was an increased rate of HSG cell apoptosis, but when caspase-1 was knocked down by small interfering RNA in the THP-1 cells, the rate of apoptosis in HSG cells was reversed back to normal (Bulosan et al. 2009). These data indicate that the increased caspase-11 expression in macrophages and dendritic cells present in the salivary glands of 8 week old C57BL/6.NOD-*Aec1Aec2* mice may increase apoptotic cell death of surrounding acinar cells by activating capase-1, resulting in the secretion of pro-inflammatory cytokines IL-1β and IL-18. In other words, inflammatory caspases are essential in promoting a pro-inflammatory microenvironment and influencing salivary gland cell death prior to disease onset.

2.4.3 Altered microRNA expression in SS

MicroRNAs (miRNAs) are small non-coding RNA molecules that post-transcriptionally regulate gene expression by binding to the 3′ untranslated regions of specifc mRNAs and blocking translation or causing degradation. Recently, miRNAs have been implicated in a number of diseases including autoimmune disorders. In 2011, it is becoming clear that miRNAs may also play a role in SS, although that specific role has yet to be determined. Alevizos, et al. demonstrated that miRNA expression patterns can accurately distinguish salivary glands from control subjects and SS patients, and that comparing miRNA from patients with preserved or low saliva flow identified a set of differentially expressed miRNAs, indicating a potential role for miRNAs in secretory dysfunction of the salivary glands (Alevizos et al. 2011). Later in 2011, we reported that miR-146a is significantly overexpressed in the PBMCs of SS patients compared to healthy controls and in the salivary glands and PBMCs of 8 week old C57BL/6.NOD-*Aec1Aec2* female mice compared to wild-type mice (Pauley et al. 2011). It is particularly interesting that miR-146a is upregulated in the target tissues (salivary glands) at 8 weeks of age since this is prior to disease onset in this mouse model. These data suggest that miR-146a could play a role in early disease pathogenesis in SS or could be a result of altered glandular homeostasis prior to disease onset.

Taken together, it is becoming increasingly clear that innate differences in the salivary glands of SS contribute to disease onset and/or loss of secretory function. Developmental defects, altered glandular homeostasis in the absence of immune cell infiltrates, and a tendency towards a proinflammatory environment are all evident in the salivary glands of SS mouse models, sometimes even prior to disease onset. It remains to be seen how these changes develop, but one hypothesis is that chronic stimulation by pathogens can lead to subclinical changes in the glands. In this case, it will be critical to identify the signatures left behind by these pathogens, such as viral or bacterial footprints, in order to use them as early disease markers to detect individuals susceptible to developing SS.

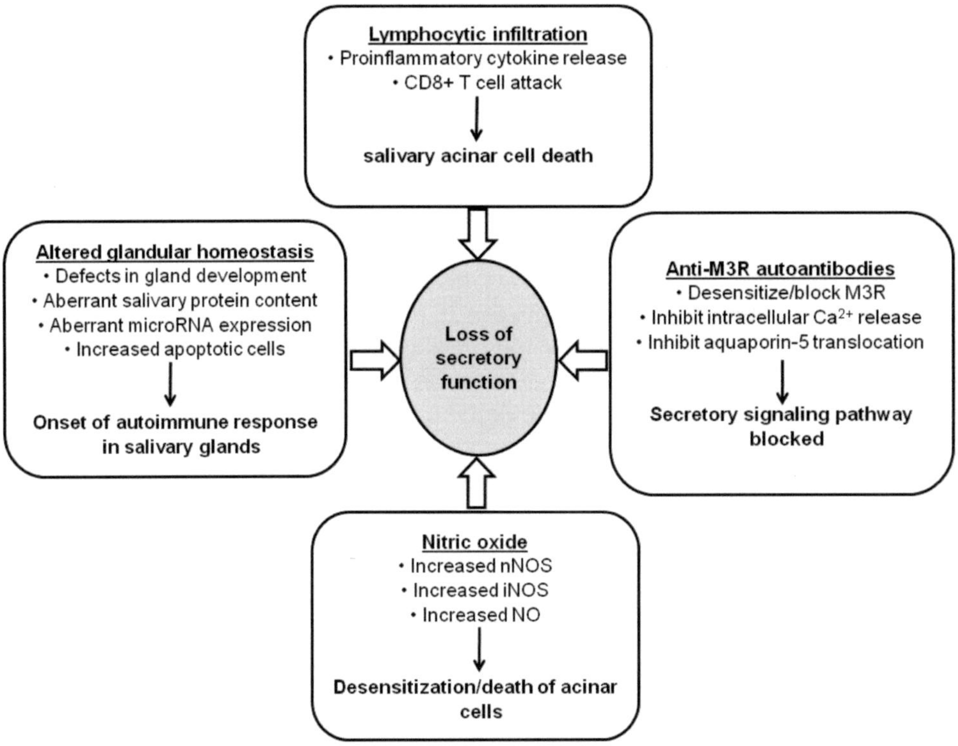

Fig. 4. Mechanisms contributing to secretory dysfunction in SS salivary glands.

3. Conclusion

In conclusion, it is evident that numerous mechanisms contribute to salivary gland dysfunction in SS. The initial trigger of autoimmune reactivity and which of these mechanisms, if any, are more important in SS pathogenesis remains to be seen. Also, it is unclear whether pre-existing genetic factors predetermine certain individuals to develop SS, or if there is a specific environmental or immunological trigger. It would be interesting and very informative to transplant the salivary glands of a pre-disease SS-prone mouse to a wild-type mouse to see if the recipient would still develop SS. This would identify whether a systemic environment or a glandular environment is critical for the onset of SS. Hopefully, ongoing research in the field of SS will lead to a better understanding of how the different mechanisms of secretory hypofunction discussed here can be prevented or circumvented to improve the quality of life of SS patients. There is a great need for potential new therapeutic strategies that can either turn off the autoimmune reaction in the exocrine tissue or preserve/replace the glandular tissue to restore secretory function.

4. Acknowledgment

The authors wish to acknowledge Mr. Yunjong Park for collecting latest articles on cytokines and summarized them for this chapter.

5. References

Alevizos, I., S. Alexander, R. J. Turner, and G. G. Illei. (2011). MicroRNA expression profiles as biomarkers of minor salivary gland inflammation and dysfunction in Sjogren's syndrome. *Arthritis Rheum,* Vol.63, No.2, pp. 535-44. ISSN: 1529-0131

Bacman, S., L. Sterin-Borda, J. J. Camusso, R. Arana, O. Hubscher, and E. Borda. (1996). Circulating antibodies against rat parotid gland M3 muscarinic receptors in primary Sjogren's syndrome. *Clin Exp Immunol,* Vol.104, No.3, pp. 454-9. ISSN: 0009-9104

Baker, O. J. (2010). Tight junctions in salivary epithelium. *J Biomed Biotechnol,* Vol.2010, pp. 278948. ISSN: 1110-7251

Beroukas, D., J. Hiscock, R. Jonsson, S. A. Waterman, and T. P. Gordon. (2001). Subcellular distribution of aquaporin 5 in salivary glands in primary Sjogren's syndrome. *Lancet,* Vol.358, No.9296, pp. 1875-6. ISSN: 0140-6736

Bikker, A., J. M. van Woerkom, A. A. Kruize, M. Wenting-van Wijk, W. de Jager, J. W. Bijlsma, F. P. Lafeber, and J. A. van Roon. (2010). Increased expression of interleukin-7 in labial salivary glands of patients with primary Sjogren's syndrome correlates with increased inflammation. *Arthritis and rheumatism,* Vol.62, No.4, pp. 969-77. ISSN: 1529-0131

Billiau, A. (1996). Interferon-gamma: biology and role in pathogenesis. *Advances in immunology,* Vol.62, pp. 61-130. ISSN: 0065-2776

Bodis, S., and A. Haregewoin. (1993). Evidence for the release and possible neural regulation of nitric oxide in human saliva. *Biochem Biophys Res Commun,* Vol.194, No.1, pp. 347-50. ISSN: 0006-291X

Bombardieri, M., F. Barone, V. Pittoni, C. Alessandri, P. Conigliaro, M. C. Blades, R. Priori, I. B. McInnes, G. Valesini, and C. Pitzalis. (2004). Increased circulating levels and salivary gland expression of interleukin-18 in patients with Sjogren's syndrome: relationship with autoantibody production and lymphoid organization of the periductal inflammatory infiltrate. *Arthritis Res Ther,* Vol.6, No.5, pp. R447-56. ISSN: 1478-6362

Bulosan, M., K. M. Pauley, K. Yo, E. K. Chan, J. Katz, A. B. Peck, and S. Cha. (2008). Inflammatory caspases are critical for enhanced cell death in the target tissue of Sjogren's syndrome before disease onset. *Immunol Cell Biol,* pp. ISSN: 0818-9641 (

Cai, F. Z., S. Lester, T. Lu, H. Keen, K. Boundy, S. M. Proudman, A. Tonkin, and M. Rischmueller. (2008). Mild autonomic dysfunction in primary Sjogren's syndrome: a controlled study. *Arthritis Res Ther,* Vol.10, No.2, pp. R31. ISSN: 1478-6362

Caulfield, V. L., C. Balmer, L. J. Dawson, and P. M. Smith. (2009). A role for nitric oxide-mediated glandular hypofunction in a non-apoptotic model for Sjogren's syndrome. *Rheumatology,* Vol.48, No.7, pp. 727-33. ISSN: 1462-0332

Cha, S., J. Brayer, J. Gao, V. Brown, S. Killedar, U. Yasunari, and A. B. Peck. (2004). A dual role for interferon-gamma in the pathogenesis of Sjogren's syndrome-like autoimmune exocrinopathy in the nonobese diabetic mouse. *Scand J Immunol,* Vol.60, No.6, pp. 552-65. ISSN: 0300-9475

Cha, S., H. Nagashima, V. B. Brown, A. B. Peck, and M. G. Humphreys-Beher. (2002). Two NOD Idd-associated intervals contribute synergistically to the development of autoimmune exocrinopathy (Sjogren's syndrome) on a healthy murine background. *Arthritis Rheum,* Vol.46, No.5, pp. 1390-8. ISSN: 0004-3591

Cha, S., E. Singson, J. Cornelius, J. P. Yagna, H. J. Knot, and A. B. Peck. (2006). Muscarinic acetylcholine type-3 receptor desensitization due to chronic exposure to Sjogren's syndrome-associated autoantibodies. *J Rheumatol,* Vol.33, No.2, pp. 296-306. ISSN: 0315-162X

Cha, S., S. C. van Blockland, M. A. Versnel, F. Homo-Delarche, H. Nagashima, J. Brayer, A. B. Peck, and M. G. Humphreys-Beher. (2001). Abnormal organogenesis in salivary gland development may initiate adult onset of autoimmune exocrinopathy. *Exp Clin Immunogenet,* Vol.18, No.3, pp. 143-60. ISSN: 0254-9670

Chan, E. K., J. C. Hamel, J. P. Buyon, and E. M. Tan. (1991). Molecular definition and sequence motifs of the 52-kD component of human SS-A/Ro autoantigen. *J Clin Invest,* Vol.87, No.1, pp. 68-76. ISSN: 0021-9738

Cheema, G. S., V. Roschke, D. M. Hilbert, and W. Stohl. (2001). Elevated serum B lymphocyte stimulator levels in patients with systemic immune-based rheumatic diseases. *Arthritis and rheumatism,* Vol.44, No.6, pp. 1313-9. ISSN: 0004-3591

Dawson, L. J., P. C. Fox, and P. M. Smith. (2006). Sjogrens syndrome--the non-apoptotic model of glandular hypofunction. *Rheumatology,* Vol.45, No.7, pp. 792-8. ISSN: 1462-0324

Denninger, J. W., and M. A. Marletta. (1999). Guanylate cyclase and the .NO/cGMP signaling pathway. *Biochim Biophys Acta,* Vol.1411, No.2-3, pp. 334-50. ISSN: 0006-3002

Dinarello, C. A. (1997). Proinflammatory and anti-inflammatory cytokines as mediators in the pathogenesis of septic shock. *Chest,* Vol.112, No.6 Suppl, pp. 321S-329S. ISSN: 0012-3692

Doreau, A., A. Belot, J. Bastid, B. Riche, M. C. Trescol-Biemont, B. Ranchin, N. Fabien, P. Cochat, C. Pouteil-Noble, P. Trolliet, I. Durieu, J. Tebib, B. Kassai, S. Ansieau, A. Puisieux, J. F. Eliaou, and N. Bonnefoy-Berard. (2009). Interleukin 17 acts in synergy with B cell-activating factor to influence B cell biology and the pathophysiology of systemic lupus erythematosus. *Nature Immunology,* Vol.10, No.7, pp. 778-85. ISSN: 1529-2916

Ewert, P., S. Aguilera, C. Alliende, Y. J. Kwon, A. Albornoz, C. Molina, U. Urzua, A. F. Quest, N. Olea, P. Perez, I. Castro, M. J. Barrera, R. Romo, M. Hermoso, C. Leyton, and M. J. Gonzalez. (2010). Disruption of tight junction structure in salivary glands from Sjogren's syndrome patients is linked to proinflammatory cytokine exposure. *Arthritis and rheumatism,* Vol.62, No.5, pp. 1280-9. ISSN: 1529-0131

Fox, R. I., and H. I. Kang. (1992). Pathogenesis of Sjogren's syndrome. *Rheum Dis Clin North Am,* Vol.18, No.3, pp. 517-38. ISSN: 0889-857X

Galione, A., H. C. Lee, and W. B. Busa. (1991). Ca(2+)-induced Ca2+ release in sea urchin egg homogenates: modulation by cyclic ADP-ribose. *Science,* Vol.253, No.5024, pp. 1143-6. ISSN: 0036-8075

Galione, A., A. White, N. Willmott, M. Turner, B. V. Potter, and S. P. Watson. (1993). cGMP mobilizes intracellular Ca2+ in sea urchin eggs by stimulating cyclic ADP-ribose synthesis. *Nature,* Vol.365, No.6445, pp. 456-9. ISSN: 0028-0836

Gao, J., S. Killedar, J. G. Cornelius, C. Nguyen, S. Cha, and A. B. Peck. (2006). Sjogren's syndrome in the NOD mouse model is an interleukin-4 time-dependent, antibody isotype-specific autoimmune disease. *J Autoimmun,* Vol.26, No.2, pp. 90-103. ISSN: 0896-8411

Gao, Juehua, Seunghee Cha, Roland Jonsson, Jeffrey Opalko, and Ammon B Peck. (2004). Detection of anti-type 3 muscarinic acetylcholine receptor autoantibodies in the sera of Sjögren's syndrome patients by use of a transfected cell line assay. *Arthritis Rheum,* Vol.50, No.8, pp. 2615-21.

Groom, J., S. L. Kalled, A. H. Cutler, C. Olson, S. A. Woodcock, P. Schneider, J. Tschopp, T. G. Cachero, M. Batten, J. Wheway, D. Mauri, D. Cavill, T. P. Gordon, C. R. Mackay, and F. Mackay. (2002). Association of BAFF/BLyS overexpression and altered B cell differentiation with Sjogren's syndrome. *The Journal of clinical investigation,* Vol.109, No.1, pp. 59-68. ISSN: 0021-9738

Haneji, N., T. Nakamura, K. Takio, K. Yanagi, H. Higashiyama, I. Saito, S. Noji, H. Sugino, and Y. Hayashi. (1997). Identification of alpha-fodrin as a candidate autoantigen in primary Sjogren's syndrome. *Science,* Vol.276, No.5312, pp. 604-7. ISSN: 0036-8075

Harmer, A. R., D. V. Gallacher, and P. M. Smith. (2001). Role of Ins(1,4,5)P3, cADP-ribose and nicotinic acid-adenine dinucleotide phosphate in Ca2+ signalling in mouse submandibular acinar cells. *Biochem J,* Vol.353, No.Pt 3, pp. 555-60. ISSN: 0264-6021

Hu, Y., K. R. Purushotham, P. Wang, R. Dawson, Jr., and M. G. Humphreys-Beher. (1994). Downregulation of beta-adrenergic receptors and signal transduction response in salivary glands of NOD mice. *Am J Physiol,* Vol.266, No.3 Pt 1, pp. G433-43. ISSN: 0002-9513

Kassan, S. S., and H. M. Moutsopoulos. (2004). Clinical manifestations and early diagnosis of Sjogren syndrome. *Arch Intern Med,* Vol.164, No.12, pp. 1275-84. ISSN: 0003-9926

Katsifis, G. E., S. Rekka, N. M. Moutsopoulos, S. Pillemer, and S. M. Wahl. (2009). Systemic and local interleukin-17 and linked cytokines associated with Sjogren's syndrome immunopathogenesis. *The American journal of pathology,* Vol.175, No.3, pp. 1167-77. ISSN: 1525-2191

Kendall, H. K., H. R. Haase, H. Li, Y. Xiao, and P. M. Bartold. (2000). Nitric oxide synthase type-II is synthesized by human gingival tissue and cultured human gingival fibroblasts. *J Periodontal Res,* Vol.35, No.4, pp. 194-200. ISSN: 0022-3484

Kendall, H. K., R. I. Marshall, and P. M. Bartold. (2001). Nitric oxide and tissue destruction. *Oral Dis,* Vol.7, No.1, pp. 2-10. ISSN: 1354-523X

Killedar, S. J., S. E. Eckenrode, R. A. McIndoe, J. X. She, C. Q. Nguyen, A. B. Peck, and S. Cha. (2006). Early pathogenic events associated with Sjogren's syndrome (SjS)-like disease of the NOD mouse using microarray analysis. *Lab Invest,* Vol.86, No.12, pp. 1243-60. ISSN: 0023-6837

Kimura-Shimmyo, A., S. Kashiwamura, H. Ueda, T. Ikeda, S. Kanno, S. Akira, K. Nakanishi, O. Mimura, and H. Okamura. (2002). Cytokine-induced injury of the lacrimal and salivary glands. *J Immunother,* Vol.25 Suppl 1, pp. S42-51. ISSN: 1524-9557

Knowles, R. G., and S. Moncada. (1994). Nitric oxide synthases in mammals. *Biochem J,* Vol.298 (Pt 2), pp. 249-58. ISSN: 0264-6021

Kong, L., C. P. Robinson, A. B. Peck, N. Vela-Roch, K. M. Sakata, H. Dang, N. Talal, and M. G. Humphreys-Beher. (1998). Inappropriate apoptosis of salivary and lacrimal gland epithelium of immunodeficient NOD-scid mice. *Clin Exp Rheumatol,* Vol.16, No.6, pp. 675-81. ISSN: 0392-856X

Konttinen, Y. T., L. A. Platts, S. Tuominen, K. K. Eklund, N. Santavirta, J. Tornwall, T. Sorsa, M. Hukkanen, and J. M. Polak. (1997). Role of nitric oxide in Sjogren's syndrome. *Arthritis Rheum,* Vol.40, No.5, pp. 875-83. ISSN: 0004-3591

Konttinen, Y. T., E. K. Tensing, M. Laine, P. Porola, J. Tornwall, and M. Hukkanen. (2005). Abnormal distribution of aquaporin-5 in salivary glands in the NOD mouse model for Sjogren's syndrome. *J Rheumatol,* Vol.32, No.6, pp. 1071-5. ISSN: 0315-162X

Kovacs, L., M. Papos, R. Takacs, R. Roka, Z. Csenke, A. Kovacs, T. Varkonyi, L. Pajor, L. Pavics, and G. Pokorny. (2003). Autonomic nervous system dysfunction involving the gastrointestinal and the urinary tracts in primary Sjogren's syndrome. *Clin Exp Rheumatol,* Vol.21, No.6, pp. 697-703. ISSN: 0392-856X

Lee, Byung Ha, Mauro A Tudares, and Cuong Q Nguyen. (2009). Sjögren's syndrome: an old tale with a new twist. *Arch. Immunol. Ther. Exp.,* Vol.57, No.1, pp. 57-66.

Li, J., Y. M. Ha, N. Y. Ku, S. Y. Choi, S. J. Lee, S. B. Oh, J. S. Kim, J. H. Lee, E. B. Lee, Y. W. Song, and K. Park. (2004). Inhibitory effects of autoantibodies on the muscarinic receptors in Sjogren's syndrome. *Lab Invest,* Vol.84, No.11, pp. 1430-8. ISSN: 0023-6837

Liew, F. Y. (1994). Regulation of nitric oxide synthesis in infectious and autoimmune diseases. *Immunol Lett,* Vol.43, No.1-2, pp. 95-8. ISSN: 0165-2478

Locksley, R. M. (1993). Interleukin 12 in host defense against microbial pathogens. *Proceedings of the National Academy of Sciences of the United States of America,* Vol.90, No.13, pp. 5879-80. ISSN: 0027-8424

Looms, D. K., S. Dissing, K. Tritsaris, A. M. Pedersen, and B. Nauntofte. (2000). Adrenoceptor-activated nitric oxide synthesis in salivary acinar cells. *Adv Dent Res,* Vol.14, pp. 62-8. ISSN: 0895-9374

Looms, D. K., K. Tritsaris, B. Nauntofte, and S. Dissing. (2001). Nitric oxide and cGMP activate Ca2+-release processes in rat parotid acinar cells. *Biochem J,* Vol.355, No.Pt 1, pp. 87-95. ISSN: 0264-6021

Looms, D., K. Tritsaris, A. M. Pedersen, B. Nauntofte, and S. Dissing. (2002). Nitric oxide signalling in salivary glands. *J Oral Pathol Med,* Vol.31, No.10, pp. 569-84. ISSN: 0904-2512

Mackay, F., S. A. Woodcock, P. Lawton, C. Ambrose, M. Baetscher, P. Schneider, J. Tschopp, and J. L. Browning. (1999). Mice transgenic for BAFF develop lymphocytic disorders along with autoimmune manifestations. *The Journal of experimental medicine,* Vol.190, No.11, pp. 1697-710. ISSN: 0022-1007

Manoussakis, M. N., S. Boiu, P. Korkolopoulou, E. K. Kapsogeorgou, N. Kavantzas, P. Ziakas, E. Patsouris, and H. M. Moutsopoulos. (2007). Rates of infiltration by macrophages and dendritic cells and expression of interleukin-18 and interleukin-12 in the chronic inflammatory lesions of Sjogren's syndrome: correlation with certain features of immune hyperactivity and factors associated with high risk of lymphoma development. *Arthritis and rheumatism,* Vol.56, No.12, pp. 3977-88. ISSN: 0004-3591

Mosaad, Y. M., S. S. Metwally, F. A. Auf, E. L. Samee E. R. Abd, B. el-Deek, N. I. Limon, and F. A. el-Chennawi. (2003). Proinflammatory cytokines (IL-12 and IL-18) in immune rheumatic diseases: relation with disease activity and autoantibodies production. *The Egyptian journal of immunology / Egyptian Association of Immunologists,* Vol.10, No.2, pp. 19-26. ISSN: 1110-4902

Nathan, C., and Q. W. Xie. (1994). Nitric oxide synthases: roles, tolls, and controls. *Cell,* Vol.78, No.6, pp. 915-8. ISSN: 0092-8674

Nguyen, C. Q., H. Yin, B. H. Lee, W. C. Carcamo, J. A. Chiorini, and A. B. Peck. (2010). Pathogenic effect of interleukin-17A in induction of Sjogren's syndrome-like disease using adenovirus-mediated gene transfer. *Arthritis research & therapy,* Vol.12, No.6, pp. R220. ISSN: 1478-6362

Nguyen, C. Q., H. Yin, B. H. Lee, J. A. Chiorini, and A. B. Peck. (2011). IL17: potential therapeutic target in Sjogren's syndrome using adenovirus-mediated gene transfer. *Laboratory investigation; a journal of technical methods and pathology,* Vol.91, No.1, pp. 54-62. ISSN: 1530-0307

Nguyen, Cuong Q, Jue-hua Gao, Hyuna Kim, Daniel R Saban, Janet G Cornelius, and Ammon B Peck. (2007). IL-4-STAT6 signal transduction-dependent induction of the clinical phase of Sjögren's syndrome-like disease of the nonobese diabetic mouse. *J Immunol,* Vol.179, No.1, pp. 382-90.

Nguyen, Cuong Q, Min H Hu, Yi Li, Carol Stewart, and Ammon B Peck. (2008). Salivary gland tissue expression of interleukin-23 and interleukin-17 in Sjögren's syndrome: findings in humans and mice. *Arthritis Rheum,* Vol.58, No.3, pp. 734-43.

Nguyen, K. H., J. Brayer, S. Cha, S. Diggs, U. Yasunari, G. Hilal, A. B. Peck, and M. G. Humphreys-Beher. (2000). Evidence for antimuscarinic acetylcholine receptor antibody-mediated secretory dysfunction in nod mice. *Arthritis Rheum,* Vol.43, No.10, pp. 2297-306. ISSN: 0004-3591

Ogawa, N., T. Kawanami, K. Shimoyama, L. Ping, and S. Sugai. (2004). Expression of interferon-inducible T cell alpha chemoattractant (CXCL11) in the salivary glands of patients with Sjogren's syndrome. *Clinical immunology,* Vol.112, No.3, pp. 235-8. ISSN: 1521-6616

Ogawa, N., L. Ping, L. Zhenjun, Y. Takada, and S. Sugai. (2002). Involvement of the interferon-gamma-induced T cell-attracting chemokines, interferon-gamma-inducible 10-kd protein (CXCL10) and monokine induced by interferon-gamma (CXCL9), in the salivary gland lesions of patients with Sjogren's syndrome. *Arthritis and rheumatism,* Vol.46, No.10, pp. 2730-41. ISSN: 0004-3591

Ohashi, M., M. Iwase, and M. Nagumo. (1999). Elevated production of salivary nitric oxide in oral mucosal diseases. *J Oral Pathol Med,* Vol.28, No.8, pp. 355-9. ISSN: 0904-2512

Pacher, P., J. S. Beckman, and L. Liaudet. (2007). Nitric oxide and peroxynitrite in health and disease. *Physiol Rev,* Vol.87, No.1, pp. 315-424. ISSN: 0031-9333

Palmer, R. M., A. G. Ferrige, and S. Moncada. (1987). Nitric oxide release accounts for the biological activity of endothelium-derived relaxing factor. *Nature,* Vol.327, No.6122, pp. 524-6. ISSN: 0028-0836

Park, K., R. V. Haberberger, T. P. Gordon, and M. W. Jackson. (2011). Antibodies interfering with the type 3 muscarinic receptor pathway inhibit gastrointestinal motility and cholinergic neurotransmission in Sjogren's syndrome. *Arthritis Rheum,* Vol.63, No.5, pp. 1426-34. ISSN: 1529-0131

Pauley, K. M., C. M. Stewart, A. E. Gauna, L. C. Dupre, R. Kuklani, A. L. Chan, B. A. Pauley, W. H. Reeves, E. K. Chan, and S. Cha. (2011). Altered miR-146a expression in Sjogren's syndrome and its functional role in innate immunity. *Eur J Immunol,* pp. ISSN: 1521-4141

Reksten, T. R., M. V. Jonsson, E. A. Szyszko, J. G. Brun, R. Jonsson, and K. A. Brokstad. (2009). Cytokine and autoantibody profiling related to histopathological features in primary Sjogren's syndrome. *Rheumatology,* Vol.48, No.9, pp. 1102-6. ISSN: 1462-0332

Robinson, C. P., J. Brayer, S. Yamachika, T. R. Esch, A. B. Peck, C. A. Stewart, E. Peen, R. Jonsson, and M. G. Humphreys-Beher. (1998). Transfer of human serum IgG to nonobese diabetic Igmu null mice reveals a role for autoantibodies in the loss of secretory function of exocrine tissues in Sjogren's syndrome. *Proc Natl Acad Sci U S A,* Vol.95, No.13, pp. 7538-43. ISSN: 0027-8424

Robinson, C. P., J. Cornelius, D. E. Bounous, H. Yamamoto, M. G. Humphreys-Beher, and A. B. Peck. (1998). Characterization of the changing lymphocyte populations and cytokine expression in the exocrine tissues of autoimmune NOD mice. *Autoimmunity,* Vol.27, No.1, pp. 29-44. ISSN: 0891-6934

Robinson, C. P., S. Yamachika, C. E. Alford, C. Cooper, E. L. Pichardo, N. Shah, A. B. Peck, and M. G. Humphreys-Beher. (1997). Elevated levels of cysteine protease activity in saliva and salivary glands of the nonobese diabetic (NOD) mouse model for Sjogren syndrome. *Proc Natl Acad Sci U S A,* Vol.94, No.11, pp. 5767-71. ISSN: 0027-8424

Robinson, C. P., H. Yamamoto, A. B. Peck, and M. G. Humphreys-Beher. (1996). Genetically programmed development of salivary gland abnormalities in the NOD (nonobese diabetic)-scid mouse in the absence of detectable lymphocytic infiltration: a potential trigger for sialoadenitis of NOD mice. *Clin Immunol Immunopathol,* Vol.79, No.1, pp. 50-9. ISSN: 0090-1229

Sakai, A., Y. Sugawara, T. Kuroishi, T. Sasano, and S. Sugawara. (2008). Identification of IL-18 and Th17 cells in salivary glands of patients with Sjogren's syndrome, and amplification of IL-17-mediated secretion of inflammatory cytokines from salivary gland cells by IL-18. *J Immunol,* Vol.181, No.4, pp. 2898-906. ISSN: 1550-6606

Sarih, M., V. Souvannavong, and A. Adam. (1993). Nitric oxide synthase induces macrophage death by apoptosis. *Biochem Biophys Res Commun,* Vol.191, No.2, pp. 503-8. ISSN: 0006-291X

Soinila, J., K. Nuorva, and S. Soinila. (2006). Nitric oxide synthase in human salivary glands. *Histochem Cell Biol,* Vol.125, No.6, pp. 717-23. ISSN: 0948-6143

Steinfeld, S., E. Cogan, L. S. King, P. Agre, R. Kiss, and C. Delporte. (2001). Abnormal distribution of aquaporin-5 water channel protein in salivary glands from Sjogren's syndrome patients. *Lab Invest,* Vol.81, No.2, pp. 143-8. ISSN: 0023-6837

Stohl, W., S. Metyas, S. M. Tan, G. S. Cheema, B. Oamar, D. Xu, V. Roschke, Y. Wu, K. P. Baker, and D. M. Hilbert. (2003). B lymphocyte stimulator overexpression in patients with systemic lupus erythematosus: longitudinal observations. *Arthritis and rheumatism,* Vol.48, No.12, pp. 3475-86. ISSN: 0004-3591

Takeda, I., Y. Kizu, O. Yoshitaka, I. Saito, and G. Y. Yamane. (2003). Possible role of nitric oxide in radiation-induced salivary gland dysfunction. *Radiat Res,* Vol.159, No.4, pp. 465-70. ISSN: 0033-7587

Tapinos, N. I., M. Polihronis, A. G. Tzioufas, and F. N. Skopouli. (1998). Immunopathology of Sjogren's syndrome. *Annales de medecine interne,* Vol.149, No.1, pp. 17-24. ISSN: 0003-410X

Tobin, G., D. Giglio, and O. Lundgren. (2009). Muscarinic receptor subtypes in the alimentary tract. *J Physiol Pharmacol,* Vol.60, No.1, pp. 3-21. ISSN: 1899-1505

Tsubota, K., S. Hirai, L. S. King, P. Agre, and N. Ishida. (2001). Defective cellular trafficking of lacrimal gland aquaporin-5 in Sjogren's syndrome. *Lancet,* Vol.357, No.9257, pp. 688-9. ISSN: 0140-6736

Vitali, C., S. Bombardieri, R. Jonsson, H. M. Moutsopoulos, E. L. Alexander, S. E. Carsons, T. E. Daniels, P. C. Fox, R. I. Fox, S. S. Kassan, S. R. Pillemer, N. Talal, and M. H. Weisman. (2002). Classification criteria for Sjogren's syndrome: a revised version of the European criteria proposed by the American-European Consensus Group. *Ann Rheum Dis,* Vol.61, No.6, pp. 554-8. ISSN: 0003-4967

Vosters, J. L., M. A. Landek-Salgado, H. Yin, W. D. Swaim, H. Kimura, P. P. Tak, P. Caturegli, and J. A. Chiorini. (2009). Interleukin-12 induces salivary gland dysfunction in transgenic mice, providing a new model of Sjogren's syndrome. *Arthritis and rheumatism,* Vol.60, No.12, pp. 3633-41. ISSN: 0004-3591

Wanchu, A., M. Khullar, A. Sud, and P. Bambery. (2000). Elevated nitric oxide production in patients with primary Sjogren's syndrome. *Clin Rheumatol,* Vol.19, No.5, pp. 360-4. ISSN: 0770-3198

Wang, F., M. W. Jackson, V. Maughan, D. Cavill, A. J. Smith, S. A. Waterman, and T. P. Gordon. (2004). Passive transfer of Sjogren's syndrome IgG produces the pathophysiology of overactive bladder. *Arthritis Rheum,* Vol.50, No.11, pp. 3637-45. ISSN: 0004-3591

Wang, Y., A. Shnyra, C. Africa, C. Warholic, and C. McArthur. (2009). Activation of the extrinsic apoptotic pathway by TNF-alpha in human salivary gland (HSG) cells in vitro, suggests a role for the TNF receptor (TNF-R) and intercellular adhesion molecule-1 (ICAM-1) in Sjogren's syndrome-associated autoimmune sialadenitis. *Archives of oral biology,* Vol.54, No.11, pp. 986-96. ISSN: 1879-1506

Waterman, S. A., T. P. Gordon, and M. Rischmueller. (2000). Inhibitory effects of muscarinic receptor autoantibodies on parasympathetic neurotransmission in Sjogren's syndrome. *Arthritis Rheum,* Vol.43, No.7, pp. 1647-54. ISSN: 0004-3591

Willmott, N., J. K. Sethi, T. F. Walseth, H. C. Lee, A. M. White, and A. Galione. (1996). Nitric oxide-induced mobilization of intracellular calcium via the cyclic ADP-ribose signaling pathway. *J Biol Chem,* Vol.271, No.7, pp. 3699-705. ISSN: 0021-9258

Yamamoto, H., N. E. Sims, S. P. Macauley, K. H. Nguyen, Y. Nakagawa, and M. G. Humphreys-Beher. (1996). Alterations in the secretory response of non-obese diabetic (NOD) mice to muscarinic receptor stimulation. *Clin Immunol Immunopathol,* Vol.78, No.3, pp. 245-55. ISSN: 0090-1229

Zhang, J., V. Roschke, K. P. Baker, Z. Wang, G. S. Alarcon, B. J. Fessler, H. Bastian, R. P. Kimberly, and T. Zhou. (2001). Cutting edge: a role for B lymphocyte stimulator in systemic lupus erythematosus. *Journal of immunology,* Vol.166, No.1, pp. 6-10. ISSN: 0022-1767

11

Sjögren's Syndrome: The Proteomic Approaches

Laura Giusti, Chiara Baldini, Laura Bazzichi,
Stefano Bombardieri and Antonio Lucacchini
Department of Psychiatry, Neurobiology, Pharmacology and Biotechnology,
Department of Internal Medicine, University of Pisa,
Italy

1. Introduction

Sjögren's syndrome (SS) is a chronic autoimmune disease characterised by epithelial cell destruction and by peri-epithelial B and T lymphocytic infiltration of multiple organ targets, and particularly of the exocrine glands. Salivary and lachrymal glands are emblematically involved, with dry mouth (xerostomia) and dry eyes (xerophtalmia) representing the clinical hallmarks of the disease. Moreover, despite the dominance of T cells in the glandular lesions, B cell activation plays a very prominent role as demonstrated by the presence of serum hypergammaglobulinemia, by the occurrence of a wide spectrum of autoantibodies (i.e., antinuclear antibodies, anti-Ro/SSA and anti-La/SSB antibodies, and Rheumatoid factor) and, in some cases, by the development of B cell lymphomas. High-throughput mass spectrometry approaches coupled with different separation techniques have been applied to several human rheumatic diseases in order to discover biomarkers and therapeutic targets by studying the proteome of biological fluids. We will describe our results obtained up to now on the proteomic analysis of whole saliva, particularly on how to distinguish primary and secondary SS manifestations. Moreover, we will report on the state of the art of proteomic studies of other biological fluids and of parotid gland tissues, focusing on the potentiality of proteomic applications in defining a panel of biomarkers useful in the diagnosis and therapy strategy of SS.

2. Clinical aspects

SS is a chronic inflammatory disease characterised by an autoimmune exocrinopathy of the lachrymal and salivary glands due to lymphocytic infiltrations. SS typically presents as dry eyes (xerophthalmia) and dry mouth (xerostomia). This process can manifest either as the independent phenomenon of primary SS or as a secondary when found in the context of another autoimmune process, most commonly rheumatoid arthritis, systemic lupus erythematosus or systemic sclerosis (Ramos-Casals et al., 2005a; Kassan & Moutsopoulos, 2004). Given the overlap of SS with many other rheumatic disorders, it is sometimes difficult to determine whether a clinical manifestation is a consequence of only SS or is due to one of its overlapping disorders.

2.1 Incidence and causes of Sjögren's syndrome

With a population prevalence ranging from 0.5 to 3%, SS appears to be a rather common disease (Binard et al., 2007). SS can develop at any age, but is most common in elderly people. Onset typically occurs in the fourth to fifth decade of life. It is frequent in women, who account for 9 out of 10 cases. The cause of SS remains unknown, but there is growing scientific support for genetic (inherited) and environmental factors. The presence of activated salivary gland epithelial cells expressing Major Histocompatibility Complex class II molecules and the identification of inherited susceptibility markers suggest that environmental or endogenous antigens trigger a self-perpetuating inflammatory response in susceptible individuals. Viruses are possible candidates for environmental triggers since Sjögren-like syndromes are seen in patients infected with HIV, hepatitis C and HTLV-1.

Damage and/or cell death due to viral infection or other causes may provide triggering antigens to Toll-like receptors in or on dendritic or epithelial cells, which, by recognising pathogen-associated patterns, are activated and begin producing cytokines, chemokines, and adhesion molecules. As T and B lymphocytes migrate into the gland, they themselves become activated by dendritic and epithelial cells, thereafter acting as antigen-presenting cells (Fox, 2005). Expressed antigens include SSA/Ro, SSB/La, alpha-fodrin and beta-fodrin, or cholinergic muscarinic receptors (Gottenberg et al., 2003). Recent studies suggest that the disease process of SS has a neuroendocrine component. Proinflammatory cytokines released by epithelial cells and lymphocytes may impair neural release of acetylcholine. In addition, Bolstad and colleagues (Bolstad et al., 2003) have focused on the role of apoptotic mechanisms in the pathogenesis of primary SS. A defect in Fas-mediated apoptosis, which is necessary for down-regulation of the immune response, can result in a chronic inflammatory destruction of the salivary gland, resembling SS.

2.2 Symptoms of Sjögren's syndrome

Symptoms of SS can involve the glands and /or other organs of the body (extra glandular manifestations). Glandular or exocrine manifestations of SS result from the periepithelial lymphocytic infiltration of the salivary and lacrimal glands. Inflammation of the salivary glands can lead to mouth dryness, swallowing difficulties, dental decay, cavities, gum disease, mouth sores and swelling, and stones and/or infection of the parotid gland. Dry lips often accompany the mouth dryness. Extraglandular problems in SS include joint pain or inflammation, Raynaud's phenomenon, lung inflammation, lymph node enlargement, and kidney, nerve and muscle disease. A rare serious complication of SS is inflammation of the blood vessels (vasculitis), which can damage body tissues supplied by these vessels. A common disease that is occasionally associated with SS is autoimmune thyroiditis (Hashimoto's thyroiditis), while a small percentage of patients with SS develop cancer of the lymph glands (lymphoma).

2.3 Diagnosis of Sjögren's syndrome and classification criteria

At present, the diagnosis of SS is based upon the combination of several clinical, serological, histological, and instrumental elements suggestive of both exocrine gland involvement and of typical laboratory abnormalities (antibodies anti-Ro/SSA and La/SSB). From a practical point of view, the diagnosis can be made according to the "American-European Consensus

Group Revised Classification Criteria, which were published in 2002 (Vitali et al., 2002) and revised in 2010 (Seror et al., 2010). Before their elaboration, there were several different concomitant criteria sets, varying in their emphasis, mostly on laboratory tests, on clinical features of dry eye and dry mouth, or on both. At that time, there was no uniform agreement on the diagnosis of primary SS, with substantial confusion in research publications and clinical-trial reports. The Revised Criteria exhibit approximately 95% sensitivity and specificity for SS, and due to their high specificity and sensitivity, they can be used as diagnostic criteria. They encompass the presence of subjective and objective sicca manifestations, antibodies to Ro/SS-A and La/SS-B antigens, and characteristic histopathologic findings in minor salivary glands with an average of 50 or more lymphocytes (focus) per 4 mmq of minor salivary gland samples. Of the 6 given criteria, 4 must be present to establish a diagnosis of SS, with 1 of the 4 being an objective measurement (i.e., by histopathologic examination or antibody screening) (Vitali et al., 2002). In their present state, the Classification Criteria are insufficient to make a clear diagnosis, and a certain proportion of patients may be misclassified, particularly in the early stages of the disorder, when the typical signs and symptoms are often lacking or are not entirely expressed. On the other hand, early diagnosis is crucial in avoiding destructive processes that frequently lead to a poor quality of life and early invalidity (Gran, 2002). Moreover, there is quite a weak correlation between clinical symptoms and the exocrinopathy measurements, and the assessment of organ involvement is currently limited to general markers of inflammation or organ function and needs profound improvement (Hay et al., 1998). Finally, no specific predictive factors of flares, disease relapses or disease outcomes have been described yet, even if unfavourable predictors have been thoroughly investigated, especially for lymphoproliferative disorders, which are the most serious complication in patients with SS (Gran, 2002; Manganelli et al., 2006; Voulgarelis et al., 1999).

2.4 Extra-glandular Sjögren's syndrome involvement

SS involves primarily the exocrine glands. Extraglandular involvement falls into two general categories. Peri-epithelial infiltrative processes include interstitial nephritis, liver involvement, and bronchiolitis, and generally follow a benign course. Extra-epithelial extra-glandular involvement in SS is related to B-cell hyper-reactivity, hyper-gammaglobulinemia, and immune complex formation, and includes palpable purpura, glomerulonephritis, and peripheral neuropathy. These latter manifestations occur later in the course of SS and are associated with a higher risk of transformation to lymphoma (Tzioufas & Voulgarelis, 2007). The incidence of systemic vasculitis manifestation in SS is approximately 5-10% of patients with SS (Ramos-Casals et al., 2005b). Skin involvement mainly manifests in the form of vasculitis cutaneous purpura. These lesions are clinically identical to those found in patients affected by systemic lupus erythematosus. In addition, Raynaud's phenomenon is a vascular condition with an incidence of 13% in patients with SS (Bayetto & Logan, 2010).

3. Applicability of proteomic to study rheumatic diseases

Proteomic approaches are expanding our ability to determinate changes in protein expression, and the technology used has rapidly evolved over the last decade allowing for more accurate quantitation of the differentially expressed proteins (Vanarsa & Mohan,

2010). In rheumatology, the application of proteomic in the search for potential biomarkers of the disease has produced a high number of reports concerning different diseases such as rheumatoid arthritis, systemic lupus erythematosus, ankylosing spondylitis, osteoarthritis, 333systemic sclerosis, and SS. Depending on the nature of the rheumatic disease, the choice of samples include saliva, serum, synovial fluid, urine, blood cells, cell lines (chondrocytes, synoviocytes, fibroblasts) or tissues (parotid glands, articular tissue, cartilage). Moreover, new applications have been found such as cerebro-spinal fluid in multiple sclerosis, peritoneal dialysate and haemodialysis fluid, broncoalveolar lavage fluid in interstitial lung disease. The aims have been to add new information about the disease pathogenesis and to identify protein biomarkers for non-invasive diagnosis, staging, and monitoring. A list of proteomic studies performed in rheumatic diseases in the last ten years is shown in table 1. Together, these studies underline the potentiality and applicability of proteomic in the study of rheumatic diseases. Unfortunately, there have not been any studies so far that have identified a panel of biomarkers with high specificity and sensitivity able to diagnose and predict rheumatic diseases.

Rheumatic diseases	References	Samples	Proteomic approach
Osteoartritis	De Ceuninck et al., 2005	cartilage	2DE/tandem MS
	Ruiz-Romero et al., 2005	chondrocytes	2DE/MALDI-TOF
	Gobezie et al., 2007	synovial fluid	1DE/electrospray ionization tandem MS (LC-ESI-MS)
	Wu et al., 2007	cartilage	2DE/nano-LC-tandem MS
	Guo et al., 2008	cartilage	2DE/linear ion trap-Fourier transform ion cyclotron resonance mass spectrometry
	Lambrecht et al., 2008	cartilage	2DE/tandem MS
	Rosenthal et al., 2011	cartilage	nano-LC-tandem MS
	de Seny et al., 2011	serum	SELDI-TOF-MS
	Ma et al., 2011	cartilage	2DDIGE/MALDI/TOF/MS
Spondyloarthritis	Tilleman et al., 2005	synovium	2DE/MALDI-TOF-ESI, tandem MS
	Wright et al., 2009	monocytes	2-DE/MALDI-TOF-MS
	Liu et al., 2007	serum	ESI-Q-TOF MS/MS
	Li et al., 2010	serum	2-DE/MALDI-TOF-MS
	Li et al., 2010	peripheral blood mononuclear cells	2-DE/MALDI-TOF-MS
Rheumatoid Arthritis	Sinz et al., 2002	serum, synovial fluid	2DE/MS

Rheumatic diseases	References	Samples	Proteomic approach
	Liao et al., 2004	serum, synovial fluid	LC/MS/MS
	Drynda et al., 2004	serum, synovial fluid	2DE/MS
	de Seny et al., 2005	serum	SELDI-TOF-MS
	Hueber et al., 2005	serum	antigen-microarrays
	Kim et al., 2006	synovial fluid	2DE/MALDI-TOF
	Matsuo et al., 2006	synovium	2DE/MALDI-TOF
	Schulz et al., 2007	peripheral blood mononuclear cells	2DE/MALDI-TOF
	Hueber et al., 2007	serum	antigen- microarrays
	de Seny et al., 2008	serum	SELDI-TOF-MS
	Zheng et al., 2009	plasma	capillary reversed-phase - HPLC/ion trap-FT-MS
	Chang et al., 2009	synovial tissues	2DE/MALDI-TOF
	Bo et al., 2009	synovial fibroblasts	2DE/MALDI-TOF-MS
	Giusti et al., 2010	saliva	2DE/MALDI-TOF-MS
	Li et al., 2010	serum	2DE/MALDI-TOF-MS
	Baillet et al., 2010	synovial fluid	SELDI-TOF-MS
	Matsuo et al., 2011	synoviocytes	phoshoproteomic
Wegener's Granulomatosis	Stone et al., 2005	serum	SELDI-TOF-MS
Systemic Sclerosis	Fietta et al., 2006	bronchoalveolar fluid	2DE/MALDI-TOF LC/MS/MS
	Giusti et al., 2007	saliva	2DE/MALDI-TOF
	Aden et al., 2008	skin	2DE /MALDI-TOF
	Scambi et al., 2010	serum	2DE/MALDI-TOF-MS
+ *Lupus erithematosus systemic*	Carlsson et al., 2011	serum	antibody microarray
Lupus erithematosus systemic	Pavon et al., 2006	plasma	2DE/MALDI-TOF-MS
	Mosley et al., 2006	urine	SELDI-TOF-MS

Rheumatic diseases	References	Samples	Proteomic approach
	Zhang et al., 2008	urine	SELDI-TOF-MS
	Dai et al., 2008	peripheral blood mononuclear cells	2DE/MALDI-TOF-MS
	Dai et al., 2010	serum	magnetic beads-based weak cation exchange chromatography/ MALDI-TOF-MS
	Lood et al., 2010	platelets	antigen- microarrays
	Wang et al., 2010	peripheral blood mononuclear cells	Isobaric tagging for relative and absolute protein quantification (iTRAQ)-multiple chromatographic fractionation and tandem mass spectrometry
Sjogren'Syndrome	Tomosugi et al., 2005	tears	SELDI-TOF-MS
	Ryu et al., 2006	parotid saliva	SELDI-TOF-MS/2D-DIGE
	Giusti et al., 2007	whole saliva	2DE/MALDI-TOF
	Stea et al., 2007	parotid glands	SDS-PAGE
	Peluso et al., 2007	whole saliva	HPLC-ESI/MS
	Hu et al., 2007b	whole saliva	2DE/MALDI-TOF-MS/LC-MS/MS
	Fleissig et al., 2009	whole saliva	2DE/MALDI-TOF-MS
	Hjelmervik et al., 2009	minor salivary glands	LC-ESI/MS-MS; 2DE/MALDI-TOF-MS
	Hu et al.2011	whole Saliva	protein microarrays
Fybromialgia	Bazzichi et al., 2009	whole saliva	2DE/MALDI-TOF
+ Chronic Fatigue Syndrome	Baraniuk et al., 2005	cerebrospinal fluid	capillary chromatography, quadrupole-time-of-flight mass spectrometry

Table 1. Proteomics in Rheumatology

4. Proteomic and Sjogren's syndrome

The majority of proteomic studies concerning SS chose saliva as the biological fluid (6 papers), and only a limited number used tears (1 paper) or salivary gland tissue (3 paper).

4.1 Tears

Histological and functional changes of the lachrymal gland might be reflected in proteomic patterns in tear fluids. In SS, a reduced production of aqueous tear was clarified when examined by the Schirmer test. Reduction of tear film stability as shown by the tear film break-up time test seems to be responsible for a disturbance of the quality of the mucus layer composition. However, there was no screening test for the changes in quality of tear components, which should accurately reflect the physiologic state of the lachrymal gland and the level of its function. The first proteomic trial for carrying out a determination of the disease biomarkers in tear fluid for SS was performed by Tomosugi and co-workers (Tomosugi et al., 2005). The authors, using surface-enhanced laser desorption/ionisation time-of-flight mass spectrometry, identified 10 potential novel proteins that differed between SS patients and control subjects. Seven were down regulated, and three correlated significantly with SS scores and epithelial damage of the ocular surface. Although these investigators have not yet identified the proteins, this study clearly demonstrates how such techniques can be applied in identifying specific protein profiles involved in the pathophysiological processes associated with SS.

4.2 Parotid glands tissue

Proteomic analysis has been applied not only to the study of salivary and lachrymal fluids, but also to the study of gland tissues because SS directly affects the glands and because autoantibodies characterising SS (anti-Ro/SSA and anti-La/SSB) are produced mainly in these affected tissues. Parotid gland extracts of SS patients were then analysed by combining conventional immunological methods (2DE and immunoblot) with mass spectrometry in order to evaluate modifications of known autoantigens (i.e., La/SSB), and in order to determine other targets of the autoimmune response in the parotid glands of SS patients. In the work by Stea and co-workers (Stea et al., 2007), in order to identify the isoforms of La/SSB in parotid glands of SS patients, an immunoblot with purified anti-La antibodies was performed after 2DE of parotid gland extracts from two SS patients. An extract from a human salivary gland epithelial cell line and a parotid gland extract from a patient with mixed parotid tumour were used as controls. The results of the study revealed that SS salivary glands contained high levels of post-translationally modified La/SSB autoantigen, degraded from 48 kDa to 34 kDa. The 48 kDa form of the protein was faintly recognised, in contrast to normal controls. Moreover, only five distinct La/SSB isoforms were detected in SS patients' specimens, in contrast to seven isoforms in controls. Finally, a new potential autoantigen was identified in the parotid glands of SS. A protein at around 45 kDa was recognised as a target of autoantibodies by the SS sera. This protein was identified as human actin by combining conventional immunological methods and mass spectrometry. Moreover, Hjelmervik and colleagues (Hjelmervik et al., 2009) conducted a large-scale mapping of the minor salivary gland proteome, applying two complementary methods: the LC-ESI-MS/MS and 2DE. The main objective of their work was to achieve a large-scale delineation of the minor salivary gland proteome in samples from both SS patients and non-SS controls. Heat shock proteins, mucins, carbonic anhydrases, enolase, vimentin, and cyclophillin B were among the proteins identified. Six proteins were exclusively identified in SS patients with respect the controls in particular alpha defensin 1 and calmodulin. A system biology approach has been used by Hu and co-workers (Hu et al., 2009) to study parotid gland tissue samples obtained from patients with primary SS, from patients with SS /MALT lymphoma, and from subjects without primary SS. The tissue samples were assessed by gene-expression microarray profiling and proteomics analysis. The authors defined a panel of 8 candidate genes for distinguishing primary SS/MALT lymphoma from primary SS. Among the 115 proteins showing >3-fold elevated levels, 20 proteins were up-regulated in primary SS parotid gland tissue samples as compared with non- primary SS control and primary SS/MALT lymphoma parotid gland tissue samples. Twenty-five proteins were up regulated in both primary SS and primary SS/MALT lymphoma samples as compared with non–primary SS control samples, and 70 proteins were up-regulated in primary SS/MALT lymphoma samples as compared with both non–primary SS control and primary SS samples. From a functional point of view, the proteins overexpressed in SS were related to the immune/defence response, apoptosis, cell-cell adhesion, and anti-oxidative stress, whereas many of the proteins with high expression in primary SS/MALT lymphoma were related to signal transduction, gene regulation, apoptosis, the immune response, and oxidative stress.

4.3 Saliva

Human saliva contains a large number of proteins and peptides, which have several important biological functions and potentially reflect both oral and systemic health conditions. Compared to blood, saliva possesses a smaller amount of proteins with a minor risk of non-specific interference. Saliva is an attractive medium for proteomic analysis for many different reasons. One of its major advantages is that salivary fluid can be obtained by using a non-invasive, simple, safe, and stress-free procedure that can be applied to large groups of subjects. The simple nature of saliva collection allows for repetition and multiple collection of saliva useful in early diagnosis, monitoring disease progression or treatment responses. Finally, this fluid undoubtedly reflects the salivary gland involvement that characterises SS disease (primary and secondary), which directly involves the oral cavity (Streckfus et al., 2007; Hu et al., 2007a).

Six studies have been performed in SS, and they are quite different in their principal goals as well as in their general methodologies (Ryu et al., 2006; Giusti et al., 2007; Hu et al., 2007b; Peluso et al., 2007; Flesseig et al., 2009; Hu et al., 2011). Whole saliva or individual glands saliva have been examined, and samples were collected both in stimulated and unstimulated conditions. Moreover, differences were present in salivary protein preparation and separation. However, although the collection protocol was different, many common biomarkers for SS have been found from the five different papers such as actin, Ig gamma-1 chain C region, beta-2 microglobulin, salivary amylase, carbonic anhydrase VI, prolactin inducible protein, calgranulins A and B, and fatty acid binding protein. Table 2 reports the proteomic studies performed up to now in saliva, distinguishing the source of this biofluid, and the type of proteomic approach. A list of potential biomarkers defined by these studies is also shown.

First, we will report the results obtained in other studies, and then in the following paragraph we will discuss our findings.

Study	Samples/Patients	Methods	Proteins differentially expressed
Ryu et al., 2006	stimulated parotid saliva/ primary Sjogren's syndrome	SELDI-TOF-MS/2D-DIGE	β2-microglobulin, lactoferrin, Ig □ light chain, l, polymeric Ig receptor (PIGR), lysozyme C, cystatin C, proline-rich proteins (PRPs), α-amylase, carbonic anhydrase VI
Giusti et al., 2007	unstimulated whole saliva primary Sjogren's syndrome	2DE/MALDI-TOF	carbonic anhydrase VI, cystatin S, cystatin C, cystatin D, calgranulin B, cyclophillin A, lipocalin-1, phosphatidylethanolammine-binding protein (PEPB), IgkC protein, zinc-α-glycoprotein, fatty acid binding protein (FABP), ACTB, β-actin fragment, leukocyte elastase inhibitor, glutathione-S-transferase, α-amylase precursor, cystatin SN precursor, keratin 6L, prolactine-inducible protein precursor
Peluso et al., 2007	unstimulated whole saliva primary and secondary Sjogren's syndrome	HPLC-ESI-MS	acidic and basic proline-rich proteins (PRPs), statherins, histatins, and cystatins, α-defensin 1, β-defensin 2, statherins
Hu et al.,2007b	Stimulated whole saliva/ parotid, submandibular, sublingual saliva primary Sjogren's syndrome	2DE/MALDI-TOF-MS/LC-MS-MS	carbonic anhydrase VI, polymeric immunoglobulin receptor, lysozime C, prolactin inducible protein, Von Ebner's gland protein, cystatin C, cystatin SN, cystatin D, cystatin S, cystatin SA, calgranulin A, calgranulin B, psoriasin, hemoglobin β-chain, hemoglobin α-1-globin chain, fatty acid binding protein epidermal, Ig-γ-1 chain C, Ig μ chain C region (IGHM), α-enolase, salivary α-amylase, fructose-biphosphate aldolase A, carbonic anhydrase I, carbonic anhydrase II, caspase 14, β2-microglobulin, actin, serum albumin
Fleissig et al.,2009	unstimulated whole saliva primary and secondary Sjogren's syndrome	2DE/ESI-MS-MS	calgranulin B, calgranulin A, Ig-γ-1 chain C, β-actin, serum albumin, keratine type I cytoskeletal, α-actin-1, α-amylase, vitamin D, polymeric-immunoglobulin receptor

Study	Samples/Patients	Methods	Proteins differentially expressed
Hu S et al., 2011	unstimulated whole saliva primary Sjogren's syndrome	protein microarrays	24 saliva autoantibodies: Bcl2 modifying factor, cardiolipin, chromosome X orf56, hypothetical protein DKFZp761G2113, Jun dimerization protein p21SNFT, La/SS-B, Lectin galactoside binding soluble 3, Lectin galactoside binding soluble 7, Megacaryocite-associated tyrosine Kinase, melanoma antigen family B 4, mesenchyme homeobox 1, NEFA-interacting nuclear protein, olfactory receptor family 6 N2, outer dense fiber of sperm tails 2, plasma membrane proteolipid, protein kinase C, ribosomal protein S6 kinase, Ro52/SS-A, SERPINA 3, small inducible cytokine subfamily E1, testis specific 10, TAO kinase 3, transglutaminase, Unfrac whole histone

Table 2. Saliva and Proteomic studies of Sjogren's syndrome.

The pilot study of proteomic applied to SS saliva was performed in 2006 by Ryu and co-workers. Using SELDI-TOF and 2D difference gel electrophoresis (2D-DIGE), they analysed stimulated parotid saliva from five healthy volunteers, 41 primary SS patients, and 20 non-SS subjects, including 15 non-SS subjects with complaints of xerostomia who, nonetheless, did not meet the diagnostic criteria for SS. Combining these two approaches, the authors focused their attention on ten differentially expressed proteins and, in particular, they identified significant increases of β-2 microglobulin, lactoferrin, Ig κ-light chain, polymeric Ig receptor, lysozyme C, and cystatin C. They also found in the patient group a reduction of amylase, carbonic anhydrase VI and of two presumed proline-rich proteins. Moreover, they found no association between the focus score and any biomarker. Lactoferrin and β2-microglobulin showed the greatest increases, but because their levels have been reported to increase also in other inflammatory diseases affecting salivary glands, the authors related these proteins to aspecific salivary gland inflammatory activity. More intriguingly, the increased levels of Ig κ-light chains were explained by the authors as being related to the increase in the intra-glandular immunoglobulin synthesis of the disease. Finally, the decrease of the two proline-rich proteins and α-amylase were ascribed to acinar parenchymal damage, while the reduction in carbonic anhydrase VI was reported as in line with a recent report on its decreased gene expression in SS minor gland biopsies.

Next, a profile of potential salivary proteomic and genomic biomarkers for SS was depicted by Hu and co-workers (Hu et al., 2007b). Sixteen WS proteins were found to be down-regulated, and 25 WS proteins were found to be up-regulated in SS patients compared with matched healthy control subjects. Moreover, using gene chip followed by real time PCR analysis of whole saliva, Hu and co-workers revealed factors such as interferon (IFN) and IFN-inducible protein G1P2 specifically expressed in SS patients. One of the important findings of this study was that many up-regulated genes were involved in the IFN pathway, suggesting the involvement of viral infection in SS pathogenesis.

Peluso and colleagues (Peluso et al., 2007) analysed the differences in the salivary protein profiles of primary SS and secondary SS patients, and of control subjects using HPLC-ESI-MS. The authors collected whole saliva specimens from 9 primary SS patients, 9 secondary SS patients (3 Rheumatoid Arthritis-2° SS; 3 systemic sclerosis-2° SS; 3 systemic lupus erythematosus-2° SS), and 10 healthy controls, and they analysed the levels and frequencies of 62 proteins. The analysis focused mainly on low molecular weight proteins represented by acid and basic proline-rich proteins, statherins, histatins, cystatins, lysozyme, and defensins. In the second part of the study, the authors examined the effect of pilocarpine on the salivary peptide and protein profiles in a subgroup of 6 primary SS patients. They found that the basic and acid proline-rich proteins and the statherins had the best response to the pilocarpine treatment, while the salivary cystatin and histatin protein classes were modified less. In the comparison between primary and secondary SS salivary profiles, the researchers outlined that patients with secondary SS showed a protein profile that was intermediate between that of the primary SS patients and the healthy subjects. In particular, salivary cystatins (C, S, S2, SA, and SN) and histatins (2, 3, 4, 7, 9, 11 and 12) were less frequently identifiable in primary and secondary SS patients versus controls. On the other hand, 3 proteins (IB-6, P-B Des1-4, and α-defensin 2) were identifiable in a significantly higher percentage of secondary SS patients than in the controls. In particular, α-defensin 2 was found in 6 of the primary SS patients, in 3 of the 9 secondary SS patients, and in none of the controls. Finally, IB-1 and statherin showed significantly lower levels in secondary SS than in the controls.

Additional information was reported by Flesseig and colleagues (Flesseig et al., 2009), who in a preliminary individual saliva sample analysis showed that SS patients (six SS patients as well as one symptomatic subject not fulfilling the criteria completely, and one who had developed follicular lymphoma) exhibited two patterns of protein expression with an indirect relation to the clinical serological or histological severity of disease.

Recently, Hu and co-workers (Hu et al., 2011) have demonstrated the potential of the high-throughput protein microarray approach in the discovery of autoantibody biomarkers for the non-invasive diagnosis of SS. Saliva autoantibodies present in patients with SS or systemic lupus erythematosus and healthy control subjects were profiled with protein microarrays. After comparison with controls (systemic lupus erythematosus and healthy subjects), statistical analysis of the microarray data revealed 24 autoantibody biomarkers that could differentiate SS from both control groups. A validation of four of these autoantibodies (anti-SSA, anti-SSB, anti-transglutamine, anti-histone) was performed using commercial ELISA kits. Although these are known autoantibodies in SS, they were usually tested in serum samples. The authors suggest that testing these autoantibodies in saliva may be valuable for the diagnosis of SS. Therefore, up to now a wide spectrum of proteins has been identified that might include both "true" disease biomarkers, as well as specific markers of tissue damage (i.e., actin) or inflammation (calgranulins). Therefore, we can hypothesise that further studies might shed some light on this aspect.

4.3.1 Our results

In 2005, we began to study rheumatic diseases using a proteomic approach. In our studies, whole saliva was chosen as the biological fluid to discover specific disease biomarkers for primary and secondary manifestations of SS and also of other correlated rheumatic diseases such as systemic sclerosis (Giusti et al., 2007; Baldini et al., 2008), fybromialgia (Bazzichi et al., 2009) and rheumatoid arthritis (Giusti et al., 2010). In our work on SS, we analysed the whole saliva of 12 primary SS patients in comparison with 12 healthy controls by using quantitative 2DE experiments combined with MALDI-TOF-MS for protein identification (Giusti et al., 2007). In particular, in this study, by comparing the SS with control classes, we found that 4 proteins were unique to the control samples (carbonic anhydrase VI, cystatins S, C precursor and cystatin D), and 6 proteins were unique to the SS samples (calgranulin B, cyclophilin A, lipocalin-1 precursor, phosphatidyl ethanolammine binding protein, Ig kappa chain C region (IGKC), protein and Zinc-α-2 glycoprotein precursor). Moreover, in evaluating the mean ± SD of the percentage of the volume of each single protein of the analytical (not synthetic) gels, the authors also discovered that 10 protein spots were up-regulated with > 2-fold changes (fatty acid binding protein (E-FABP), ACTB protein, α-actin fragment, leukocyte elastase inhibitor, glutathione-S-transferase (GST), and 5 unidentified proteins). On the other hand, 4 were down regulated (α-amylase precursor, cystatin SN precursor, keratin 6L, prolactin-inducible protein precursor) in SS patients compared with controls. These results confirmed the decrease of some of the typical acinar proteins and the increase of many inflammatory proteins. Moreover, they outlined the relevance of proteins not previously described i.e., PIP, keratin 6L, and lipocalin, as markers of acinar damage and oral environment alteration. This study was the basis for further investigations aimed at characterising possible differences in salivary protein profiles in patients who have connective tissue diseases associated with secondary SS. Therefore, we extended the study to refine the diagnostic power of a panel of candidate salivary biomarkers described in SS with respect to both healthy volunteers and pathological controls (sicca syndrome). Moreover, the aim of the study was also to explore the biological and pathogenetic functions of the putative salivary proteomic biomarkers, both in the local exocrinopathy and in the systemic inflammatory autoimmune systemic processes of SS. Our preliminary results, to be published, suggest that novel, non-invasively-collected salivary proteomic biomarkers might be helpful in an early and accurate characterisation of primary and secondary SS. In addition, some of the secondary SS identified biomarkers apparently reflected not only the SS component, but also the concomitant systemic autoimmune disorders, shedding new light on the potential diagnostic role of saliva in autoimmune diseases irrespectively of salivary gland involvement.

The capacity of whole saliva to reflect systemic conditions was also suggested from the preliminary unpublished results of a case study on the salivary proteome of non-Hodgkin' lymphomas. We observed that clinical and functional changes of the salivary glands driven by autoimmune and lymphoproliferative processes might be reflected in patients' whole saliva proteins, and that there was a specific correspondence between clinical improvement and proteomic changes of the salivary peptide complex. These observations indicate the potential usefulness of proteomic analysis in discovering not only diagnostic but also prognostic and therapeutic biomarkers for patients with primary SS and non-Hodgkin's lymphomas. Therefore, we speculate that during the follow-up of patients with lymphomas, proteomic analysis might be able to use the salivary biomarkers as early predictors of treatment response. From the perspective of the research, the analysis of biomarker signatures in saliva could also help to clarify the pathogenetic pathways underlying lymphoproliferation in SS, leading to the development of new methods in early diagnosis and curative therapies.

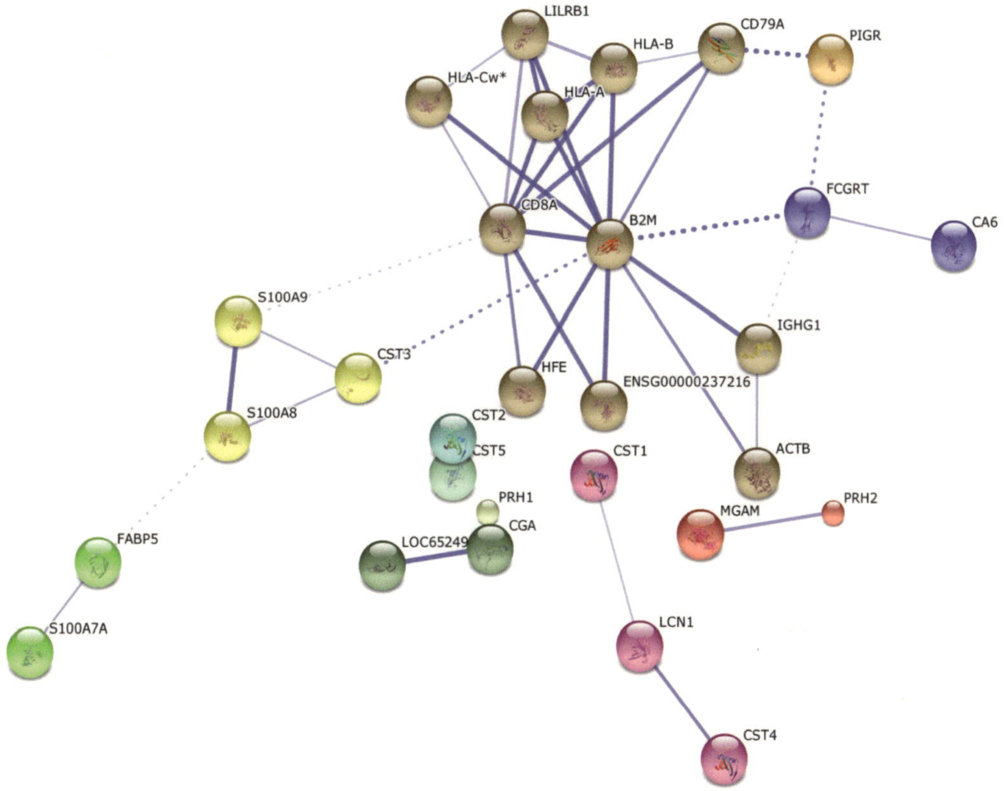

Fig. 1. Protein-protein interaction network of regulated pSS-associated proteins identified in at least two proteomic studies found differentially expressed in saliva. The STRING tool (http://string-db.org/) was used making the network with the following proteins: β-2-microglobulin, polymeric Ig receptor (PIGR), salivary acidic proline-rich phosphoprotein 1 (PRH1) and 2 (PRH2), α-amylase, carbonic anhydrase VI, Cystatin SA (CST2), Cystatin SN (CST1), Cystatin C (CST3), Cystatin S (CST4), Cystatin D (CST5), LCN1, Calgranulin A (S100A8), Calgranulin B (S100A9), Psoriasin (S100A7), Fatty acid-binding protein, epidermal (FABP5), IGKC (LOC652493), Ig γ-1 chain C region (IGHG1), β-Actin (ACTB), Fc fragment of IgG, receptor, transporter (FCGRT), leukocyte immunoglobulin-like receptor (LILRB1), HLA class I histocompatibility antigen, alpha chain G (ENSG00000237216) , major histocompatibility complex class IA (HLA-A) major histocompatibility complex class IB (HLA-B) and glycoprotein hormones, alpha polypeptide (CGA). In the figure is shown the potential interaction with additional proteins with score values ranging from 0.993 to 0.999. The different clusters are indicated by the same colour. The thickness of the connecting lines indicates the level of confidence.

5. Conclusions

SS lacks any true diagnostic criteria for primary and secondary manifestations as well as a set of activity criteria. The risk of misdiagnosis is still quite high, and it highlights the need for a more definitive set of tests and criteria to classify these patients. One possible solution is the proteomic approach, which might represent a promising tool to explore biomarkers for diagnostic aims. Until now, the studies performed have been carried out on parotid biopsies, tears, and saliva. Saliva represents an attractive medium for proteomic analysis because its composition is not complex, and it reflects more accurately the current state of the organism at any moment. Moreover, it presents many logistical advantages because the collection is not invasive, and may be repeated for monitoring over time. However, the identification of true biomarkers of primary and secondary SS is still in its infancy. The results obtained from different studies have not yet defined a conclusive panel of biomarkers useful in diagnostic purposes. Nonetheless, some conclusions can be drawn: SS patients showed a decrease of proteins of glandular origins and an increase of inflammatory proteins, while the salivary profile of secondary SS is intermediate between that of primary SS patients and healthy subjects. Figure 1 shows a representative interactive network obtained by STRING analysis among the proteins found differentially expressed in the proteomic studies performed in saliva. In addition to identifying proteins, we enlarged the network to obtain a large interactive network with more nodes. Interestingly, the figure shows that β-2 microglobulin, which is the invariant chain of the Major Histocompatibility Complex class I molecules, considered as a marker of B cell activation, is the key node of the main cluster.

6. Acknowledgement

The authors wish to thanks Dr Laura Fatuzzo for her valuable contribution in reviewing the text.

7. References

Aden, N., Shiwen, X., Aden, D., Black, C., Nuttall, A., Denton, C.P., Leask ,A., Abraham, D. & Stratton, R. (2008). Proteomic analysis of scleroderma lesional skin reveals activated wound healing phenotype of epidermal cell layer. *Rheumatology (Oxford)*, Vol. 47, No. 12, (December 2008), pp. 1754-1760, ISSN 1462-0324.

Baillet, A., Trocmé, C., Berthier, S., Arlotto, M., Grange, L., Chenau, J., Quétant, S.,Sève, M., Berger, F., Juvin, R., Morel, F. & Gaudin, P. (2010). Synovial fluid proteomic fingerprint: S100A8, S100A9 and S100A12 proteins discriminate rheumatoid arthritis from other inflammatory joint diseases. *Rheumatology (Oxford)*, Vol. 49, No. 4 (April 2010), pp. 671-682, ISSN 1462-0324.

Baldini, C., Giusti, L., Bazzichi, L., Ciregia, F., Giannaccini, G., Giacomelli, C., Doveri, M., Del Rosso, M., Bombardieri, S. & Lucacchini, A. (2008). Association of psoriasin (S100A7) with clinical manifestations of systemic sclerosis: is its presence in whole saliva a potential predictor of pulmonary involvement? *Journal of Rheumatology*, Vol. 35, No. 9, (September 2009), pp.1820-1824, ISSN 0315-162X.

Baraniuk, J.N., Casado, B., Maibach, H., Clauw, D.J., Pannell, L.K. & Hess, S.S. (2005). A Chronic Fatigue Syndrome-related proteome in human cerebrospinal fluid. *BMC Neurology*, Vol. 5, No. 22, (December 2005), ISSN 1471-2377.

Bayetto, K. & Logan, R.M. Sjögren's syndrome: a review of aetiology, pathogenesis, diagnosis and management. (2010). *Australian Dental Journal*, Vol. 55, No 1, (June 2010), pp. 39-47, ISSN 0045-0421

Bazzichi, L., Ciregia, F., Giusti, L., Baldini, C., Giannaccini, G., Giacomelli, C., Servissi, F., Bombardieri, S. & Lucacchini, A. (2009). Detection of potential markers of primary fibromyalgia syndrome in human saliva. *Proteomics Clinical Applications*, Vol. 3, No. 11, (November 2009), pp. 1296-1304, ISSN 1862-8346.

Binard, A., Devauchelle-Pensec, V., Fautrel, B., Jousse, S., Youinou, P. & Saraux, A. Epidemiology of Sjögren's syndrome: where are we now? (2007). *Clinical and Experimental Rheumatology*, Vol. 25, No. 1, (January 2007), pp. 1-4, ISSN 0392-856X.

Bo, G.P., Zhou, L.N., He, W.F., Luo, G.X., Jia, X.F., Gan, C.J., Chen, G.X., Fang, Y.F., Larsen, P.M. & Wu, J. (2009). Analyses of differential proteome of human synovial fibroblasts obtained from arthritis. *Clinical Rheumatology*, Vol. 28, No. 2, (February 2009), pp. 191-199, ISSN 0770-3198.

Bolstad, A.I., Eiken, H.G., Rosenlund, B., Alarcón-Riquelme, M.E. & Jonsson, R. Increased salivary gland tissue expression of Fas, Fas ligand, cytotoxic T lymphocyte-associated antigen 4, and programmed cell death 1 in primary Sjögren's syndrome. (2003). *Arthritis and Rheumatism*, Vol. 48, No.1, (January 2003), pp. 174-185, ISSN 0004-3591.

Carlsson, A., Wuttge, D.M., Ingvarsson, J., Bengtsson, A.A., Sturfelt, G., Borrebaeck, C.A. & Wingren, C. Serum protein profiling of systemic lupus erythematosus and systemic sclerosis using recombinant antibody microarrays. (2011). *Molecular Cellular Proteomics*, Vol. 10, No. 5, (May 2011), doi: 10.1074/mcp.M110.005033, ISSN 1535-9476.

Chang, X., Cui, Y., Zong, M., Zhao, Y., Yan, X., Chen, Y. & Han, J. Identification of proteins with increased expression in rheumatoid arthritis synovial tissues. (2009). *Journal of Rheumatology*, Vol. 36, No. 5, (May 2009), pp. 872-880, ISSN 0315-162X.

Dai, Y., Hu, C., Huang, Y., Huang, H., Liu, J. & Lv, T. A proteomic study of peripheral blood mononuclear cells in systemic lupus erythematosus. (2008). *Lupus*, , Vol. 17, No. 9, (September 2008), pp. 799-804, ISSN 0961-2033.

Dai, Y., Hu, C., Wang, L., Huang, Y., Zhang, L, Xiao, X. & Tan, Y. Serum peptidome patterns of human systemic lupus erythematosus based on magnetic bead separation and MALDI-TOF mass spectrometry analysis. (2010). *Scandinavian Journal of Rheumatology*, Vol. 39, No. 3, (May 2010), pp. 240-246, ISSN 0300-9742.

De Ceuninck, F., Marcheteau, E., Berger, S., Caliez, A., Dumont, V., Raes, M., Anract, P., Leclerc, G., Boutin, J.A. & Ferry, G. (2005). Assessment of some tools for the characterization of the human osteoarthritic cartilage proteome. *Journal Biomolecular Techniques*, Vol. 16, No. 3, (September 2005), pp. 256-265, ISSN: 1524-0215.

de Seny, D., Fillet, M., Meuwis, M.A., Geurts, P., Lutteri, L., Ribbens, C., Bours, V., Wehenkel, L., Piette, J., Malaise, M. & Merville, M.P. (2005). Discovery of new rheumatoid arthritis biomarkers using the surface-enhanced laser desorption/ionization time-of-flight mass spectrometry ProteinChip approach. *Arthritis and Rheumatism*, Vol.52, No.12, (December 2005), pp. 3801-3812, ISSN 0004-3591.

de Seny, D., Fillet, M., Ribbens, C., Marée, R., Meuwis, M.A., Lutteri, L., Chapelle, J.P., Wehenkel, L., Louis, E., Merville, M.P. & Malaise, M. Monomeric calgranulins measured by SELDI-TOF mass spectrometry and calprotectin measured by ELISA as biomarkers in arthritis. (2008). *Clinical Chemistry*, Vol. 54, No. 6, (June 2008), pp.1066-1075, ISSN 0009-9147.

de Seny, D., Sharif, M., Fillet, M., Cobraiville, G., Meuwis, M.A., Marée, R., Hauzeur, J.P., Wehenkel, L., Louis, E., Merville, M.P., Kirwan, J., Ribbens, C. & Malaise, M. Discovery and biochemical characterisation of four novel biomarkers for osteoarthritis. (2011). *Annals of Rheumatic Diseases.* Vol. 70, No. 6 (June 2011), pp.1144-1152, ISSN 0003-4967.

Drynda, S., Ringel, B., Kekow, M., Kühne, C., Drynda, A., Glocker, M.O., Thiesen, H.J. & Kekow, J. Proteome analysis reveals disease-associated marker proteins to differentiate RA patients from other inflammatory joint diseases with the potential to monitor anti-TNF-alpha therapy. (2004). *Pathology Research and Practice,* Vol. 200, No. 2, pp. 165-171, ISSN 0344-0338.

Fietta, A., Bardoni, A., Salvini, R., Passadore, I., Morosini, M., Cavagna, L., Codullo, V., Pozzi, E., Meloni, F. & Montecucco, C. (2006). Analysis of bronchoalveolar lavage fluid proteome from systemic sclerosis patients with or without functional, clinical and radiological signs of lung fibrosis. *Arthritis Research & Therapy,* Vol. 8, No 6, (June 2006), pp. R160, ISSN 1478-6354.

Fleissig, Y, Deutsch, O., Reichenberg, E., Redlich, M., Zaks, B., Palmon, A. & Aframian, D.J. Different proteomic protein patterns in saliva of Sjögren's syndrome patients. (2009). *Oral Diseases,* Vol. 15, No. 1, (January 2009), pp. 61-68, ISSN 1354-523X.

Fox, R.I. Sjogren's Syndrome. (2005). *Lancet,* Vol. 366, No. 9482, (July 2005), pp. 321-331, ISSN 0140-6736.

Giusti, L., Baldini, C., Bazzichi, L., Ciregia, F., Tonazzini, I., Mascia, G., Giannaccini, G., Bombardieri, S.& Lucacchini, A. Proteome analysis of whole saliva: a new tool for rheumatic diseases--the example of Sjögren's syndrome. (2007) *Proteomics,* Vol. 7, No. 10, (May 2007), pp. 1634-1643, ISSN 1615-9853.

Giusti, L., Baldini, C., Ciregia, F., Giannaccini, G., Giacomelli, C., De Feo, F., Delle Sedie, A., Riente, L., Lucacchini, A., Bazzichi, L, & Bombardieri, S. Is GRP78/BiP a potential salivary biomarker in patients with rheumatoid arthritis? (2010). *Proteomics Clinical Application,* Vol. 4, No. 3, (March 2010), pp. 315-324, ISSN 1862-8346.

Giusti, L., Bazzichi, L., Baldini, C., Ciregia, F., Mascia, G., Giannaccini, G., Del Rosso, M., Bombardieri, S. & Lucacchini, A. Specific proteins identified in whole saliva from patients with diffuse systemic sclerosis. (2007). *Journal of Rheumatology,* Vol. 34, No. 10, (October 2007), pp. 2063-2069, ISSN 0315-162X.

Godezie, R., Kho, A., Krastins, B., Saracino, D.A., Thornhill, T.S., Chase, M., Millett, P.J. & Lee, D.M. High abundance synovial fluid proteome: distinct profiles in health and osteoarthritis. (2007). *Arthritis Research & Therapy,* Vol. 9, No. 2, (February 2007), pp. R36, ISSN 1478-6354.

Gottenberg, J.E., Busson, M., Loiseau, P., Cohen-Solal, J., Lepage, V., Charron, D., Sibilia, J. & Mariette, X. In primary Sjögren's syndrome, HLA class II is associated exclusively with autoantibody production and spreading of the autoimmune response. (2003). *Arthritis and Rheumatism,* Vol. 48, No. 8, (August 2003), pp. 2240-2245, ISSN 0004-3591.

Gran, J.T. Diagnosis and definition of primary Sjögren's syndrome. *Scandinavian Journal of Rheumatology,* Vol. 31, No. 2, (February 2002), pp. 57-59 (2002), ISSN 0300-9742.

Guo, D., Tan, W., Wang, F., Lv, Z., Hu, J., Lv, T., Chen, Q., Gu ,X., Wan, B. & Zhang, Z. Proteomic analysis of human articular cartilage: identification of differentially expressed proteins in knee osteoarthritis. (2008). *Joint Bone Spine,* Vol. 75, No. 4, (July 2008), pp. 439-444, ISSN 1297-319X.

Hay, E.M., Thomas, E., Pal, B., Hajer, A., Chambers, H. & Silman, A.J. Weak association between subjective symptoms and objective testing for dry eyes and mouth: results from a population based study. (1998). *Annals of Rheumatic Diseases.* Vol. 57, No.1, (January 1998), pp. 20-24, ISSN 0003-4967.

Hjelmervik, T.O., Jonsson, R.& Bolstad, A.I. The minor salivary gland proteome in Sjögren's syndrome. (2009). *Oral Diseases,* Vol. 15, No. 5, (July 2009), pp. 342-353, ISSN 1354-523X.

Hu, S., Loo, J.A. & Wong, D.T. Human saliva proteome analysis. (2007a), *Annals of the New York Academy of Sciences,* Vol. 1098, (March 2007), pp. 323-329, ISSN 0077-8923.

Hu, S., Wang, J., Meijer, J., Ieong, S., Xie, Y., Yu, T., Zhou, H., Henry, S., Vissink, A., Pijpe, J., Kallenberg, C., Elashoff, D., Loo, J.A. & Wong, D.T. Salivary proteomic and genomic biomarkers for primary Sjögren's syndrome. (2007b). *Arthritis and Rheumatism,* Vol. 56, No.11, (November 2007), pp. 3588-3600, ISSN 0004-3591.

Hu, S., Vissink, A., Arellano, M., Roozendaal, C., Zhou, H., Kallenberg, C.G. & Wong, D.T. Identification of autoantibody biomarkers for primary Sjögren's syndrome using protein microarrays. (2011). *Proteomics,* Vol. 11, No. 8, (April 2011), pp. 1499-1507, ISSN 1615-9853.

Hu, S., Zhou, M., Jiang, J., Wang, J., Elashoff, D., Gorr, S., Michie, S.A., Spijkervet, F.K., Bootsma, H., Kallenberg, C.G., Vissink, A., Horvath, S. & Wong, D.T. Systems biology analysis of Sjögren's syndrome and mucosa-associated lymphoid tissue lymphoma in parotid glands. (2009). *Arthritis and Rheumatism,* Vol. 60, No. 1, (January 2009), pp. 81-92, ISSN 0004-3591.

Hueber, W., Kidd, B.A., Tomooka, B.H., Lee, B.J., Bruce, B., Fries, J.F., Sønderstrup, G., Monach, P., Drijfhout, J.W., van Venrooij, W.J., Utz, P.J., Genovese, M.C. & Robinson, W.H. Antigen microarray profiling of autoantibodies in rheumatoid arthritis. (2005). *Arthritis and Rheumatism,* Vol. 52, No. 9 (September 2009), pp. 2645-2655, ISSN 0004-3591.

Hueber, W., Tomooka, B.H., Zhao, X., Kidd, B.A., Drijfhout, J.W., Fries, J.F., van Venrooij, W.J., Metzger, A.L., Genovese, M.C.& Robinson, W.H. Proteomic analysis of secreted proteins in early rheumatoid arthritis: anti-citrulline autoreactivity is associated with up regulation of proinflammatory cytokines. (2007). *Annals of Rheumatic Diseases,* Vol. 66, No. 6, (June 2007), pp. 712-719, ISSN 0003-4967.

Kassan, S.S. & Moutsopoulos, H.M. Clinical manifestations and early diagnosis of Sjögren's syndrome. (2004). *Archives of Internal Medicine,* Vol. 164, No. 12, (June 2004), pp. 1275-1284, ISSN 0003-9926.

Kim, C.W., Cho, E.H., Lee, Y.J., Kim, Y.H., Hah, Y.S. & Kim, D.R. Disease-specific proteins from rheumatoid arthritis patients. (2006). *Journal of Korean Medical Science,* Vol. 21, No. 3 (June 2006), pp. 478-484, ISSN 1011-8934.

Lambrecht, S., Verbruggen, G., Verdonk, P.C., Elewaut, D. & Deforce, D. Differential proteome analysis of normal and osteoarthritic chondrocytes reveals distortion of vimentin network in osteoarthritis. (2008). *Osteoarthritis and Cartilage,* Vol. 16, No. 2, (February 2008), pp. 163-173, ISSN 1063-4584.

Li, T., Huang, Z., Zheng, B., Liao, Z., Zhao, L.& Gu, J. Serum disease-associated proteins of ankylosing spondylitis: results of a preliminary study by comparative proteomics. (2010). *Clinical and Experimental Rheumatology,* Vol. 28, No. 2, (March 2010), pp. 201-207. ISSN 0392-856X.

Li, T., Zheng, B., Huang, Z., Lu, H., Lin, Q., Liao, Z., Lin, Z., Zhao, L., Wang, X. & Gu, J. Over-expression of talin 1 and integrin-linked kinase in PBMCs of patients with ankylosing spondylitis: a proteomic study. (2010). *Clinical and Experimental Rheumatology,* Vol. 28, No. 6, (November 2010), pp. 828-835, ISSN 0392-856X.

Li, T.W., Zheng, B.R., Huang, Z.X., Lin, Q., Zhao, L.K., Liao, Z.T., Zhao, J.J., Lin, Z.M. & Gu, J.R. Screening disease-associated proteins from sera of patients with rheumatoid arthritis: a comparative proteomic study. (2010). *Chinese Medical Journal (Engl).* Vol. 5, No. 123, Suppl. 5, (March 2010), pp. 537-43. ISSN 0366-6999.

Liao, H., Wu, J., Kuhn, E., Chin, W., Chang, B., Jones, M.D., O'Neil, S., Clauser, K.R., Karl, J., Hasler, F., Roubenoff, R., Zolg, W.& Guild, B.C. Use of mass spectrometry to identify protein biomarkers of disease severity in the synovial fluid and serum of patients with rheumatoid arthritis. (2004). *Arthritis and Rheumatism,* Vol. 50, No. 12 (December 2004), pp. 3792-3803, ISSN 0004-3591.

Liu, J., Zhu, P., Peng, J., Li, K., Du, J., Gu, J.& Ou, Y. Identification of disease-associated proteins by proteomic approach in ankylosing spondylitis. (2007). *Biochemical and Biophysical Research Communications,* Vol. 1, No. 357, suppl. 2, (June 2007), pp. 531-536, ISSN 0006-291X.

Lood, C., Amisten, S., Gullstrand, B., Jönsen, A., Allhorn, M., Truedsson, L., Sturfelt, G., Erlinge, D.& Bengtsson, A.A. Platelet transcriptional profile and protein expression in patients with systemic lupus erythematosus: up-regulation of the type I interferon system is strongly associated with vascular disease. (2010). *Blood.* Vol. 16, No. 116, suppl. 11, (September 2010), pp. 1951-1957, ISSN 0006-4971.

Ma, W.J., Guo, X., Liu, J.T., Liu, R.Y., Hu, J.W., Sun, A.G., Yu, Y.X. & Lammi, M.J. Proteomic changes in articular cartilage of human endemic osteoarthritis in China. (2011). *Proteomics,* Vol.11, No. 14, (July 2011), pp. 2881-2890, ISSN 1615-9853.

Manganelli, P., Fietta, P. & Quaini, F. Hematologic manifestations of primary Sjögren's syndrome. (2006). *Clinical and Experimental Rheumatology,* Vol 24, N0. 4, (July 2006), pp. 438-448, ISSN 0392-856X.

Matsuo, K., Arito, M., Noyori, K., Nakamura, H., Kurokawa, M.S., Masuko, K., Okamoto, K., Nagai, K., Suematsu, N., Yudoh, K., Beppu, M., Saito, T. & Kato, T. Arthritogenicity of annexin VII revealed by phosphoproteomics of rheumatoid synoviocytes. (2011). *Annals of Rheumatic Diseases,* Vol. 70, No. 8, (August 2011), pp. 1489-1495, ISSN 0003-4967.

Matsuo, K., Xiang, Y., Nakamura, H., Masuko, K., Yudoh, K., Noyori, K., Nishioka, K., Saito, T. & Kato, T. (2006). Identification of novel citrullinated autoantigens of synovium in rheumatoid arthritis using a proteomic approach. *Arthritis Research & Therapy,* Vol. 8, No. 6, (June 2006), pp. R175, ISSN 1478-6354.

Mosley, K., Tam, F.W., Edwards, R.J., Crozier, J., Pusey, C.D. & Lightstone, L. Urinary proteomic profiles distinguish between active and inactive lupus nephritis. (2006). *Rheumatology (Oxford),* Vol. 45, No. 12, (December 2006), pp. 1497-1504, ISSN 1462-0324.

Pavón, E.J,, Muñoz, P., Lario, A., Longobardo, V., Carrascal, M., Abián, J., Martin, A.B., Arias, S.A., Callejas-Rubio, J.L., Sola, R., Navarro-Pelayo, F., Raya-Alvarez, E., Ortego-Centeno, N., Zubiaur, M. & Sancho, J. Proteomic analysis of plasma from patients with systemic lupus erythematosus: increased presence of haptoglobin alpha2 polypeptide chains over the alpha1 isoforms. (2006). *Proteomics,* Vol. 6, suppl. 1, (April 2006), pp. S282-92, ISSN 1615-9853.

Peluso, G., De Santis, M., Inzitari, R., Fanali, C., Cabras, T., Messana, I., Castagnola & M., Ferraccioli, G.F. Proteomic study of salivary peptides and proteins in patients with Sjögren's syndrome before and after pilocarpine treatment. (2007). *Arthritis and Rheumatism,* Vol. 56, No. 7, (July 2007), pp. 2216-2222, ISSN 0004-3591.

Ramos-Casals, M., Tzioufas, A.G.& Font, J. Primary Sjögren's syndrome: new clinical and therapeutic concepts. (2005a). *Annals of Rheumatic Diseases,* Vol. 64, No. 3, (March 2005), pp. 347-354, ISSN 0003-4967.

Ramos-Casals, M., Brito-Zerón, P., Yagüe, J., Akasbi, M., Bautista, R., Ruano, M., Claver, G., Gil, V. & Font, J. Hypocomplementaemia as an immunological marker of morbidity and mortality in patients with primary Sjogren's syndrome. (2005b). *Rheumatology (Oxford),* Vol. 44, No. 1, (January 2005), pp. 89-94, ISSN 1462-0324.

Rosenthal, A.K., Gohr, C.M., Ninomiya, J. & Wakim, B.T. Proteomic analysis of articular cartilage vesicles from normal and osteoarthritic cartilage. (2011). *Arthritis and Rheumatism,* Vol. 63, No. 2, (February 2011), pp. 401-411, ISSN 0004-3591.

Ruiz-Romero, C., López-Armada, M.J. & Blanco, F.J. Proteomic characterization of human normal articular chondrocytes: a novel tool for the study of osteoarthritis and other rheumatic diseases. (2005). *Proteomics,* Vol. 5, No. 12, (August 2005), pp. 3048 -3059, ISSN 1615-9853.

Ryu, O.H,, Atkinson, J.C., Hoehn, G.T., Illei, G.G. & Hart, T.C. Identification of parotid salivary biomarkers in Sjögren'ssyndrome by surface-enhanced laser desorption/ionization time-of flight mass spectrometry and two-dimensional difference gel electrophoresis. (2006). *Rheumatology (Oxford),* Vol. 45, No. 9, (September 2006), pp. 1077-1086, ISSN 1462-0324.

Scambi, C., La Verde, V., De Franceschi, L., Barausse, G., Poli, F., Benedetti, F., Sorio, M., Deriu, F., Roncada, P., Bortolami, O., Turrini, F., Caramaschi, P., Stranieri, C., Bambara, L.M. & Biasi, D. Comparative proteomic analysis of serum from patients with systemic sclerosis and sclerodermatous GVHD. Evidence of defective function of factor H. (2010). *PLoS One,* Vol. 13, No. 5, suppl. 8(August 2010), pp. e12162, ISSN 1932-6203.

Schulz, M., Dotzlaw, H., Mikkat, S., Eggert, M. & Neeck, G. Proteomic analysis of peripheral blood mononuclear cells: selective protein processing observed in patients with rheumatoid arthritis. (2007). *Journal of Proteome Research,* Vol. 6, No. 9, (September 2007), pp. 3752-3759, ISSN 1535-3893.

Seror, R., Ravaud, P., Bowman, S.J., Baron, G., Tzioufas, A., Theander, E., Gottenberg, J.E., Bootsma, H., Mariette, X., Vitali, C. & EULAR Sjögren's Task Force. EULAR Sjogren's syndrome disease activity index: development of a consensus systemic disease activity index for primary Sjogren's syndrome. (2010). *Annals of Rheumatic Diseases,* Vol. 69, No. 6, (June 2010), pp. 1103-1109, ISSN 0003-4967.

Sinz, A., Bantscheff, M., Mikkat, S., Ringel, B., Drynda, S., Kekow, J., Thiesen, H.J. & Glocker, M.O. Mass spectrometric proteome analyses of synovial fluids and plasmas from patients suffering from rheumatoid arthritis and comparison to reactive arthritis or osteoarthritis. (2002). *Electrophoresis,* Vol. 23, No. 19, (September 2002), pp. 3445-3456, ISSN 0173-0835.

Stea, E.A., Routsias, J.G., Samiotaki, M., Panayotou, G., Papalambros, E., Moutsopoulos, H.M. & Tzioufas, A.G. (2007). Analysis of parotid glands of primary Sjögren's syndrome patients using proteomic technology reveals altered autoantigen composition and novel antigenic targets. (2007). *Clinical Experimental Immunology,* Vol. 147, No. 1, (January 2007), pp. 81-89, ISSN 0009-9104.

Stone, J.H., Rajapakse, V.N., Hoffman, G.S., Specks, U., Merkel, P.A., Spiera, R.F., Davis, J.C., St Clair, E.W., McCune, J., Ross, S., Hitt, B.A., Veenstra, T.D., Conrads, T.P., Liotta, L.A. & Petricoin, E.F. 3rd. Wegener's Granulomatosis Etanercept Trial Research Group. A serum proteomic approach to gauging the state of remission in

Wegener's granulomatosis. (2005). *Arthritis and Rheumatism,* Vol. 52, No. 3, (March 2005), pp. 902-910, ISSN 0004-3591.

Streckfus, C.F. & Dubinsky, W.P. Proteomic analysis of saliva for cancer diagnosis. (2007), *Expert Review of Proteomics,* Vol. 4, No. 3, (June 2007), 329-332, ISSN 1478-9450.

Tilleman, K., Van Beneden, K., Dhondt, A., Hoffman, I., De Keyser, F., Veys, E., Elewaut, D. & Deforce, D. Chronically inflamed synovium from spondyloarthropathy and rheumatoid arthritis investigated by protein expression profiling followed by tandem mass spectrometry. (2005). *Proteomics,* Vol. 5, No. 8, (May 2005), pp. 2247-2257, ISSN 1615-9853.

Tomosugi, N., Kitagawa, K., Takahashi, N., Sugai, S. & Ishikawa, I. Diagnostic potential of tear proteomic patterns in Sjögren's syndrome. (2005). *Journal of Proteome Research,* Vol. 4, No. 3, (May 2005), pp. 820-825, ISSN 1535-3893.

Tzioufas, A.G. & Voulgarelis, M. Update on Sjögren's syndrome autoimmune epithelitis: from classification to increased neoplasias. (2007). *Best Practice & Research in Clinical Rheumatology.* Vol. 21, No. 6, (December 2007), pp. 989-1010, ISSN 1521-6942.

Vanarsa, K. & Mohan, C. Proteomics in rheumatology: the dawn of a new era. (2010). *F1000 Medicine Report,* Vol. 8, No. 2, (December 2010), pp. 87, ISSN 1757-5931.

Vitali, C., Bombardieri, S., Jonsson, R., Moutsopoulos, H.M., Alexander, E.L., Carsons, S.E., Daniels, T.E., Fox, P.C., Fox, R.I., Kassan, S.S., Pillemer, S.R., Talal, N., Weisman, M.H.& European Study Group on Classification Criteria for Sjögren's Syndrome. Classification criteria for Sjögren's syndrome: a revised version of the European criteria proposed by the American-European Consensus Group.(2002). *Annals of Rheumatic Diseases,* Vol. 61, No. 6, (June 2002), pp. 554-558, ISSN 0003-4967.

Voulgarelis, M., Dafni, U.G., Isenberg, D.A.& Moutsopoulos, H.M. Malignant lymphoma in primary Sjögren's Syndrome: a multicenter, retrospective, clinical study by the European Concerted Action on Sjögren's Syndrome. (1999). *Arthritis and Rheumatism,* Vol. 42, No. 8, (August 1999), pp. 1765-1772, ISSN 0004-3591.

Wang, L., Dai, Y., Qi, S., Sun, B., Wen, J., Zhang, L. & Tu, Z. Comparative proteome analysis of peripheral blood mononuclear cells in systemic lupus erythematosus with iTRAQ quantitative proteomics. (2010). *Rheumatology International,* doi 10.1007/s00296-010-1625-9, ISSN 0172-8172.

Wright, C., Edelmann, M., diGleria, K., Kollnberger, S., Kramer, H., McGowan, S., McHugh, K., Taylor, S., Kessler, B.& Bowness, P. Ankylosing spondylitis monocytes show upregulation of proteins involved in inflammation and the ubiquitin proteasome pathway. (2009). *Annals of Rheumatic Diseases,* Vol. 68, No. 10, (October 2009), pp. 1626-1632, ISSN 0003-4967.

Wu, J., Liu, W., Bemis, A., Wang, E., Qiu, Y., Morris, E.A., Flannery, C.R. & Yang, Z. Comparative proteomic characterization of articular cartilage tissue from normal donors and patients with osteoarthritis. (2007). *Arthritis and Rheumatism,* Vol. 56, No. 11, (November 2007), pp. 3675-3684, ISSN 0004-3591.

Zhang, X., Jin, M., Wu, H., Nadasdy, T., Nadasdy, G., Harris, N., Green-Church, K., Nagaraja, H., Birmingham, D.J., Yu, C.Y., Hebert, L.A. & Rovin, B.H. Biomarkers of lupus nephritis determined by serial urine proteomics. (2008) *Kidney International,* Vol. 74, No. 6, (September 2008), pp. 799-807, ISSN 0085-2538.

Zheng, X., Wu, S.L., Hincapie, M. & Hancock, W.S. Study of the human plasma proteome of rheumatoid arthritis. (2009). *Journal of Chromatography A,* Vol. 17, No. 1216, suppl. 16, (April 2009), 3538-3545, ISSN 0021-9673.

Part 3

Psychosocial Considerations in Rheumatic Disease

12

The Pathogenetic Link Between Stress and Rheumatic Diseases

O. Malysheva and C.G.O. Baerwald
Rheumatology Unit, Medical Clinic II, University Hospital Leipzig
Germany

1. Introduction

1.1 Definition of stress

Hans Selye was the first to define stress as a non-specific response of the body to any demand made upon it (1936). It has been demonstrated that Selye's theory about the effects of stress is applicable to any type of stress (Stojanovich & Marisavljevich, 2008). Key organ of stress processes is the brain. It determines what individuals will experience as stressful, it orchestrates how individuals will cope with stressful experiences, and it changes both functionally and structurally as a result of stressful experiences (McEwen & Gianaros, 2011).

Stress begins with a stimulus (stressor) that causes a reaction in the brain (stress perception), which subsequently activates physiologic systems in the body (stress response). The stress response system reacts with the release of neurotransmitters (norepinephrine etc.) and hormones (cortisol etc.) which serve to send an efferent message from the brain to the periphery in order to modulate the stressful event (Cutolo & Straub, 2006).

It is clear that stress, originating in the cortex of the brain, must be converted into somatic signals, which can modulate the immune system or pain perception. These somatic signals typically start off in the highest centres of the autonomic nervous system (ANS) and the endocrine system within the hypothalamus (Cutolo & Straub, 2006). Selye was the first to describe the system by which the body copes with stress: the hypothalamus-pituitary-adrenal system (HPA) (Stojanovich & Marisavljevich, 2008). The hypothalamus has close connections to the limbic system, which is responsible for the emotionalisation of psychological stress (whether it is perceived as positive eustress or negative distress). The major neuroendocrine response mediating stress adaptation relies on the activation of the HPA axis by stimulating corticotropin releasing hormone (CRH) and vasopressin (VP) from parvocellular neurons of the hypothalamic paraventricular nucleus. This leads in turn to stimulation of pituitary aderocorticotropic hormone (ACTH) secretion and increases in glucocorticoid secretion from the adrenal cortex. Basal production of glucocorticoids and its hypothalamic regulators together with transient increases during stress are essential for neuronal plasticity and normal brain function. While activation of the HPA axis is essential for survival during stress, chronic exposure to stress hormones can predispose to psychological, metabolic and immune alterations (Aguilera et al., 2011).

Selye is considered to be the first to demonstrate the existence of a particular stress disease, the stress syndrome, or the general adaptation syndrome (Stojanovich & Marisavljevich, 2008). These processes can be adaptive in the short term and may contribute to the dysregulation of the hormone status if persisting for a longer time. Moreover, they are involved in bidirectional signalling between the brain and the body as well as in stress-related mental and physical health conditions (McEwen & Gianaros, 2011). The chronic stress-induced dysregulation appears to be of sufficient magnitude to impact health (Gouin et al., 2008).

Recent advances in psychoneuroimmunology have provided insight into the complex mechanisms by which stressors might affect the homeostasis and the body's immune system (de Brouwer et al., 2010). Stress challenges the organism's homeostatic mechanisms, triggering a cascade of events that should, normally, maintain or allow a return to equilibrium (Pêgo et al., 2010). Psychological stress can influence immunoregulatory circuits and the course of an inflammatory disease (Marshall GD Jr, 1997). Furthermore, cytokines generated by the immune system influence hormonal secretion and the central nervous system, producing specific behavioural changes accompanying infectious and inflammatory diseases (Straub et al., 2008). Psychological distress and immune dysregulation have been linked to each other in chronic stress, in disease and other major life events.

It was shown that psychological stress is also thought to contribute to the aetiology, maintenance and exacerbation of rheumatic diseases (de Brouwer et al., 2010). Stress has been studied in several autoimmune rheumatic diseases, including systemic lupus erythematosus (SLE), rheumatoid arthritis (RA) and juvenile idiopathic arthritis (JIA) (Cutolo & Straub, 2006). Growing evidence supports the hypothesis that alterations of the stress response and interactions between the neuroendocrine and immune systems contribute to the pathogenesis of rheumatic diseases (Chikanza et al., 1992).

2. Neurotransmitter-cytokine relationship

The stress response is mediated by the sympathetic nervous system and it results in the release of some neurotransmitters (epinephrine, norepinephrine) that regulates the immune system at regional, local, and systemic levels (Felten et al., 1988).

Immune organs including thymus, spleen, and lymph nodes are innervated by sympathetic nerves (Felten et al., 1988). Interruption of sympathetic innervation of immune organs has been shown to modulate the outcome of, and susceptibility to, inflammatory and infectious disease. Denervation of noradrenergic fibres of lymph nodes is associated with exacerbation of inflammation (Lorton et al., 1996), whereas systemic sympathectomy or denervation of joints is associated with decreased severity of inflammation (Eskandari et al., 2005).

Immune cells also express neurotransmitter receptors, such as adrenergic receptors (alpha- or beta- subtype) on lymphocytes that allow them to respond to sympathetic neurotransmitters (Elenkov & Chrousos, 1999). Neural influences on the immune response may be due to direct synapse-like nerve-lymphocyte connections (Mix et al., 2007). Through stimulation of adrenergic receptors locally released norepinephrine or circulating catecholamines affect lymphocyte traffic, circulation, and proliferation, and, in turn, modulate cytokine production as well as functional activity of various lymphoid cells (Elenkov et al., 2000; Straub et al., 2000; Madden et al., 2001).

Cytokines are important factors connecting and modulating the immune and neuroendrocrine systems (Elenkov, 2005). Furthermore, cytokines and their receptors are expressed in the neuroendocrine system and exert their effects both centrally and peripherally (Benveniste et al., 1998). Systemic cytokines can affect the brain through several mechanisms, including active transport across the blood-brain barrier, through leaky areas in the blood-brain barrier in the circumventricular organs or through the activation of neural pathways such as the vagal nerve (Eskandari, 2005). For example, IL-6 and tumour necrosis factor (TNF)-a, released during an immune response and inflammation activate the central components of the stress system, alter neurotransmitter networks activity and induce fever, sleepiness, fatigue, loss of appetite and decreased libido. In addition, they activate the hepatic synthesis of acute phase proteins—changes referred to as 'sickness behavior' and 'acute-phase response', respectively (Elenkov, 2005).

Otherwise, administration of interleukin (IL)-1 in the periphery increases the turnover of norepinephrine in the hypothalamus; intracerebroventricular and peripheral injection of interferon (IFN)-α or IL-1β produces a long-lasting increase of the sympathetic activity of the splenic nerve and an increased turnover of norepinephrine in the spleen (Elenkov, 2000). Furthermore, it was shown that monoamine neurotransmitters, released in stress situations, represent a tonic sympathetic control on cytokine production and on the balance of pro-inflammatory/anti-inflammatory cytokines (Szelényi & Vizi, 2007).

Autoimmune diseases are characterized by common alterations of the T-helper (Th)1 versus Th2 cells and a shift towards pro-inflammatory cytokines. In RA the balance is skewed towards Th1 and an excess of IL-12 and TNF-α production, whereas Th2 activity and the production of IL-10 appear to be deficient (Segal et al., 1998).

Neurotransmitters, through stimulation of the beta 2-adrenoreceptors (b2AR)-cAMP-protein kinase A pathway, inhibit the production of type 1/proinflammatory cytokines, such as IL-12, TNF-alpha, and IFN-gamma by antigen-presenting cells and Th1 cells, whereas they stimulate the production of type 2/anti-inflammatory cytokines such as IL-10 and transforming growth factor-beta. Through these mechanisms endogenous catecholamines may cause a selective suppression of Th1 responses and cellular immunity and a Th2 shift towards dominance of humoral immunity (Madden et al., 1995, Elenkov et al., 2000). On the other hand, in certain local responses and under certain conditions, catecholamines may actually boost regional immune responses through induction of IL-1, TNF-α, and IL-8 production. Thus, activation of the sympathetic nervous system during an immune response might be aimed to confine the inflammatory response on the local level through induction of neutrophil accumulation and stimulation of more specific humoral immune responses. However, systemically the SNS may suppress Th1 responses and thus protect the organism from the detrimental effects of pro-inflammatory cytokines and other products of activated macrophages (Elenkov et al., 2000). Otherwise, norepinephrine and epinephrine, through stimulation of classic cytoplasmic/nuclear glucocorticoid receptors and β2-AR, respectively, suppress the production of IL-12 by antigen presenting cells (APCs) being the main inducer of Th1 responses (Elenkov et al., 2005). It was shown that an increase in disease activity among RA patients was associated with an increase in the level of stress experienced by these patients, suggesting that a stress induced increase in norepinephrine release might activate naive Th1 cells and/or increase their activity (Kin & Sanders, 2007).

Since β2-ARs are expressed on Th1 cells, but not on Th2 cells (Sanders et al., 1997), catecholamines do not affect directly the cytokine production by Th2 cells. In murine and human systems β2-AR agonists inhibit IFN-gamma production by Th1 cells, but do not affect IL-4 production by Th2 cells (Borger et al., 1998; Wahle et al., 2006). However, neurotransmitters through stimulation of β2-AR up-regulate the production of the anti-inflammatory cytokine IL-6 and IL-10 by APCs (Elenkov, 2005). Administration of a β2AR antagonist or a β2AR agonist prior to or during the development of arthritis inhibits or exacerbates disease pathology, suggesting that NE stimulating β2AR on naive T and/or Th1 cells modulate IFN-gamma production. As with the in vitro findings, the in vivo effects were found to depend on the time point when norepinephrine was released during the course of a disease (Kin & Sanders, 2007). The increased responsiveness of T cells from RA patients to β2AR stimulation following NE exposure might exacerbate IFN-gamma production and promote conditions for RA development and progression. Therefore, NE, which normally participates in a CD4- T cell response to maintain homeostasis by enhancing the baseline immune cell-regulated IFN-gamma response, may cause disease progression when the regulatory conditions controlling sympathetic nervous system/ β2AR activity have changed (Kin & Sanders, 2007).

Otherwise, between RA patients and controls there was a highly significant distortion in the distribution of the beta2AR polymorphisms at codon 16 and to a lower extent at codon 27 contributing together with the human leuokocyte antigen (HLA)-DR alleles to the genetic background of RA. Furthermore, polymorphisms of the beta2R gene may modulate the expression of anti citrullinated peptide (anti-CCP) antibodies further supporting the close interplay between the autonomic nervous system and the immune system (Malysheva et al., 2008). Single nucleotide polymorphisms have been found to be associated with the β2AR expressed by cells of RA patients, suggesting that a change in the β2AR structure on a naive T and/or Th1 cell may heighten the level of cell responsiveness to NE (Kin & Sanders, 2007).

In patients with RA, experimental stress did not change levels of inflammatory markers (IL-2, soluble IL-2 receptor, IL-4, IL-10 and IFN-γ) but TNF-α. Results for IL-6 were inconsistent (S.de Brouwer, 2010). In patients with SLE, experimental stress did not change levels of cytokines and other inflammatory markers (IL-2, IL-6, IL-10, IFN-γ, β-adrenoceptors), although levels of IL-4 increased after stress (Jocobs et al., 2001). Patients with SLE differed from controls in their response to stress, having a larger increase in IL-4, smaller IL-10 and IFN-γ responses, and fewer β-adrenoceptors on monocytes (S. de Brouwer, 2010). In patients with JIA, stress did not affect IL-8 production, but increased IL-6 production (Roupe et al., 2000). However, in healthy subjects stress increased IFN gamma and IL-10 levels (Jacobs et al., 2001; Motivala et al., 2008). Thus, although experimental stress does not seem to influence levels of certain cytokines and inflammatory markers in patients with rheumatic diseases (for example, sIL-2, IL-8, IL-10, IFN-γ, β-adrenoceptors), it does cause specific changes in c-reactive protein (CRP) and TNF-α in patients with RA, changes in IL-4 in patients with SLE, and changes in IL-6 in patients with JIA. These changes are not observed in controls (S. de Brouwer, 2010). Finally, the pharmacological manipulation of the sympathetic-immune interface is reviewed with focus on new therapeutic strategies using selective alpha(2)- and beta(2)-AR agonists and antagonists and inhibitors of phosphodiesterase type IV in the treatment of experimental models of autoimmune diseases (Elenkov et al., 2000).

3. Integration of stress hormones, cytokines and neurotransmitters

Perception of an external stressful stimulus prompts the activation of various physiological systems that together define the body's stress response, which is aimed at re-establishing homeostasis (S. de Brouwer, 2010). Central to the maintenance of homeostasis is an appropriate response of the HPA axis as well as the sympathetic nervous system (Dunn & Swiergiel, 2008; Eskandari et al., 2003,). From animal models of arthritis as well as from clinical studies in RA patients a central role of the HPA axis in onset and severity of RA was suggested (Chikanza, 1992). In these patients an inadequate secretion of cortisol in the setting of a sustained inflammatory disease has been observed (Vassilopoulos & Mantzoukis, 2006). A hypoactive stress system may facilitate or sustain the Th1 shift in Th1-mediated RA. A suboptimal production of cortisol is involved in the onset and/or progression of RA. Patients with RA have "inappropriately normal" or low plasma cortisol levels in the setting of severe, chronic inflammation, characterized by increased production of TNF-a, IL-1 and IL-6. This may actually facilitate or sustain the pro-inflammatory shift in this disease (Elenkov, 2005). The HPA axis has been evaluated in multiple forms in former studies of RA patients. Assuming that an inflammatory process up-regulates HPA axis function, cortisol levels are inappropriately normal in RA patients when cytokine levels are increased (Straub et al., 2008). The proposed defect could reside at various levels of the HPA axis, i.e. the hypothalamic level, the pituitary, and the adrenal gland. However, results of HPA axis tests in RA patients were inconclusive since steroid treatment, drugs including disease modifying antirheumatic drugs (DMARD) and disease duration might interfere with the results leading to conflicting results for ACTH levels and cortisol response in RA patients (Eijsbouts, 2005).

Experimental psychosocial stress consistently increased autonomic activity, blood pressure and catecholamine levels in patients with RA and SLE, and increased neuroendocrine variables (cortisol and ACTH]) in patients with RA. Furthermore, after such stress exposure an increase in IL-4 level in patients with SLE, an increase in TNF-α in RA patients, and inconsistent findings for IL-6 were observed (S. de Brouwer, 2010). Exercise stress was characterised by decreased levels of cortisol whereas ACTH levels and growth hormone levels increased. Moreover, this stress elicited a different cytotoxic T cell response in patients with RA and SLE (Pool et al., 2004; Kurtais et al., 2006).

The stress hormones, supposedly acting via β- and α-adrenergic as well as glucocorticoid receptors, down-regulate immune and inflammatory processes; however, these processes also influence the central nervous system (Ader et al., 1995; MacEwen, 1998). Circulating cytokines and activated immune cells, markers of inflammation, activate both (intermediates of) the HPA axis and the autonomic nervous system. Chronically elevated levels of cytokines, as occur during long-term inflammation, might lead to changes in HPA axis and ANS activity (Chrousos, 1995). Otherwise, circulating hormones or locally released neurotransmitters regulate major immune functions, such as antigen presentation, antibody production, lymphocyte activity, proliferation and traffic, and the secretion of cytokines including the modulation of Th1 or Th2 cytokine responses. During inflammation, activation of the stress system, through induction of a Th2 shift protects the organism from systemic "overshooting" with Th1/pro-inflammatory cytokines. Under certain conditions, however, stress hormones, substance P, adenosine triphosphate (ATP) and the activation of CRH/substance P-histamine axis may actually facilitate inflammation, through induction of

IL-1, IL-6, IL-8, IL-18, TNF-alpha and CRP production. Thus, a dysfunctional neuroendocrine-immune interface associated with abnormalities of the 'systemic anti-inflammatory feedback' and/or 'hyperactivity' of the local pro-inflammatory factors may play a role in the pathogenesis of autoimmune diseases (Elenkov, 2008).

Cytokines signalling to the brain can not only activate the HPA axis but also facilitate pain and induce a series of mood and behavioural responses generally termed sickness behaviour (Watkins & Maier, 2000). Cytokines, such as IL-1, IL-6, and TNF-alpha, are also produced in the brain (Sebire, 1993). These brain-derived cytokines can stimulate the HPA axis. For example, IL-1 stimulates the expression of the gene encoding CRH and thereby the release of the hormone from the hypothalamus, the release of AVP from the hypothalamus, and the release of ACTH from the anterior pituitary, IL-2 stimulates AVP secretion from the hypothalamus, IL-6 and TNF-alpha also stimulate ACTH secretion. Otherwise, in chronic inflammation there seems to be a shift from CRH-driven to arginine vasopressin (AVP)-driven HPA axis response (Eskandari, 2005).

CRH is the strongest known activator of the HPA axis which has been functionally implicated in the regulation of many endocrine functions, such as glucocorticoid release from the adrenal gland and associated endocrine-immune responses (Elenkov, 2008). CRH not only activates the pituitary-adrenal axis but also sets in motion a coordinated series of behavioural and physiologic responses, suggesting that the central nervous system may coordinate both behavioural and immunologic adaptation during stressful situations (Stermberg, 1992; O'Connor, 2000). CRH is positively regulated by catecholaminergic system (Eskandari, 2005). During an immune response certain cytokines, such as IL-1, IL-6, and TNF-a can signal the brain, which via a complex CRH-dependent pathway, triggers activation of both the SNS and the HPA axis (Elenkov, 2000).

Recently several polymorphisms in the highly conserved regulatory region of the CRH gene were described with the gene being located on chromosome 8q13. Three polymorphisms co-segregated absolutely resulting in two alleles *A1* and *A2* with a further polymorphism being assigned as alleles *B1* and *B2*. Population investigations demonstrated a distortion in the distribution of the resulting compound alleles A1B1, A2B1 and A2B2 between RA patients and healthy controls (Baerwald et al., 1997). In vitro studies revealed a different regulation of the CRH gene by these polymorphisms (Wagner et al., 2006). Furthermore, it was shown that the stress induced response of cortisol is differentially modulated by CRH promoter polymorphisms in RA patients. Thus, during insulin hypoglycemia test RA patients bearing the A2B2 allele exhibited an earlier CRH as well as ACTH peak compared to A1B1 positive patients. The integrated cortisol response to hypoglycemia expressed as area under the curve was significantly lower in RA patients with the A1B1 allele than in RA patients with the A2B2 allele. Moreover, there was a significant difference in the molar ratio cortisol to ACTH between controls and RA patients underlining the dissociation of the pituitary and the adrenal gland in patients with RA (Malysheva et al., 2011).

4. Environmental factors in stress – disease interaction

The concept of environment included different factors that could disturb the homeostatic state of health (Parniapour, 1990). A growing body of research in rheumatic diseases highlights the importance of environmental influences to the contribution of stress on disease activity of rheumatic diseases. These influences include factors such as emotional distress, coping, and familial factors (Anthony & Schanberg, 2007), diet, and some socio-economic factors (such as level of education, area of residence and income) may affect levels of pain and physical disability experienced by rheumatic patients (Symmons, 2003; Kobayshi et al., 2008).

4.1 Family factors

It was shown that the family environment is important in juvenile rheumatic diseases. Thus, diagnosis of a rheumatic disease in children was associated with depression in the mother and a composite measure of parental (mother and father) distress and passive coping. Children's emotional and behavioural functioning was not related to medical diagnosis, however, a mother's depression and parental distress were associated with a child's behavioural problems. This kind of distress was associated with child functioning and interventions to ameliorate parental distress may have beneficial effects on the children's behaviour and on parent's reactions to their children (Frank et al, 1998). Furthermore, the social environment was found to operate on the core health outcome, i.e. pain severity in rheumatic diseases. Not only the status of being married but also the quality of the relationship in terms of long-term stress and emotional support may be useful prognostic factors in rheumatic diseases. Patient reports of negative spouse behaviour (such as avoidance and critical remarks) and baseline depression predicted worse pain outcome, and this association remained significant in analyses controlling for baseline pain. The level of formal education showed a weak correlation to disability, emotional support, and pain. Daily emotional support and social life domains associated with positive affect had an indirect influence on outcome. The absence of strong rather than weak social ties was the component of the loneliness construct linked to pain. These associations between social prognostic factors and pain severity, however, were mediated by psychological functioning at baseline (Waltz et al., 1999).

4.2 Socioeconomic status

One more important factor of environment is socioeconomic status. Although RA occurrence is more frequent in lower socioeconomic parts of the population, it was not identified as a significant risk factor in RA (Damjanovic et al., 2009). Otherwise, there is a lack of good quality studies of the epidemiology of rheumatic diseases in developing countries. It appears that a threshold level where higher socio-economic status is associated with reduced prevalence of rheumatic disease is not reached in developing countries. Therefore, differences in the prevalence between socio-economic groups can be undetected. A similar case can be made for overcrowding (Steer et al., 2002). However, the education level as risk factor is significantly related to RA occurrence (Damjanovic et al., 2009). Furthermore, socioeconomic disparities in patients with chronic musculoskeletal complains leading to increased pain may be attributable to both greater frequency of stressful financial events as well as greater vulnerability to economic hardship for those at the lower end of the socioeconomic spectrum. Conditions of economic hardship and daily ratings of financial worry both had significant detrimental effects on daily pain. Participants with greater levels of economic hardship reported greater pain severity in response to daily financial worries than their counterparts with little or no economic hardship. Further, participants in the sample who were not employed and who reported higher levels of economic hardship exhibited the most pain reactivity in response to daily financial worries. Economic hardship was associated not only with greater exposure to daily financial worries but also with greater vulnerability to pain on days when daily financial worries were experienced (Rios & Zautra, 2011). A prospective cohort study (1958 British Birth Cohort Study) demonstrated that the prevalence of shoulder, forearm, low back, knee and chronic widespread pain at 45 years generally increased with lower social class. Persons in the lowest social class (compared to the highest) experienced nearly a threefold increase in the risk of chronic widespread pain (relative risk: 2.9, 95% CI 1.8 to 4.6). Social class during childhood also demonstrated a relationship with most regional pain and chronic widespread pain. With the exception of forearm pain, the magnitude of effect of childhood social status on reporting of pain in adulthood was less than that of adult social status. On multivariable analysis these relationships were partly explained by poor adult mental health, psychological distress, adverse life events and lifestyle factors (Macfarlane, 2009). Furthermore, there was an association between socioeconomic status, occupation, and hospitalization for RA. A total of 13,820 male and 14,509 female hospitalizations for RA were analysed during the study. Men and women with an education level > 12 years had a significantly decreased incidence ratio. Occupation also played a role in these items studied with an increased incidence ratio among farmers, miners and quarry workers, electrical workers, other construction workers, and engine and motor operators for men. Among women, assistant nurses and religious, juridical, and other social-science-related workers had significantly increased incidence ratio in all 3 cohorts (Li et al, 2008).

4.3 Education and life style

It was proposed that such environmental factor as level of education was significantly inversely associated with the risk of RA, with a 2-fold lower risk of RA among those with the highest education compared with those having the lowest level of education. On the other hand, it is hypothesised that RF-positive and RF-negative RA have different "aetiologies" with factors related to educational level predominantly associated with the risk of RF-positive RA (Pedersem et al., 2006).

Diet and food life style could also be an important environmental factor contributing to rheumatic diseases. For example, diet, nutrition, and weight loss have shown promise in alleviating some of rheumatic burden. These lifestyle changes may give patients a feeling of control over their disease as well as a non-pharmacologic means of treatment. In particular the role of the Mediterranean diet has to be recognised as a protective factor against RA (Li & Micheletti, 2011). The goals of dietary therapy in rheumatic diseases are alleviation of under- and malnutrition, inhibition of inflammation, prophylaxis of osteoporosis, as well as recognition and treatment of nutrient sensitivities or intolerances. Inhibition of inflammation in these patients is improved by modulating the omega-3/omega-6 fatty acids ratio in the diet. Reduction of dietary arachidonic acid is recommended. This polyunsaturated fatty acid is the main precursor of pro-inflammatory mediators which interact with chemokines und cytokines. Simultaneously, intake of anti-inflammatory omega-3 fatty acids is increased. Studies have shown that this dietary regimen results in an amelioration of symptoms in patients with inflammatory rheumatic diseases (Adam et al., 2009).

The role of other types of environmental stress was studied in patients with different autoimmune diseases as well. For example, cognitive stressors elicited changes in leukocyte/lymphocyte counts, subsets of lymphocytes, and CRP levels in patients with RA (Geenen, 1998; Veldhuijzen van Zanten, 2005), and changes in leucocyte counts and cytoxic T cell numbers in patients with SLE (Hinrichsen, 1992). It has recently been demonstrated that thermal stress (Spa therapy) induces a reduction in the circulating levels of prostaglandin E2 (PGE2), leukotriene B4 (LTB4), IL-1β and TNF-α, important mediators of inflammation and pain in patients with rheumatic diseases (Fioravanti, 2011). It was shown that environmental desiccating stress can be involved in the pathogenesis of chronic dry eye syndrome by exposing shared epitopes in the cornea, conjunctiva, and the lacrimal gland that induce pathogenic CD4+T cells leading to lacrimal keratoconjunctivitis, which under normal circumstances is restrained by CD4(+)CD25(+) forkhead/winged helix transcription factor(+) regulatory T cells (Niederkorn et al., 2006).

4.4 Climate conditions

Some other environmental factors such as weather conditions and climate could be also important in rheumatic pain. For example, persons with osteoarthritis in urban Chicago exhibited more weather sensitivity than their rural counterparts in Grand Forks, North Dakota. Multiple regression analysis revealed that precipitation affected pain for urban subjects who identified weather as a pain-generating factor; barometric pressure, relative humidity and sunshine were significant factors influencing pain-related stress. Wind speed correlated with pain and pain-related stress; relative humidity and precipitation correlated with pain-related stress for urban subjects who did not perceive weather as a problem. Specific weather variables were not identified as affecting rural subjects' pain. However, temperature and barometric pressure affected pain-related stress in rural subjects who perceived weather as a problem (Laborde et al., 1986). However, one systematic review of nine longitudinal observational studies (up to September 2009) dealing with the association of weather variables (temperature, relative humidity and atmospheric pressure) and severity of pain in RA could not demonstrate any significant effects. Individual analyses from two studies indicate that pain reporting in a minority (< 25%) of RA patients is influenced by temperature, relative humidity or atmospheric pressure. The studies to date do not show any consistent group effect of weather conditions on pain in RA. There is, however, evidence suggesting that pain in some individuals is more affected by the weather than in others, and that patients react in different ways to various weather conditions. Thus, the hypothesis that weather changes might significantly influence pain reporting in clinical care and research in some patients with RA cannot be rejected (Smedslund & Hagen, 2011). Otherwise, one population-based study demonstrated that pain is not an inevitable consequence of climatic conditions. Persons were less likely to report pain on days with > 5.8 h of sunshine and with average temperature of > 17.5°C underlining a strong relationship between lack of sunshine, lower temperatures and pain reporting (Macfarlane et al, 2010). Interestingly, 84% of RA patients believe in an association between weather and rheumatism, while 57% claimed to have ability to forecast weather. The maximum contribution of weather on symptoms was 17.1 %. Of interest, the belief about a presence of an association between weather and arthritis was found to be stronger than its statistical power (Cay et al., 2011).

4.5 Cultural difference

In addition, cultural differences in experiencing individual stress in RA patients were observed. In one study covering Polish and German RA patients it was demonstrated that in both countries, mental as well as physical health deteriorated resulting in about 50% of patients requiring support in everyday activities. 95% of Polish and 62% of German patients felt rejected from social activities. For the psychological stress perceived, functional capacity class 3 and male gender were shown to be predictive in Polish patients and living in a small town in German patients. In the Polish group, the tertiary/bachelor level of education was linked with lower distress level. RA has a serious impact on the mental health owing to a great disease burden (Bugajska et al., 2010).

4.6 Other factors

Interestingly, during a 15-year follow-up study of 74 female patients with RA two categories of RA were identified: a disease form less connected with genetic factors and more influenced by major psychodynamic conflict situations ('major conflict group') and a second form more associated with hereditary predisposition and less influenced by environmental psychosocial changes ('non-conflict group') (Rimón & Laakso,1985). In addition, a patient's perspective of the causes and consequences of RA could underline the role of environmental factors in disease. Two descriptive categories of patient's understanding of disease could be identified: the category 'consequences beyond personal control' comprised not having a clue, being exposed to climatic change, being genetically exposed and unexpected effects of events; the category 'overloaded circumstances' involved work and family-related strain. Consequences beyond personal control implied that the patients could not prevent the disease and expressed their lack of understanding as to why they contracted it. Overloaded circumstances were described as strained situations that were both work and family factors related and could be influenced by the patient. Reasoning along these lines it is concluded that understanding the patients' own view of disease is needed in order to achieve a more successful medical care model (Bergsten et al., 2009). Identifying of how these factors contribute to the development of autoimmune diseases may further lead to better explaining the pathogenesis of rheumatic diseases (Symmons, 2003; Kobayshi et al., 2008).

Finally, in one recent study of patients with psoriatic arthritis environmental factors such as lifting heavy loads of at least 100 pounds/hr (OR 2.8, 95% CI 1.51-5.05), infections that required antibiotics (OR 1.7, 95% CI 1.00-2.77), and injuries (OR 2.1, 95% CI 1.11-4.01) were associated with the occurrence of arthritis. No association was found between psoriasis arthritis and alcohol consumption, vaccination, and female hormonal exposures (Eder et al., 2011).

5. Rheumatic diseases as a model of stress induced disease

Despite more than twenty years of stress research in rheumatology, it is not completely understood whether stress induced neuroimmune dysfunctions play a causal role in the aetiology of rheumatic diseases or, in turn, rheumatic disease could change the stress reaction and thereby changing disease activity and worsening the outcome. However, epidemiological research increasingly suggests that exposure to traumatic stressors and psychological trauma is related to increased health care utilisation, adverse health outcomes, the onset of specific diseases including rheumatic diseases, and premature death (Boscarino et al., 2004; Sommershof et al., 2009).

5.1 Stress as pathogenetic factor of autoimmune diseases

From results of 27 studies evaluating more than 3,000 patients with RA it was recognised that stress is an important risk factor in the pathogenesis of autoimmune diseases. Major life events (e.g. death of a spouse, severe long-term illness of a spouse, loss of a parent, divorce of parents, death of a parent or severe disease of a parent) lead to an intense release of stress mediators (large time integral of released neurotransmitters and hormones), whereas in minor life events (daily hassles with small intensity) only short-lived surges of neurotransmitters and hormones are expected. Therefore, it is suggested that neurotransmitters such as norepinephrine or stress hormones such as cortisol might have different effects on immune/inflammatory responses at high and low concentrations present during short or extended periods of time, respectively. Long-lasting (chronic) stress may lead to pro-inflammatory effects since no adequate long-term responses of stress axes (anti-inflammatory) are to be expected (Cutolo & Straub, 2006). Furthermore, major life events and chronic minor stress seem to be important factors in juvenile chronic arthritis and are significantly associated with the onset of the rheumatic disease. With respect to RA, stress may be a provoking factor. However, during the course of the disease, minor stress could aggravate SLE and RA (Herrmann et al., 2000). In contrast, strong major stress, which is likely accompanied by a large and long-lived release of stress axes mediators, was associated with a decrease in disease activity (Cutolo & Straub, 2006).

5.1.1 Early life stress

One study (follow up 1980 till 1996) examining the risk of RA in parents after the death of a child does not support an association between severe psychological stress and RA. The relative risk of first hospitalisation for RA was 0.88 [95% CI 0.63-1.24]. The risk was close to 1 throughout the 18 years of follow-up (Li et al., 2005). Recent findings are consistent on the impact of early life stress on subsequent inflammatory responses. A predominant role for parent distress in children's adjustment to juvenile rheumatic disease was shown (Ryan et al., 2010). In one retrospective cohort study (follow-up 1995/1997 through 2005) of 15,357 adults it could be demonstrated that 64% adults reported early life stress with at least one adverse childhood experience (ACE), including childhood physical, emotional, or sexual abuse; witnessing domestic violence; growing up with household substance abuse, mental illness, parental divorce, and/or an incarcerated household member. The event rate (per 10,000 person-years) for a first hospitalization with any autoimmune disease was 31.4 in women and 34.4 in men. First hospitalizations for any autoimmune disease increased with increasing number of ACEs ($p < 0.05$). Persons with equal or more than 2 ACEs were at a 100 % increased risk for rheumatic diseases compared to persons without any ACE ($p < 0.05$) (Dube et al., 2009). Patients with juvenile idiopathic arthritis reported having pain, stiffness, and fatigue on > 70% of days, with significant variability in symptom levels. Furthermore, significant same-day relationships between stress, mood, and disease symptoms were revealed. Specifically, daily fluctuations in both stress and mood were predictive of increased pain, stiffness, and fatigue. Increases in daily stress, mood, and disease symptoms were also significantly related to decreased participation in social activities on a day-to-day basis (Schanberg et al., 2005). However, one study does not support the hypothesis that stressful life events and adverse childhood experiences play an aetiologic role in the development of rheumatic disease. The number and timing of occurrence of stressful life events, as well as their subjective immediate impact, did not differ between participants who developed RA and their matched controls. Termination of pregnancy was the only specific event individually associated with a higher risk of developing RA (OR 3.74; 95% CI 1.4-9.9). Negative childhood experiences were not associated with the risk of RA. However, RA cases reported significantly slower adaptation to the effects of adverse events than controls (Carette et al., 2000).

5.1.2 Posttraumatic stress disorder

Some studies have demonstrated a link between the traumatic stress exposures and posttraumatic stress disorder (PTSD) to rheumatic disorders. Recent finding indicate that victims of PTSD exhibit higher numbers of circulating T-cell lymphocytes and lower cortisol levels, suggesting that chronic sufferers of PTSD may be at risk for autoimmune diseases. In addition, patients with comorbid PTSD were more likely to have clinically higher T-cell counts, hyper-reactive immune responses on standardized delayed cutaneous hypersensitivity tests, higher immunoglobulin-M levels, and lower dehydroepiandrosterone levels (Stojanovich, 2008). It was also suggested that PTSD symptoms, as measured by impact of events scale, are strongly linked to chronic widespread pain (Arguelles, 2006). Otherwise, in one twin pair's study it was shown that PTSD symptoms were associated with onset of adult RA. Even after adjustment for familial/genetic factors and other confounders, an association between PTSD symptoms and RA remained (Boscarino et al., 2010). Furthermore, cross-sectional data from the 2002 National Health Interview Survey, an in-person household interview survey, in adults with (n = 6,829) and without (n = 20,676) arthritis demonstrated that the prevalence of severe psychological distress (SPD) in adults with arthritis is significantly higher than in adults without arthritis (5.6 % vs. 1.8 % and 26.2 % vs. 10.7 %, $P < 0.001$, respectively). In adults with arthritis, SPD was significantly associated with younger age, lower socioeconomic status, divorce/separation, recurrent pain, physical inactivity, having functional or social limitations, and having comorbid medical conditions. Adults aged 18 to 44 years were 6.5 times more likely to report SPD than those 65 years or older, and adults with recurrent pain were 3 times more likely to report SPD than those without recurrent pain. Serious psychological distress affects persons with arthritis and should be addressed in their treatment. Younger adults with arthritis, and those with recurrent pain or either functional or social limitations, may be at higher risk for SPD (Shih M, et al., 2006).

5.2 Stress and modulation of rheumatic disease activity

It was shown that perceived stress could be a predictor of rheumatic activity (Curtis et al., 2005). Otherwise, psychological stress is thought to aggravate disease activity in RA, although the physiologic mechanisms are not clear. Thus it was shown that brief psychological stress can trigger increased production of TNF-alpha of stimulated monocytes in RA patients. The use of TNF-alpha antagonists protects against stress activation of cellular markers of inflammation in RA patients (Motivala et al., 2008). In two prospective studies on RA, disease flare-ups were linked to a higher number of interpersonal minor stressors few days prior to the visit (Cutolo & Straub, 2006). In addition, it was shown that stress is a potentially important risk factor for the onset of adult Still's disease. Stressful life events (OR 2.56; 95% CI 1.18 to 5.52) in the year preceding the onset was significantly associated with increased risk for adult Still's disease (Sampalis et al., 1996). Likewise, a longitudinal study over a period of 5 years showed that RA patients with a higher daily stress level at baseline had a poorer outcome and significantly more bony erosions after 5 years. Therefore, long-lasting (chronic) stress may lead to proinflammatory effects because no adequate long-term responses of stress axes (HPA - anti-inflammatory) are to be expected. Only 5 studies on about 150 RA patients did not support the link between minor stress and disease flares (Cutolo & Straub, 2006). However, it was shown that psychological distress and social support are more important than objectively assessed disease status in determining marital and sexual satisfaction in patients with RA (vam Lankfeld et al., 2004).

In RA patients pain was the predominantly perceived stressor followed by limitation in mobility, difficulties in carrying out activities of daily living, helplessness, dependency on others, threat to self-esteem, interference in social activity, interference in family relationships, difficulties performing at work, and discomfort of the treatment (Mahat, 1997). Interestingly, perceived stress had the strongest relationship with psychological well-being of rheumatic patients (Treharne et al., 2007).

In a large population-based case-control study (1996–2003) with incident cases of RA (1,221 cases and 1,454 controls) it could be shown that high psychological stress of job demands tended to be associated with a decreased risk of RA (OR = 0.8; 95 % CI = 0.6 - 1.0). Interestingly, low decision latitude was associated with an increased risk of RA (self-reported data: OR = 1.6; 95 % CI = 1.2 - 2.2). Self-reported job strain was associated with a 30% higher risk of RA, compared with relaxed working conditions (Benggsson et al., 2009).

Similarly, in patients with osteoarthritis the relationship between social support, stress and functional status was of major importance. Thus, physical disability was associated with being older and having less tangible support; psychological disability was correlated with being younger, caucasian, and having less support; and pain was associated with being younger, caucasian and having less education. Self-esteem appeared to be the most, and appraisal the least, consistent social support dimension when predicting functional status. While exposure to stressors negatively affected functional status, its impact was greatest with respect to psychological disability (Weinberger et al., 1990).

6. Therapeutic interventions

Rheumatic diseases represent an important public health burden. To reduce the social and economic impact of these pathologies, an appropriate management of these conditions should be encouraged based on the use of established intervention strategies, including stress reduction approaches (Ottonello, 2007).

6.1 Psychological approach

In a recent metaanalysis of efficacy of psychological interventions in the treatment of RA patients 31 studies with 2021 patients could be included. There is consistent supportive evidence for the efficacy of disclosure therapy and cognitive behavioural therapy followed by maintenance therapy. Similarly, there is an evidence for improvement with behavioural therapy (> 6 weeks duration) in the short-term but conflicting evidence for its long-term efficacy. While there is some evidence for improvement with biofeedback-based interventions and relaxation therapy, there is conflicting evidence for the benefits of counselling, psychotherapy, mindfulness and meditation, and behavioural therapy of less than 6 weeks duration (Dissanayake & Bertouch, 2010).

One possibility to reduce stress for patients with rheumatic diseases is cognitive-behavioural therapy aimed at minimisation of pain episodes and stressful events, improving quality of life and involving education, training in various types of relaxation approaches and other coping skills. Ideally the application of these skills includes the patient's home and work environment. It was shown that cognitive-behavioural therapy and stress management may be useful adjuvant therapy when treating the disease symptoms of children with polyarticular arthritis (Schanberg et al., 2005). Otherwise, patients with RA under greater perceived stress who do not use active coping strategies appear to be at risk of psychological comorbidity and may therefore benefit from interventions teaching specific active coping strategies (Treharne et al., 2007). A significant relationship between specific stressors and utilisation of coping strategies could be demonstrated: interference in family relationships and use of evasive coping strategies ($p < 0.05$), threat to self-esteem and use of both evasive and emotive coping strategies (Mahat, 1997). Interestingly, an active behavioural coping buffered an association of stress with depression, while active cognitive coping buffered the effect of baseline stress on life satisfaction after 6 months of intervention. Patients with RA under greater perceived stress who do not use active coping strategies appear to be at risk of psychological comorbidity and may therefore benefit from interventions teaching specific active coping strategies (Treharne et al., 2007). Optimistic and confronting coping strategies were found most frequently and perceived to be most effective against distress (Herrmann et al., 2000). Furthermore, a sample of patients with RA who completed a stress management training program (such as self-efficacy, coping strategies, and helplessness) had a decrease of pain and depression due to beneficial changes in the arenas of self-efficacy (the belief that one can perform a specific behaviour or task in the future), coping strategies (an individual's confidence in his or her ability to manage pain), and helplessness (perceptions of control regarding arthritis) (Rhee, 2000).

Moreover, several studies suggest that the cognitive-behavioural approach is efficacious in RA and osteoarthritis in improving not only the psychological adjustment during the course of the disease but also physical function (Ottonello, 2007). It was demonstrated that psychosocial intervention (conventional psychotherapy or assertion/relaxation training) leads to improvement in functional status or disease activity of RA patients (Strauss et al., 1986). Moreover, cognitive-behavioural therapy and mindfulness interventions that target responses to chronic stress, pain, and depression reduce pain and the pro-inflammatory IL-6 improving the quality of everyday life for adults with RA (Zautra et al., 2008).

Otherwise, cognitive behavioural interventions to facilitate patient adjustment could usefully include not only management of stress and its appraisal but also utilisation of social support resources (Curtis et al., 2005). Several longitudinal studies have demonstrated that stress appraisal and resultant coping responses affect health outcome and health-related quality of life in women. In addition to problem-focused coping, women often use distraction methods, seeking social support and faith or religious coping. Psychological interventions in chronic medical conditions need to move beyond education and incorporate more cognitive behavioural components, at the same time addressing women's specific needs. Coping behaviours in response to the negative threat of a chronic or severe medical illness serve to reduce psychological distress (Rao, 2009). One of the important factors to sustain a psychological well-being is the social background; in particular functioning of the family is of outstanding importance for clinical and psychological outcomes (Herrmann et al., 2000). On the other hand, personality and social relationships play an important role in almost every aspect of stress and coping. Daily process methods are particularly useful in elucidating how these factors might influence both responses to and outcomes of stress (DeLongis & Holtzman, 2005). Furthermore, a randomized clinical trial to evaluate a psychological intervention and social support program in RA patients showed that the psychological intervention produced significant reductions in patients' pain behaviour and disease activity. Significant reductions were also observed in trait anxiety after treatment and at 6-month follow-up. The social support program produced a significant reduction in trait anxiety after treatment only (Bradlex et al., 1987). Moreover, in the European Research on Incapacitating Diseases and Social Support cohort of patients with early RA it was demonstrated that patients with a greater amount of specific social support or a stronger specific support network experienced less functional limitation and less psychological distress (Demange et al., 2004). Controlled studies of RA patients demonstrated that the ability of self-management behaviours (accommodation, active remediation, perseverance) can decrease impact of RA-related stressors (pain, fatigue, physical limitations, joint changes, and symptom unpredictability) to perform life activities ($p < 0.01 - 0.0001$) (Katz et al., 2005).

6.2 Muscle relaxation training

Otherwise, supervised muscle relaxation training exercised 30 minutes, twice a week for 10 weeks in individuals with RA indicated improvements in the training group regarding self-care according to the Arthritis Impact Measurement Scales 2, and in recreation and pastimes according to the Sickness Impact Profile-RA ($p < 0.05$) directly after the intervention. Mobility and arm function ($p < 0.01$) according to the Arthritis Impact Measurement Scales 2, and muscle function of the lower limbs ($p < 0.05$) were improved after six months of training (Lundgren & Stenström, 1999). There has been an increasing interest in meditation as a mind-body approach, given its potential to alleviate emotional distress and promote improved well-being in a variety of populations (Young, 2011). A randomized, waitlist-controlled pilot study of 4 month's Mindfulness-Based Stress Reduction program showed a significant decrease of psychological distress and strengthening well-being in patients with RA (Pradhan, 2007).

6.3 Tai chi

It was also shown that Tai chi is beneficial in stress inhibition increasing daily activities in RA patients. Tai Chi is a traditional Chinese art which combines a multimodal, complex intervention that may include interaction of physical, cognitive, and ritualistic components (including, for example, elements of musculoskeletal efficiency, breathing, mindfulness, psychosocial interactions, rituals, and environment) (Wayne & Kaptchuk, 2008). Two randomised clinical trials (RCTs) and three non-randomized clinical trials about efficacy of

Tai chi in RA were published. The included RCTs reported some positive findings for Tai chi on disability index, quality of life, depression and mood for RA patients. Two RCTs assessed pain outcomes and did not demonstrate effectiveness on pain reduction compared with education plus stretching exercise and usual activity control. Currently there are few trials testing the effectiveness of Tai chi in the management of RA (Lee et al., 2007). It was demonstrated that Tai chi practice lead to improved lower-limb muscle function, confidence in moving, balance and less pain during exercise and in daily life, stress reduction, increased body awareness at the end of intervention and at 12 weeks follow-up in patients with RA (Uhlig et al., 2010). Furthermore, in one randomised controlled trial there was an ACR20 (American College Rheumatology) response of 50 % in the Tai chi group compared with 0% in the control at 12 weeks ($p = 0.03$). Tai chi had greater improvements in the disability index ($p = 0.01$), vitality subscale of the Medical Outcome Study Short Form 36 ($p = 0.01$) and the depression index ($p = 0.003$). Similar trends to improvement were also observed for disease activity, functional capacity and health-related quality of life. It was concluded that Tai Chi appears safe and may be beneficial for functional class I or II RA (Wang, 2008). Despite certain limitations this exercise showed reduction of stress and improved quality of life and it can be recommended to patients with osteoarthritis and RA as a complementary and alternative medical approach (Wang, 2011). However, in the treatment of chronic conditions such as rheumatic diseases, particularly when it comes to complementary modalities such as tai chi, therapies are often used and studied in conjunction with other treatments. Although these heterogeneous interventions may better represent how care is delivered in real-world settings, they sometimes create problems when it comes to interpreting research findings (Yeh, 2008). Otherwise, the studies that are available are of low methodological quality. Taken together, evidence is not convincing enough to suggest that Tai chi is an effective treatment for RA. The value of Tai chi for this indication therefore remains unproven (Lee et al., 2007).

6.4 Yoga

Over the last 10 years, a growing number of research studies have shown that the practice of yoga can improve strength and flexibility, and may help control such physiological variables as blood pressure, respiration and heart rate, and metabolic rate to improve overall exercise capacity finally resulting in a benefit of yoga for people compromised by musculoskeletal disease (Raub, 2002). For example, it was demonstrated that 10-week yoga interventions in patients with RA significantly decreased the disability index, perception of pain and depression, and improved balance (Bosch et al., 2009). Another study of yoga showed improvements in mental health, vitality, and self-efficacy in a group of young patients with RA (age 18-36 years). Interviews demonstrated improvement in RA symptoms and functioning but uncertainty about whether the intervention affected pain (Ewans et al., 2010). Otherwise, it was indicated that 12 sessions of Raj yoga carried out bi-weekly might improve significantly disease activity and disability index (Badsha et al., 2009). Furthermore, hand grip strength of both hands, measured with a grip dynamometer, increased in normal adults and children as well as in RA patients, but not in the corresponding control groups. Adult female volunteers and patients showed a greater improvement than corresponding adult males. This gender-based difference was not observed in children (Dash & Telles, 2001). One pilot study of 8-week course of yoga in patients with osteoarthritis suggests that yoga may provide a feasible treatment option for previously yoga-naive, obese patients > 50 years of age and offers potential reductions in pain and disability. Statistically significant reductions in Western Ontario and McMaster Universities Osteoarthritis Index (WOMAC) Pain, WOMAC Physical Function, and Arthritis Impact Measurement Scales, patient and physician global assessments were demonstrated (Kolasinski et al., 2005).

6.5 Acupuncture

Acupuncture, which originated with traditional Chinese medicine, is another therapy option that reduces stress, relieves pain and promotes an increase in quality of life. Several systematic reviews have assessed the effectiveness of acupuncture for rheumatic conditions, often with contradictory conclusions. Relatively clear evidence emerged to suggest that acupuncture is effective for osteoarthritis, low back pain and lateral elbow pain to warrant positive recommendations of this therapy in routine care for such patients but being ineffective for RA (Ernst & Lee, 2010). In another systematic review it was shown that acupuncture with duration of 11 weeks results in a decrease in pain compared to controls; the mean or median changes of acupuncture-decreased tenderness of joints ranged from 1.5 to 6.5. In addition, a significant reduction of morning stiffness (mean change - 29 minutes) was noted, but the difference was not statistically significant versus controls. With regard to inflammatory markers, a reduction in erythrocyte sedimentation ratio (mean change - 3.9 mm/hour) and a CRP level reduction (mean change - 2.9 mg/dl) was observed. Despite some favourable results in active-controlled trials, conflicting evidence exists in placebo-controlled trials concerning the efficacy of acupuncture for RA (Wang et al., 2008). Regarding anaesthesia, supportive acupuncture treatment is performed for postoperative pain based on promising results of rigorous randomised trials. Many unresolved questions remain, such as regarding specificity of concepts, indications, and optimum dose (Stör & Irnich, 2009).

Individuals who are at risk to develop an autoimmune disease should be advised to refrain from lifestyle and activities that endanger their future health and quality of life. Different stress reactions should be discussed with patients, and obligatory questionnaires about trigger factors should include psychological stress in addition the usual suspects such as infection and trauma (Stojanovich et al., 2008). Stress reduction interventions can have a positive therapeutic effect in autoimmune disease patients leading to a reduction in the social and economic impact of rheumatic diseases. An appropriate management of these conditions should be encouraged based on the use of established intervention strategies. Physicians and patients should recognize the potential of stress to impact autoimmune diseases and that stress management should be integrated in a multidimensional treatment approach (McCray & Agarwal, 2011).

7. Conclusion

Rheumatic diseases are chronic inflammatory disorders of unknown aetiology and variable severity. It is now well known that several risk factors are contributing to aetiology and pathophysiology of rheumatic diseases, including genetic factors, sex hormones and environmental factors, e.g. infections and stress. An increasing number of studies could demonstrate that psychological stress and stress-related hormones are involved in immune modulation, which ultimately may result in autoimmune disease. Stress related hormones exert numerous effects on various immune functions, e.g. chronic mild stress (family or occupational stress) lead to proinflammatory effects thereby increasing disease activity. Emotional stress could be shown to modulate pain reception and to modify quality of life in patients with rheumatic diseases. Furthermore, a positive correlation between stress levels and the onset of rheumatic diseases could be demonstrated. Unfortunately, not only stress causes disease, but the disease itself also causes significant stress in the patients disturbing the physiological stress response. In this respect, it could be demonstrated that coping strategies reduce stress episodes with a positive impact on disease activity in patients with rheumatic diseases. However, more studies are warranted to further explore the pathophysiological implications of stress on onset and activity of chronic autoimmune diseases. In particular stress is now recognised as an important risk factor for the onset and even more for the modulation of disease activity in different rheumatic diseases.

8. References

Adam, O.; Fasse, S. & Ditrich, O. (2009). Diet in rheumatic disease. *Z. Rheumat*, Vol.68, No.7 (September 2010), pp. 549-58, quiz 559

Ader, R.; Cohen, N. & Felten, D. (1995). Psychoneuroimmunology: interactions between the nervous system and the immune system. *Lancet*, Vol. 345, No. 345 (14.01.1995), pp. 99-103

Aguilera, G. (2011). HPA axis responsiveness to stress: implications for healthy aging. *Exp Gerontol*, Vol.46, No. 2 - 3 (Februar - March 2011) , pp. 90-95

Anthony, K. & Schanberg L. (2007). Assessment and management of pain syndromes and arthritis pain in children and adolescents. *Rheum Dis Clin North Am.*, Vol. 33, No. 3 (August 2007), pp. 25-60

Arguelles, L.M.; Afari, N., Buchwald, D.S., Clauw, D.J., Furner, S., Goldberg, J. (2006). A twin study of posttraumatic stress disorder symptoms and chronic widespread pain. *Pain*, Vol.124, No.1 - 2 (September 2006), pp. 150-157

Badsha, H., Chhabra, V., Leibman, C., Mofti, A., Kong, K.O. (2009). The benefits of yoga for rheumatoid arthritis: results of a preliminary, structured 8-week program. *Rheumatol Int*, Vol.29, No.12 (October 2009), pp. 1417-1421

Baerwald, C.G.; Panayi, G.S. & Lanchbury, J.S. (1997). Corticotropin releasing hormone promoter region polymorphisms in rheumatoid arthritis. *J Rheumatol*, Vol.24, No. 1 (Januar 1997), pp. 215-216

Bengtsson, C.; Theorell T., Klareskog, L., Alfredsson, L. (2009). Psychosocial stress at work and the risk of developing rheumatoid arthritis: results from the Swedish EIRA study. *Psychother Psychosom*, Vol.78, No.3 (March 2009), pp. 193-194

Benveniste, E.N. (1998). Cytokine actions in the central nervous system. *Cytokine Growth Factor Rev*, Vol.9, No.3-4 (September-December 1998), pp. 259-275

Bergsten, U.; Bergman, S., Fridlund, B., Alfredsson, L., Berglund, A., Petersson, I.F., Arvidsson, B. (2009). EIRA Study Group. Patients' conceptions of the cause of their rheumatoid arthritis: a qualitative study. *Musculoskeletal Care*, Vol.7, No.4 (December 2009), pp. 243-255

Borger, P., Hoekstra, Y., Esselink, M.T., Postma, D.S., Zaagsma, J., Vellenga, E., Kauffman, H.F. (1998). Beta-adrenoceptor-mediated inhibition of IFNgamma, IL-3, and GM-CSF mRNA accumulation in activated human T lymphocytes is solely mediated by the beta2-adrenoceptor subtype. *Am. J. Respir. Cell Mol. Biol,* Vol.19, No.3 (September 1998), pp. 400–407

Boscarino, J.A. (2004). Posttraumatic stress disorder and physical illness: results from clinical and epidemiologic studies *Ann N Y Acad Sci,* Vol.1032 (December 2004), pp. 141-153

Bosch, P.R.; Traustadóttir, T., Howard, P., Matt, K.S. (2009). Functional and physiological effects of yoga in women with rheumatoid arthritis: a pilot study. *Altern Ther Health Med,* Vol.15, No.4 (Juli - August 2009), pp. 24-31

Bradley, L.A., Young, L.D., Anderson, K.O., Turner, R.A., Agudelo, C.A., McDaniel, L.K., Pisko, E.J., Semble, E.L., Morgan, T.M. (1987). Effects of psychological therapy on pain behavior of rheumatoid arthritis patients. Treatment outcome and six-month followup. *Arthritis Rheum,* Vol.30, No.10 (October 1987), pp. 1105-1114

Bugajska, J.; Brzosko, M., Jedryka-Góral, A., Głuszko, P., Zołnierczyk-Zreda, D., Sagan, A., Konarska, M., Rell-Bakalarska, M., Pazdur, J., Zeidler, H., Rihl, M.; PGG-SES-AIMs. (2010). Psychological stress in rheumatoid arthritis patients: a comparative Polish-German study: summary of the current conceptualization of the role of stress in rheumatoid arthritis. *Autoimmun Rev,* Vol.9, No.4 (Februar 2010), pp. 211-215

Carette, S., Surtees, P.G., Wainwright, N.W., Khaw, K.T., Symmons, D.P., Silman, A.J. (2000). The role of life events and childhood experiences in the development of rheumatoid arthritis. *J Rheumatol,* Vol.27, No.9 (September 2000), pp. 2123-2130

Cay, H.F.; Sezer, I., Firat, M.Z., Kaçar, C. (2011). Which is the dominant factor for perception of rheumatic pain: meteorology or psychology? *Rheumatol Int,* Vol.31, No.3 (March 2011), pp. 377-385.

Chikanza, I.C., Chrousos, G.P. & Panayi, G.S. (1992). Abnormal neuroendocrine immune communications in patients with rheumatoid arthritis. *Eur J Clin Invest,* Vol.26, No.10 (October 1992), pp. 635-637

Chikanza, I.C., Petrou, P., Kingsley, G., Chrousos, G., Panayi, G.S. (1992). Defective hypothalamic response to immune and inflammatory stimuli in patients with rheumatoid arthritis. *Arthritis Rheum,* Vol.35, No.11 (November 1992), pp. 1281-1288

Chrousos, G.P. (1995). The hypothalamic-pituitary-adrenal axis and immunemediated inflammation. *N Engl J Med,* Vol.332, No.20 (May 1995), pp. 1351-1362

Curtis, R., Groarke, A., Coughlan, R., Gsel, A. (2005). Psychological stress as a predictor of psychological adjustment and health status in patients with rheumatoid arthritis. *Patient Educ Couns,* Vol.59, No.2 (November 2005), pp.192-198

Cutolo, M. & Straub R.H. (2006). Stress as a risk factor in the pathogenesis of rheumatoid arthritis. *Neuroimmunomodulation,* Vol.13, No.5-6 (August 2006), pp. 277-282

Damjanović, V.; Vasilj, I., Vlak, T., Zelenika, D. (2009). Prevalence and risk factors of the rheumatoid arthritis in Herzegovina region in 2003-2005. *Coll Antropol,* Vol.33, Suppl. 2 (December 2009), pp. 73-77

Dash, M. & Telles, S. (2001). Improvement in hand grip strength in normal volunteers and rheumatoid arthritis patients following yoga training. *Indian J Physiol Pharmacol,* Vol.45, No.3 (Juli 2001), pp. 355-360

de Brouwer, S.J.; Kraaimaat, F.W., Sweep, F.C., Creemers, M.C., Radstake, T.R., van Laarhoven, A.I., van Riel, P.L., Evers, A.W. (2010). Experimental stress in inflammatory rheumatic diseases: a review of psychophysiological stress responses. *Arthritis Res Ther,* Vol.12, No.3 (Mai 2010), R.89

DeLongis, A. & Holtzman, S. (2005). Coping in context: the role of stress, social support, and personality in coping. *J Pers.* Vol.73, No.6 (December 2005), pp. 1633-1656

Demange, V.; Guillemin, F., Baumann, M., Suurmeijer, T.P., Moum, T., Doeglas, D., Briançon, S., van den Heuvel, W.J. (2004). Are there more than cross-sectional relationships of social support and support networks with functional limitations and psychological distress in early rheumatoid arthritis? The European Research on Incapacitating Diseases and Social Support Longitudinal Study. *Arthritis Rheum*, Vol.15, No.5 (October 2004), pp. 782-791

Dissanayake, R.K. & Bertouch, J.V. (2010). Psychosocial interventions as adjunct therapy for patients with rheumatoid arthritis: a systematic review. *Int J Rheum Dis*, Vol.13, No.4 (October 2010), pp. 324-334

Dube, S.R.; Fairweather, D., Pearson, W.S., Felitti, V.J., Anda, R.F., Croft, J.B. (2009). Cumulative childhood stress and autoimmune diseases in adults. *Psychosom Med*, Vol.71, No.2 (Februar 2009), pp. 243-250

Dunn, A.J. & Swiergiel, A.H. (2008). The role of corticotropin-releasing factor and noradrenaline in stress-related responses, and the inter-relationships between the two systems. *Eur J Pharmacol*, Vol.583, No.2-3 (07.04.2008), pp. 186-193

Eder, L.; Loo, T., Chandran, V., Kalman-Lamb, G., Shanmugarajah, S., Shen, H., Rosen, C.F., Cook, R.J., Gladman, D.D. (2011). The association between environmental factors and onset of psoriatic arthritis in patients with psoriasis. *Arthritis Care Res (Hoboken)*, (10.05.2011), doi: 10.1002/acr.20496

Eijsbouts, A.M.; van den Hoogen, F.H., Laan, R.F., Hermus, A.R., Sweep, C.G. van de Putte, L.B. (2005). Hypothalamic-pituitary-adrenal axis activity in patients with rheumatoid arthritis. *Clin Exp Rheumatol,* Vol.23, No.5 (September-October 2005), pp. 658-664

Elenkov, I.J. & Chrousos, G.P. (1999). Stress hormones, Th1/Th2 patterns, pro/anti-inflammatory cytokines and susceptibility to disease. *Trends Endocrinol Metab,* Vol.10, No.9 (November 1999), pp. 359-368

Elenkov, I.J. (2008). Neurohormonal-cytokine interactions: implications for inflammation, common human diseases and well-being. *Neurochem Int,* Vol.52, No.1-2 (Januar 2008), pp. 40-51

Elenkov, I.J.; Wilder, R.L., Chrousos, G.P., Vizi, E.S. (2000). The sympathetic nerve--an integrative interface between two supersystems: the brain and the immune system. *Pharmacol Rev,* Vol.52, No.4 (December 2000), pp. 595-638

Ernst, E. & Lee, M.S. (2010). Acupuncture for rheumatic conditions: an overview of systematic reviews. *Rheumatology (Oxford),* Vol.49, No.10 (October 2010), pp. 1957-1961

Eskandari, F.; Webster, J.I. & Sternberg, E.M. (2003). Neural immune pathways and their connection to inflammatory diseases. *Arthritis Res Ther,* 2003; Vol.5, No.6 (September 2003), pp. 251-265

Evans, S.; Moieni, M., Taub, R., Subramanian, S.K., Tsao, J.C., Sternlieb, B., Zeltzer, L.K. (2010). Iyengar yoga for young adults with rheumatoid arthritis: results from a mixed-methods pilot study. *J Pain Symptom Manage,* Vol.39, No.5 (May 2010), pp. 904-913

Felten, S.Y.; Felten, D.L., Bellinger, D.L., Carlson, S.L., Ackerman, K.D., Madden, K.S., Olschowka, J.A., Livnat, S. (1988). Noradrenergic sympathetic innervation of lymphoid organs. *Prog Allergy, Vol.* 43, pp. 14-36

Fioravanti, A.; Cantarini, L., Guidelli, G.M., Galeazzi, M. (2011). Mechanisms of action of spa therapies in rheumatic diseases: what scientific evidence is there? *Rheumatol Int,* Vol.31, No.1(Januar 2011), pp. 1-8

Frank, R.G.; Hagglund, K.J., Schopp, L.H., Thayer, J.F., Vieth, A.Z., Cassidy J.T., Goldstein, D.E., Beck, N.C., Clay, D.L., Hewett, J.E., Johnson, J.C., Chaney, J.M., Kashani, J.H. (1998). Disease and family contributors to adaptation in juvenile rheumatoid arthritis and juvenile diabetes. *Arthritis Care Res,* Vol.11, No.3 (Januar 1998), pp. 166-176

Geenen, R.; Godaert, G.L., Heijnen, C.J., Vianen, M.E., Wenting, M.J., Nederhoff, M.G., Bijlsma, J.W. (1998). Experimentally induced stress in rheumatoid arthritis of recent onset: effects on peripheral blood lymphocytes. *Clin Exp Rheumatol,* Vol.16, No.5 (September - October 1998), pp. 553-559

Gouin, J.P.; Hantsoo, L. & Kiecolt-Glaser, J.K. (2008). Immune dysregulation and chronic stress among older adults: a review. *Neuroimmunomodulation,* Vol.15, No.4-6 (November 2008), pp. 251-259

Herrmann, M.; Schölmerich, J. & Straub, R.H. (2000). Stress and rheumatic diseases. *Rheum Dis Clin North Am,* Vol.26, No.4 (November 2000), pp. 737-763

Hinrichsen, H.; Barth, J., Ruckemann, M., Ferstl, R., Kirch, W. (1992). Influence of prolonged neuropsychological testing on immunoregulatory cells and hormonal parameters in patients with systemic lupus erythematosus. *Rheumatol Int,* No.12, No.2, pp. 47-51

Jacobs, R., Pawlak, C.R., Mikeska, E., Meyer-Olson, D., Martin, M., Heijnen, C.J., Schedlowski, M., Schmidt, R.E. (2001). Systemic lupus erythematosus and rheumatoid arthritis patients differ from healthy controls in their cytokine pattern after stress exposure. *Rheumatology (Oxford),* Vol.40, No.8 (August 2001), pp. 868-875

Katz, P.P. (2005). Use of self-management behaviors to cope with rheumatoid arthritis stressors. *Arthritis Rheum,* Vol.15, No.53 (December 2005), pp. 939-949

Kin, N.W. & Sanders, V.M. (2006). It takes nerve to tell T and B cells what to do. *Leukoc Biol,* Vol.79, No.6 (Juni 2006), pp. 1093-1104

Kobayashi, S.; Momohara, S., Kamatani, N., Okamoto, H. (2008). Molecular aspects of rheumatoid arthritis: role of environmental factors. *FEBS J.* Vol.275, No.18 (September 2008), pp. 4456-4462

Kohm, A.P. & Sanders, V.M. (2000). Norepinephrine: a messenger from the brain to the immune system. *Immunol Today,* Vol.21, No.11 (November 2000), pp. 539–542

Kolasinski, S.L., Garfinkel, M., Tsai, A.G., Matz, W., Van Dyke, A., Schumacher, H.R. (2005). Iyengar yoga for treating symptoms of osteoarthritis of the knees: a pilot study. *J Altern Complement Med,* Vol.11, No.4 (August 2005), pp. 689-693

Kurtais, Y.; Tur, B.S., Elhan, A.H., Erdogan, M.F., Yalcin, P. (2006). Hypothalamic-pituitaryadrenal hormonal responses to exercise stress test in patients with rheumatoid arthritis compared to healthy controls. *J Rheumatol,* Vol.33, No.8 (August 2006), pp. 1530-1537

Laborde, J.M. & Dando , W.A. & Powers, M.J. (1986). Influence of weather on osteoarthritics. *Soc Sci Med*, Vol.23, No.6, pp. 549-554

Lee, M.S.; Pittler, M.H. & Ernst, E. (2007). Tai chi for rheumatoid arthritis: systematic review. *Rheumatology (Oxford)*, Vol.46, No.11 (November 2007), pp. 1648-1651

Li, J., Schiøttz-Christensen, B., Olsen, J. (2005) Psychological stress and rheumatoid arthritis in parents after death of a child: a national follow-up study. *Scand J Rheumatol*, Vol.34, No.6 (November-December 2005), pp. 448-450

Li, S. & Micheletti, R. (2011). Role of diet in rheumatic disease. *Rheum Dis Clin North Am*, Vol.37, No.1 (Februar 2011), pp. 119-133

Li, X.; Sundquist, J. & Sundquist, K. (2008). Socioeconomic and occupational risk factors for rheumatoid arthritis: a nationwide study based on hospitalizations in Sweden. *J Rheumatol*, Vol.35, No.6 (Juni 2008), pp. 986-991

Lorton, D.; Bellinger, D., Duclos, M., Felten, S.Y., Felten, D.L. (1996). Application of 6-hydroxydopamine into the fatpads surrounding the draining lymph nodes exacerbates adjuvant-induced arthritis. *J Neuroimmunol*, 1996, Vol.64, No.2 (Februar 1996), pp.103-113

Lundgren, S. & Stenström, C.H. (1999). Muscle relaxation training and quality of life in rheumatoid arthritis. A randomized controlled clinical trial. *Scand J Rheumatol*, Vol.28, No.1, pp. 47-53

Macfarlane, G.J.; Norrie, G., Atherton, K., Power, C., Jones, G.T. (2009). The influence of socioeconomic status on the reporting of regional and widespread musculoskeletal pain: results from the 1958 British Birth Cohort Study. *Ann Rheum Dis*, Vol.68, No.10 (October 2009), pp. 1591-1595

Macfarlane, T.V., McBeth, J., Jones, G.T., Nicholl, B., Macfarlane, G.J. (2010). Whether the weather influences pain? Results from the EpiFunD study in North West England. *Rheumatology (Oxford)*, Vol.49. No.8 (August 2010), pp. 1513-1520

Madden, K.S. (2001). Catecholamines, sympathetic nerves, and immunity. In: *Psychoneuroimmunology*, Ader, R., Felten, D.L., Cohen, N., pp. 197–216, Academic Press, ISBN 0120443147, San Diego

Madden, K.S.; Sanders, V.M. & Felten, D.L. (1995). Catecholamine influences and sympathetic neural modulation of immune responsiveness. *Annu Rev Pharmacol Toxicol*, Vol.35, pp. 417-448

Mahat. G. (1997). Perceived stressors and coping strategies among individuals with rheumatoid arthritis. *J Adv Nurs*, Vol.25, No.6 (Juni 1997). pp. 1144-1150

Malysheva, O.; Pierer, M., Wagner, U., Wahle, M., Wagner, U., Baerwald, C.G. (2008). Association between beta2 adrenergic receptor polymorphisms and rheumatoid arthritis in conjunction with human leukocyte antigen (HLA)-DRB1 shared epitope. *Ann Rheum Dis*, Vol.67, No.12 (December 2008), pp. 1759-1764

Malysheva, O.; Wagner, U., Wahle, M., Pierer, M., Wagner, U., Stalla, G.K., Baerwald, C.G. (2011). Hypothalamic-pituitary-adrenal axis stress test in patients with early RA: role of corticotropin-releasing hormone promoter polymorphisms. *Ann Rheum Dis*, (10.06.2011) [Epub ahead of print]

Marshall, G.D. Jr. (1997). The adverse effects of psychological stress on immunoregulatory balance: applications to human inflammatory diseases. *Coll Antropol*, Vol.21, No.1 (Juni 1997), pp. 17-28

McCray, C.J. & Agarwal, S.K. (2011). Stress and autoimmunity. *Immunol Allergy Clin North Am*, Vol.31, No.1 (Februar 2011), pp. 1-18

McEwen, B.S. & Gianaros, P.J. (2011). Stress- and allostasis-induced brain plasticity. *Annu Rev Med*, Vol.18, No.62 (Februar 2011), pp. 431-445

McEwen, B.S. (1998). Protective and damaging effects of stress mediators. *N Engl J Med*, Vol.338, pp. 171-179

Mix, E., Goertsches, R. & Zettl, U.K. (2007). Immunology and neurology. *J Neurol*, Vol.254, Suppl 2 (May 2007), pp. II2-117

Motivala, S.J.; Khanna, D., FitzGerald, J., Irwin, M.R. (2008). Stress activation of cellular markers of inflammation in rheumatoid arthritis: protective effects of tumor necrosis factor alpha antagonists. *Arthritis Rheum*, Vol.58, No.2 (Februar 2008), pp. 376-383

Niederkorn, J.Y., Stern, M.E., Pflugfelder, S.C., De Paiva, C.S., Corrales, R.M., Gao, J., Siemasko, K. (2006). Desiccating stress induces T cell-mediated Sjögren's Syndrome-like lacrimal keratoconjunctivitis. *J Immunol*, Vol.176, No.7 (01.04.2006), pp. 3950-3957

O'Connor, T.M.; O'Halloran, D.J. & Shanahan, F. (2000). The stress response and the hypothalamic-pituitary-adrenal axis: from molecule to melancholia. *QJM*, Vol.93, No.6 (Juni 2000), pp. 323-333

Ottonello, M. (2007). Cognitive-behavioral interventions in rheumatic diseases. *G Ital Med Lav Ergon*, Vol.29, 1 Suppl.A (Januar-March 2007), pp. A19-23

Parniapour, M.; Nordin, M., Skovron, M.L., Frankel, V.H. (1990). Environmentally induced disorders of the musculoskeletal system. *Med Clin North Am*, Vol.74, No.2 (March 1990), pp. 347-359

Pedersen, M.; Jacobsen, S., Klarlund, M., Frisch, M. (2006). Socioeconomic status and risk of rheumatoid arthritis: a Danish case-control study. *J Rheumatol*, Vol.33, No.6 (Juni 2006), pp. 1069-1074

Pêgo, J.M.; Sousa, J.C., Almeida, O.F., Sousa, N. (2010). Stress and the neuroendocrinology of anxiety disorders. *Curr Top Behav Neurosci*, Vol.2, pp. 97-117.

Pool, A.J., Whipp, B.J., Skasick, A.J., Alavi, A., Bland, J.M., Axford, J.S. (2004). Serum cortisol reduction and abnormal prolactin and CD4+/CD8+ T-cell response as a result of controlled exercise in patients with rheumatoid arthritis and systemic lupus erythematosus despite unaltered muscle energetics. *Rheumatology (Oxford)*, Vol.43, pp. 43-48

Pradhan, E.K.; Baumgarten, M., Langenberg, P., Handwerger, B., Gilpin, A.K., Magyari, T., Hochberg, M.C., Berman, B.M. (2007). Effect of Mindfulness-Based Stress Reduction in rheumatoid arthritis patients. *Arthritis Rheum*, Vol.15, No.57 (October 2007), pp. 1134-1142

Rao, K. (2009). Recent research in stress, coping and women's health. *Curr Opin Psychiatry*, Vol.22, No.2 (March 2009), pp. 188-193

Raub, J.A. (2002). Psychophysiologic effects of Hatha Yoga on musculoskeletal and cardiopulmonary function: a literature review. *J. Altern Complement Med*, Vol.8, No.6 (December 2002), pp. 797-812

Rhee, S.H.; Parker, J.C., Smarr, K.L., Petroski, G.F., Johnson, J.C., Hewett, J.E., Wright, G.E., Multon, K.D., Walker, S.E. (2000). Stress management in rheumatoid arthritis: what is the underlying mechanism? *Arthritis Care Res*, Vol.13, No.6 (December 2000), pp. 435-442

Rimón, R. & Laakso, R.L. (1985). Life stress and rheumatoid arthritis. A 15-year follow-up study. *Psychother Psychosom*, Vol.43, No.1, pp. 38-43

Rios, R. & Zautra, A.J. (2011). Socioeconomic disparities in pain: the role of economic hardship and daily financial worry. *Health Psychol*, Vol.30, No.1 (Januar 2011), pp. 58-66

Roupe van der Voort, C.; Heijnen, C.J., Wulffraat, N., Kuis, W., Kavelaars, A. (2000). Stress induces increases in IL-6 production by leucocytes of patients with the chronic inflammatory disease juvenile rheumatoid arthritis: a putative role for alpha(1)-adrenergic receptors. *J Neuroimmunol*, Vol.110, No.1-2 (October 2000), pp. 223-229

Ryan, J.L.; Ramsey, R.R., Fedele, D.A., Mullins, L.L., Chaney, J.M., Jarvis, J.N. (2010). A longitudinal examination of the parent-child distress relationship in children with juvenile rheumatic disease. *Rehabil Psychol*, Vol.55, No.3 (August 2010), pp. 286-291

Sampalis, J.S.; Medsger, T.A. Jr., Fries, J.F., Yeadon, C., Senécal, J.L., Myhal, D., Harth, M., Gutkowski, A., Carette, S., Beaudet, F., Partridge, A.J., Esdaile, J.M. (1996). Risk factors for adult Still's disease. *J Rheumatol*, Vol.23, No.12 (December 1996), pp. 2049-2054

Sanders, V.M.; Baker, R.A., Ramer-Quinn, D.S., Kasprowicz, D.J., Fuchs, B.A.,Street, N.E. (1997). Differential expression of the beta2-adrenergic receptor by Th1 and Th2 clones: implications for cytokine production and B cell help. *J. Immunol*, Vol.158, No 9 (01.05.1997), pp. 4200–4210

Schanberg, L.E.; Gil, K.M., Anthony, K.K., Yow, E., Rochon, J. (2005). Pain, stiffness, and fatigue in juvenile polyarticular arthritis: contemporaneous stressful events and mood as predictors. *Arthritis Rheum*, Vol.52, No.4 (April 2005), pp. 1196-1204

Sebire, G.; Emilie, D., Wallon, C., Hery, C., Devergne, O., Delfraissy, J.F., Galanaud, P., Tardieu, M. (1993). In vitro production of IL-6, IL-1 beta, and tumor necrosis factor-alpha by human embryonic microglial and neural cells. *J Immunol*, Vol.150, No.4 (15.02.1993), pp. 1517-1523

Segal, B.M.; Dwyer, B.K., Shevach, E.M., (1998). An interleukin (IL)-10/IL-12 immunoregulatory circuit controls susceptibility to autoimmune disease. *J. Exp. Med*, Vol.187, No.4 (16.02.1998), pp. 537–546

Shih, M., Hootman, J.M., Strine, T.W., Chapman, D.P., Brady, T.J. (2006). Serious psychological distress in U.S. adults with arthritis. *J. Gen Intern Med*, Vol.21, No.11 (November 2006), pp. 1160-1166

Smedslund, G. & Hagen, K.B. (2011). Does rain really cause pain? A systematic review of the associations between weather factors and severity of pain in people with rheumatoid arthritis. *Eur J Pain*, Vol.15, No.1 (Januar 2011), pp. 5-10

Sommershof, A.; Aichinger, H., Engler, H., Adenauer, H., Catani, C., Boneberg, E.M., Elbert, T., Groettrup, M., Kolassa, I.T. (2009). Substantial reduction of naïve and regulatory T cells following traumatic stress. *Brain Behav Immun* Vol.23, No.8 (November 2009), pp. 1117-1124

Spengler, R.N.; Chensue, S.W., Giacherio, D.A., Blenk, N., Kunkel, S.L. (1994). Endogenous norepinephrine regulates tumor necrosis factor-_production from macrophages in vitro. *J Immunol*, Vol.152, No.6 (15.03.1994), pp. 3024–3031

Steer, A.C.; Carapetis, J.R., Nolan, T.M., Shann, F. (2002). Systematic review of rheumatic heart disease prevalence in children in developing countries: the role of environmental factors. *J Paediatr Child Health*, Vol.38, No.3 (Juni 2002), pp. 229-234

Sternberg, E.M.; Chrousos, G.P., Wilder, R.L., Gold, P.W. (1992). The stress response and the regulation of inflammatory disease. *Ann Intern Med*, Vol. 117, No.10 (15.11.1992), pp. 854-866

Stojanovich, L. & Marisavljevich, D. (2008). Stress as a trigger of autoimmune disease. *Autoimmun Rev*, Vol.7, No.3 (Januar 2008), pp. 209-213

Stör, W. & Irnich, D. (2009). Acupuncture: basics, practice, and evidence. *Schmer*, Vol.23, No.4 (August 2009), pp. 405-417

Straub, R.H. & Härle, P. (2005). Stress, hormones, and neuronal signals in the pathophysiology of rheumatoid arthritis. The negative impact on chronic inflammation. *Med Klin (Munich)*. Vol.100, No.12 (15.12.2005), pp. 794-803

Straub, R.H. (2000). Tables of molecular and functional neuroendocrine immune interactions. Eching (Germany): Biozol

Straub, R.H.; Dhabhar, F.S., Bijlsma, J.W., Cutolo, M. (2005). How psychological stress via hormones and nerve fibers may exacerbate rheumatoid arthritis. *Arthritis Rheum*, Vol.52, No.1 (Januar 2005), pp. 16-26

Straub, R.H.; Pongratz, G., Cutolo, M., Wijbrandts, C.A., Baeten, D., Fleck, M., Atzeni, F., Grunke, M., Kalden, J.R., Schölmerich, J., Lorenz, H.M., Tak, P.P., Sarzi-Puttini, P. (2008). Increased cortisol relative to adrenocorticotropic hormone predicts improvement during anti-tumor necrosis factor therapy in rheumatoid arthritis. *Arthritis Rheum*, Vol.58, No.4 (April 2008), pp. 976-984

Strauss, G,D.; Spiegel, J.S., Daniels, M., Spiegel, T., Landsverk, J., Roy-Byrne, P., Edelstein, C., Ehlhardt, J., Falke, R., Hindin, L. (1986). Group therapies for rheumatoid arthritis. A controlled study of two approaches. *Arthritis Rheum*, Vol.29, No.10 (October 1986), pp. 1203-1209

Symmons, D.P. (2003). Environmental factors and the outcome of rheumatoid arthritis. *Best Pract Res Clin Rheumatol*, Vol.17, No.5 (October 2003), pp. 717-727

Szelényi, J. & Vizi, E.S. (2007). The catecholamine cytokine balance: interaction between the brain and the immune system. *Ann N Y Acad Sci*, Vol.1113 (October 2007), pp. 311-324

Treharne, G.J.; Lyons, A.C., Booth, D.A., Kitas, G.D. (2007). Psychological well-being across 1 year with rheumatoid arthritis: coping resources as buffers of perceived stress. *Br J Health Psychol*, Vol.12, Pt 3 (September 2007), pp. 323-345

Uhlig, T.; Fongen, C., Stehen, E., Christie, A., Ødegård, S. (2010). Exploring Tai Chi in rheumatoid arthritis: a quantitative and qualitative study. *BMC Musculoskelet Disord*, Vol.5, No.11 (March 2010), pp. 43

van Lankveld, W.; Ruiterkamp, G., Näring, G., de Rooij, D.J. (2004). Marital and sexual satisfaction in patients with RA and their spouses. *Scand J Rheumatol*, Vol.33, No.6, pp. 405-408

Vassilopoulos, D. & Mantzoukis, D. (2006). Dialogue between the brain and the immune system in inflammatory arthritis. *Ann N Y Acad Sci*, Vol.1088 (November 2006), pp. 132-138

Veldhuijzen van Zanten, J.J.; Ring, C., Carroll, D., Kitas, G.D. (2005). Increased Creactive protein in response to acute stress in patients with rheumatoid arthritis. *Ann Rheum Dis,* Vol.64, No.9 (September 2005), pp. 1299-1304

Wagner, U.; Wahle, M., Moritz, F., Wagner, U., Häntzschel, H., Baerwald, C.G. (2006). Promoter polymorphisms regulating corticotropin-releasing hormone transcription in vitro. *Horm Metab Res,* Vol. 38, No.2 (Februar 2006), pp. 69-75

Wahle, M.; Hanefeld, G., Brunn, S., Straub, R.H., Wagner, U., Krause, A., Häntzschel, H., Baerwald, C.G. (2006). Failure of catecholamines to shift T-cell cytokine responses toward a Th2 profile in patients with rheumatoid arthritis. *Arthritis Res Ther,* Vol. 8, No.5, R.138

Waltz, M.; Kriegel, W., van't Pad Bosch, P. (1998). The social environment and health in rheumatoid arthritis: marital quality predicts individual variability in pain severity. *Arthritis Care Res,* Vol.11, No.5 (October 1998), pp. 356-374

Wang, C. (2010). Tai chi and rheumatic diseases. *Rheum Dis Clin North Am,* Vol.37, No.1 (Februar 2011), pp. 19-32

Wang, C.; de Pablo, P., Chen, X., Schmid, C., McAlindon, T. (2008). Acupuncture for pain relief in patients with rheumatoid arthritis: a systematic review. *Arthritis Rheum,* Vol.15, No.59 (September 2008), pp. 1249-1256.

Watkins, L.R. & Maier, S.F. (2000). The pain of being sick: implications of immune-to-brain communication for understanding pain. *Annu Rev Psychol,* Vol.51, pp. 29-57

Wayne, P.M. & Kaptchuk, T.K. (2008). Challenges inherent to T'ai Chi research: part 1- T'ai Chi as a complex multicomponent intervention. *J Altern Complement Med,* Vol.14, No. 1 (Januar-Februar 2008), pp. 95-102

Weinberger, M.; Tierney, W.M., Booher, P., Hiner, S.L. (1990). Social support, stress and functional status in patients with osteoarthritis. *Soc Sci Med,* Vol.30, No.4, pp. 503-508

Yeh, G.Y. (2008). Commentary on the Cochrane review of Tai Chi for rheumatoid arthritis. *Explore (NY),* Vol.4, No.4 (Juli-August 2008), pp. 275-277

Young, L.A.(2011). Mindfulness meditation: a primer for rheumatologists. *Rheum Dis Clin North Am,* Vol.37, No.1 (Februar 2011), pp. 63-75

Zautra, A.J.; Davis, M.C., Reich, J.W., Nicassario, P., Tennen, H., Finan, P., Kratz, A., Parrish, B., Irwin, M.R. (2008). Comparison of cognitive behavioral and mindfulness meditation interventions on adaptation to rheumatoid arthritis for patients with and without history of recurrent depression. *J Consult Clin Psychol,* Vol.76, No.3 (Juni 2008), pp. 408-421

13

Pain in Rheumatic Diseases

Susette Unger and Christoph Baerwald
University Hospital Leipzig
Germany

1. Introduction

Pain is defined as "an unpleasant sensory and emotional experience associated with actual or potential tissue damage or described in terms of such a damage" (Merskey et al., 1986). It is a pivotal and the most impairing symptom in rheumatic diseases (Edwards et al., 2009; Fitzcharles et al., 2005; Sokka, 2003). Most patients consulting a rheumatologist suffer pain (Fitzcharles et al., 2005). Chronic pain influences physical and psychological status and causes impairment of quality of life as well as work disability (Dhanani et al., 2002; Kroenke et al., 2009; Skevington, 1998). For rheumatologists the assessment and treatment of pain is an integral part of daily patient care. Although remission of rheumatic diseases can be achieved with therapy with disease-modifying anti-rheumatic drugs (DMARDs) or biological pain can be still a troubling symptom. Pain is influenced by multiple factors such as genetics, experience, cultural and social background and psychological conditions (Gerez-Simon et al., 1989; Martinez et al., 1995; Mogil, 1999). Comorbid depression is associated with inflammation and worsens experience of pain (Kojima et al., 2009). Pain perception enhances the elevation of pro-inflammatory cytokines and activates a cascade of neurohumoral processes which can be dysregulated in patients with rheumatic diseases (Bingham et al., 2009; Edwards et al., 2009; Fitzcharles et al., 2005).

2. Types of pain and pathophysiology of pain in rheumatic diseases

Pain perception and the development of chronic pain is a complex process of neural integration implying response of peripheral tissue damage and transduction of information in peripheral and central nervous system (Bingham et al., 2009). Adequate pain management requires subtile differentiation of rheumatic pain. Pain can be divided into various classifications depending on anatomical origin in the musculoskeletal system or special aspects in pathophysiology. Articular pain is distinguished from extra-articular pain which can be subdivided into muscular/musculotendinous or neurogenic pain. Muscular pain is caused by muscle stress due to protective posture, impaired joint-function or malposition, myositis or cortisone-induced myopathy. Neurogenic compression syndromes or entrapement syndromes induce neurogenic pain (Engel, 2008). Figure 1 demonstrates differentiation of rheumatic diseases depending on pain localization and systemic inflammatory response. Tissue damage and chronic inflammation is not solely responsible for pain perception in rheumatic diseases. Chronic rheumatic pain can also be categorized into nociceptive/inflammatory, peripheral neuropathic and central neuropathic/functional pain (Goldenberg, 2010; Goldenberg et al., 2011; Winfield, 2008). Due to complex pathophysiology rheumatic pain is often of mixed type and the concept of central neuropathic pain is currently the focus of research, in particular in chronic pain syndromes like fibromyalgia and chronic low back pain. Classical nociceptive pain pathway/sensation starts with depolarization of Aδ and C fibers acting as primary afferent neurons (Bingham et al., 2009). Tissue damage as occurring in systemic inflammatory or degenerative rheumatic diseases as well as localized tenosynovitis, bursitis or arthritis can induce firing of peripheral neurons (Winfield, 2008). Nociceptors activate ascending dorsal horn neurons (lateral and medial spinothalamic tract) which transfer the signal to brainstem and thalamus thereby projecting to the somatosensory cortex, hypothalamus and limbic system (Bingham et al., 2009; Goldenberg, 2010; Schaible et al., 2006). Afferent sensory neurons induce the release of neurotransmitters such as glutamate, substance P and γ-aminobutyric acid (GABA) in the dorsal horn influencing pain transmission (Bingham et al., 2009; Fitzcharles et al., 2005; Goldenberg, 2010). Interneurons and descending spinal pathways like periaqueductal gray, serotonergic as well as noradrenergic systems modulate the pain pathway. Cannabinoid receptors and opioid receptors have inhibitory effects (Bingham et al., 2009). Despite dense sensory and sympathetic innervation of joint capsules, ligaments, menisci, periosteum, synovial blood vessels and subchondral bone normal joints are not innervated (Fitzcharles et al., 2005). In inflammation primary afferent neurons are sensitized and silent nociceptors start firing (Bingham et al., 2009; Fitzcharles et al., 2005; Schaible et al., 2006). Their activation threshold decreases and they are activated even by gentle and nonpainful stimuli. This process is called peripheral sensitization (Bingham et al., 2009; Edwards et al., 2009; Fitzcharles et al., 2005). Inflammatory molecules such as prostanoids, TNF, chemokines, kinins and growth factors are produced in damaged tissue and stimulate primary afferent neurons (Bingham et al., 2009; Fitzcharles et al., 2005). Vice versa activated peripheral neurons release inflammatory mediators. This neurogenic inflammation maintains a "vicious circle" of persistent activation of nociceptive and immune system causing chronic rheumatic pain (Goldenberg et al., 2011). TNF has neurostimulatory properties by inducing upregulation of expression of substance P in the central nervous system (Grassi et al. 1994; Tonussi & Ferreira, 1999). Persistent activation of nociceptors and increasing production of neurotransmitters and prostanoids results in central sensitization especially in sensory neurons of the dorsal horn (Bingham et al., 2009; Fitzcharles et al., 2005; Goldenberg, 2010; Schaible et al., 2006). Sustained local inflammation induces peripheral and central sensitization as well as pathological nerve growth with innervation of cartilage contributing to development of chronic pain in rheumatic diseases (Kidd & Urban, 2001; Niissalo, 2002). Furthermore tissue damage or entrapment can affect nociceptors and peripheral neuropathic pain can develop (Bingham et al., 2009; Goldenberg, 2010; Schaible et al., 2006). Patients complain of electrical sensations, burning pain, coldness, numbness or itching. In rheumatoid arthritis chronic inflammation denervates the synovium and may cause neuropathic pain or sensations of joint swelling (Bingham et al., 2009). Central neuropathic pain former known as functional pain is characterized by chronic widespread pain in different regions of the body as observed in fibromyalgia. Usually no structural abnormalities can be identified. This type of pain is often accompanied by symptoms like fatigue, depression, sleep disturbance and memory difficulties. Dysfunction in central nervous system and imbalance of neurotransmitters like norepinephrine, γ-aminobutyric

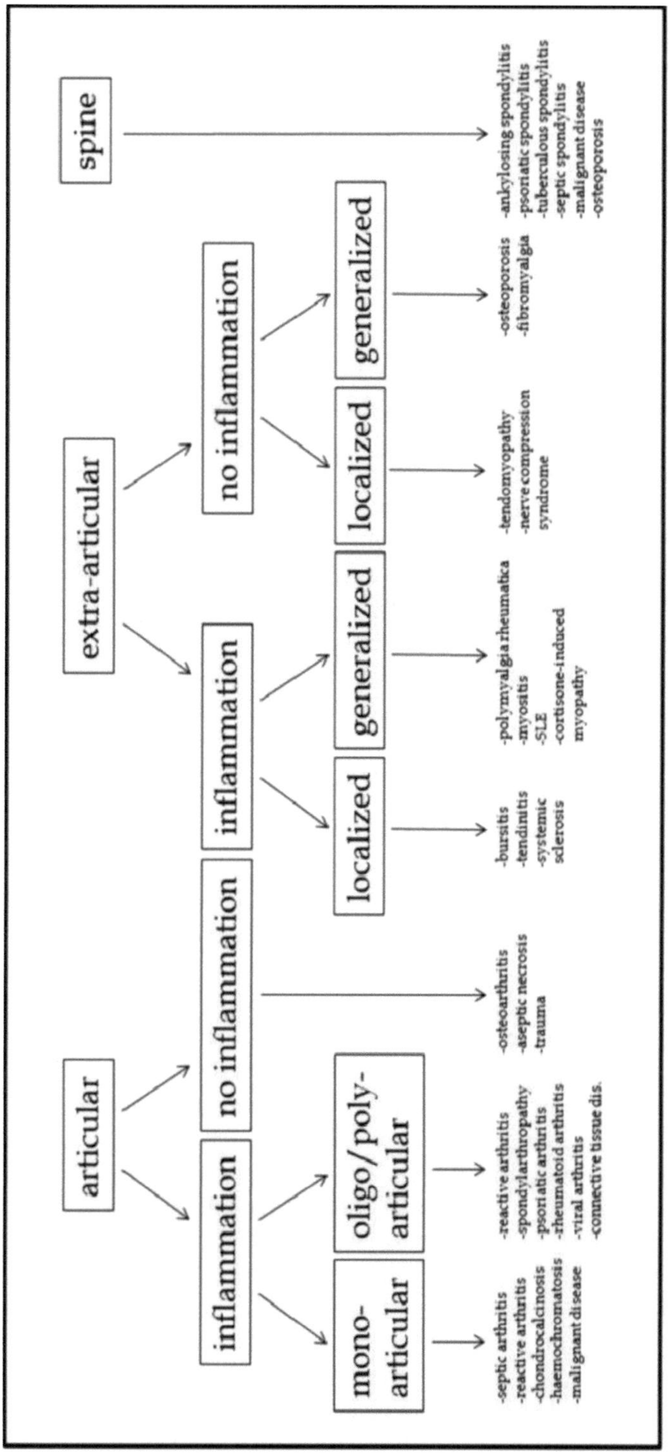

Fig. 1. Types of pain (Engel, 2008)

acid (GABA), serotonin, glutamate, and substance P can cause augmented central pain processing (Goldenberg et al., 2011). Functional neuroimaging studies could reveal that patients with central pain exhibit increased activity in brain regions involved in pain processing compared to healthy individuals (reviewed in Goldenberg et al., 2011). The stress-induced increase of cytokines like TNF could account for higher pain levels in patients with depression and anxiety (Dickens, 2002). Genetic and environmental factors like early life trauma, physical trauma, infections or emotional stress can contribute to the development of central neuropathic pain (Goldenberg et al., 2011). Central neuropathic pain is not only observed in patients with chronic pain syndromes like fibromyalgia but also seen in patients with osteoarthritis and rheumatoid arthritis (Hochman et al., 2010; Wendler et al., 2001). Patients with ankylosing spondylitis, psoriatic arthritis or osteoarthritis have a higher pain threshold compared with those of rheumatoid arthritis underlining the concept of sustained inflammation and pain perception in rheumatoid arthritis (Buskila et al., 1992; Gerecz-Simon et al., 1989). Allodynia or hyperalgesia are common sensations in patients with rheumatic diseases. Hypersensitivity to stimuli like gentle touching which are usually nonpainful is called allodynia. Hyperalgesia is defined as increased pain sensation due to lower pain threshold. The underlying pathophysiological factors are proposed to be changes in central pain processing and enhanced reactivity of immune mediators as seen in central and peripheral sensitization (Engel, 2008; Goldenberg et al., 2011; Winfield, 2008). Pain perception differs between rheumatic diseases and between individuals suffering from equal diseases making it difficult and challenging to distinguish the types of pain and to treat patients properly. The current concept of chronic rheumatic pain implies a complex, multifactorial pathophysiological model with nociceptive and neuropathic pain components called "mixed pain".

3. Pain assessment

Assessment of pain is required before the initiation of treatment to record efficacy of therapy (Fitzcharles et al., 2005; Sokka, 2003; Wendler, 2010). The patient`s pain report is subjective and depends on emotion, cognition and behavior (Fitzcharles et al., 2005; Kojima et al., 2009; Sokka, 2003). Self-reporting questionnaires provide qualitative and quantitative assessment of pain and are validated for research purposes as well as for documentation of disease activity and effectiveness of therapy (Sokka, 2003). Pain assessment should be integrated in daily practice of rheumatologists during interview and examination and includes verbal and nonverbal communication such as movements and facial expression of the patients. Verbal rating scales, numeric rating scales, visual analogue scales or pictogram analogue scales have become widely used in clinical care (Sokka, 2003; Wendler, 2010). The pain visual analogue scale (VAS) is a reliable method for assessing the intensity of pain (Jensen et al., 1998; Sokka, 2003; Wendler, 2010). It is integrated in The Health Assessment Questionnaire *(HAQ)*, a valid instrument for the measurement of functional disability, pain and global status (Fitzcharles et al., 2005; Sokka, 2003). The 10 cm scale is bordered on each side. The spectrum of pain ranges across a continuum from 0 (no pain) to 10 (very severe pain). In the numeric rating scale numbers describe the pain severity, therefore results are comparable for follow up. Figure 2 shows the visual analogue and the numeric rating scale.

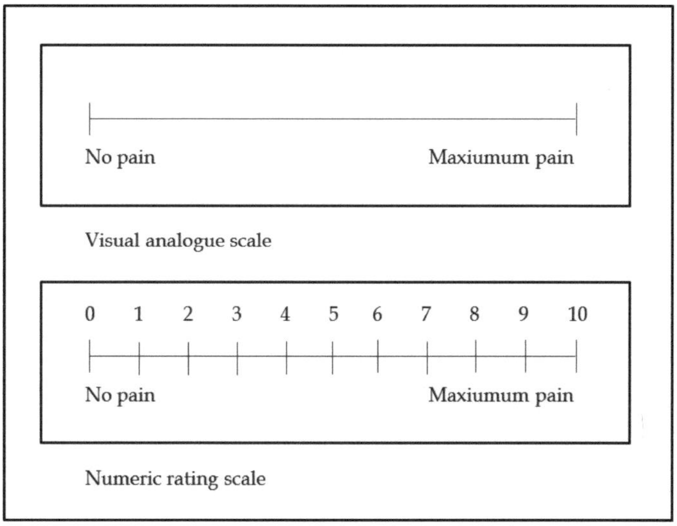

Fig. 2. Pain scales

When analyzing pain scores physicians should take into account various rheumatic diseases. In rheumatoid arthritis pain scores correlate with radiographic and laboratory results whereas fibromyalgia patients suffer severe pain in the absence of structural damage (Sokka, 2003). The first consultation of patients with pain should include a detailed interview and neurological and musculoskeletal examination of the patient (American Society of Anesthesiologists, 2010; Fitzcharles et al., 2005). A general medical history and history about the onset, quality, intensity, distribution and duration of pain, ameliorating and aggravating factors, symptoms, social and psychological impacts as well as previous therapies should be evaluated (American Society of Anesthesiologists, 2010). Body schemes, e.g. in the McGill pain questionnaire, facilitate the assessment of patients with chronic rheumatic diseases suffering from pain in various parts of the body (Wendler, 2010). Pain diaries can activate patients to document pain character and its influence in motion and function as well as to recognize effectiveness of treatment (Wendler, 2010).

4. Pain therapy in rheumatic diseases

Once the rheumatologist has assessed the patient`s pain an adequate therapy has to be initiated. Optimal pain management should encompass multimodal interventions with pharmacological and non-pharmacological treatment strategies (American Society of Anesthesiologists, 2010; Fitzcharles et al., 2005). Non-pharmacological procedures include education, psychological care, physical and/or occupational therapy as well as joint protection and/or surgery.

4.1 Non-pharmacological pain treatment

Education has a tremendous effect on sufficient pain control in patients with rheumatic diseases. Information about the disease and therapeutic options can reduce the fear of long term consequences, such as loss of function, joint damage, chronic pain, and implications on social and family life. Self-management strategies provide patients with a wide range of possibilities to influence their course of the disease. Exercise, joint protection techniques and appropriate use of pharmacological pain therapy encourage patients to cooperate with their attending physician (Goldenberg et al., 2011).

For sufficient pain control the psychological status of the patient has to be evaluated (Kojima et al., 2009). Depression can worsen the perceived pain. Therefore rheumatoid arthritis patients describing severe pain without active disease could benefit from psychological therapy (Kojima et al., 2009). Additional cognitive behavioral therapy, biofeedback, relaxation training and self-care education can improve the patient`s well-being (American Society of Anesthesiologists, 2010; Kimura & Walco, 2007).

Patients with rheumatic diseases are often physically inactive. Physiotherapy and exercise programs support mental and physical health (Kimura & Walco, 2007; Roddy et al., 2005). Patients with rheumatic diseases should always be encouraged to get exercise. Due to chronic pain they often feel weak and fatigue causes impaired activity. On the one hand patients fear exacerbation of musculoskeletal pain when moving. Consequently avoidance of exercise deteriorates muscle strength and physical condition. On the other hand excessive exercise aggravates fatigue and flares can occur. Mild exercise like walking, water aerobics, and bicycling, being appropriate for age and condition, can support physical fitness and comfort (Winfield, 2008). Physical therapy with heat or cold can reinforce therapeutic effects. In particular in nociceptive pain application of moderate heat (e.g. paraffin, packs, hydrotherapy) can improve pain control. In generalized pain syndromes sauna, baths, showers or hot mud can be effective. Cold therapy (e.g. packs, sprays or immersion) is recommended in acute pain states as seen in flares of rheumatic diseases (Winfield, 2008). Transcutaneous electrical nerve stimulation (TENS) is an independent option of physical therapy at home.

Synovectomy and arthroplasty are therapeutic options in patients with continuous pain, joint deformity and functional loss (Kimura & Walco, 2007). The role of complementary therapies in pain management needs to be further examined (Fitzcharles et al., 2005). For optimal pain management a combination of different medications is often necessary. Rheumatologists have to prove efficacy of therapy and compliance of the patient. Discontinuation of treatment is required if side effects occur or if the therapy is ineffective.

4.2 Pharmacological pain treatment

Intra-articular injections, topical applications, selective and non-selective non-steroidal anti-rheumatic drugs (NSAIDs), opioids as well as adjuvant drugs are therapeutic options for pain control. DMARDs like methotrexate, sulfasalazine, leflunomide and biologicals are prescribed to reduce disease activity and to maintain remission. Reduced disease activity is associated with improved functional status and reduced pain (Kimura & Walco, 2007). However, pain remains to be a leading symptom in patients with rheumatic diseases. Due to serious side effects of long-term application high dose corticosteroids should only be prescribed in severe, life-threatening disease. Intra-articular injections can help to reduce localized joint inflammation and pain (Kimura & Walco, 2007). The number of injections is limited to three per year (Bernau & Heeg, 2003). Avoidance of systemic side effects is an advantage of topical analgesics such as capsaicin or topical NSAIDs like diclofenac, ibuprofen, ketoprofen, and piroxicam. Although plasma concentration is low after absorption local application can reduce mild to moderate pain in arthritis (Kroenke et al., 2009; Mason et al., 2004).

4.2.1 Non-selective and selective cyclooxygenase inhibitors

Non-selective and selective cyclooxygenase inhibitors (coxibs) are potent analgesics with anti-phlogistic properties and are successfully used in the treatment of degenerative and inflammatory joint diseases (Schaible et al., 2006; Unger & Baerwald, 2010). Table 1 shows the most common selective and non-selective COX-inhibitors. Application of NSAID results in inhibition of prostaglandin synthesis which sensitizes nociceptors in inflamed joints and thereby causing pain in arthritis (Schaible et al., 2006; Unger & Baerwald, 2010). Furthermore central sensitization is followed by prostaglandin E2 (PGE2) release in the dorsal horns of the spinal cord (Bingham et al., 2009; Fitzcharles et al., 2005). However, gastrointestinal, renal, cardiovascular side effects and hepato-toxicity as well as platelet inhibition restrict their application (Kimura & Walco, 2007; Kroenke et al., 2009; Unger & Baerwald, 2010). Studies show that coxibs and traditional NSAIDs do not significantly differ in their cardiovascular side effects (reviewed in Luttosch & Baerwald, 2011; Unger & Baerwald, 2010). Therefore these agents should be administered in a low dose and for a short term only. Naproxen, paracetamol or opioids seem to be an option for pain control in patients with cardiovascular risk factors and should be preferred in these groups (Kroenke et al., 2009; Luttosch & Baerwald, 2011; Unger & Baerwald, 2010). Coxibs should be preferred in patients with risk of gastrointestinal complications due to their lower risk of developing a serious adverse event compared to non-selective cyclooxygenase-inhibitors (Unger & Baerwald, 2010). In persons 60 years or older, in those with gastrointestinal symptoms and in patients taking corticosteroids or antiplatelet agents a proton pump inhibitor should be coadministered with traditional NSAIDs, or a coxib should be prescribed (Kroenke et al., 2009).

Name	Half-time	Dose (mg)	Peculiarity	Contraindications
Etoricoxib	25 h	OA 30-60 1/day RA/SpA 90 1/day gout 120 1/day	high blood pressure is a contraindication	peptic ulcers or GI-bleeding cardio-/cerebrovascular diseases arterial occlusive disease heart failure impaired liver function crea-clear. <30 ml/min pregnancy breast-feeding Crohn`s disease
Celecoxib	12 h	OA 200 1-2/day RA 100-200 2/day SpA 100-200 2/day or 200-400 1/day	allergy against sulfonamids is a contraindication	
Diclofenac	1-2 h	50-150/day in 2-4 doses	high cardio-vascular risk	peptic ulcers, bleeding, perforation renal and liver failure
Naproxen	14 h	500-1250/day in 1-3 doses	low cardio-vascular risc	

Name	Half-time	Dose (mg)	Peculiarity	Contraindications
Piroxicam	14-160 h	10-20/day	severe skin reactions	heart failure
Indometacin	2-3 h	50 1-3/day	short term administration allergic reactions	bone marrow dysfunction ASS-induced asthma
Acemetacin	4 h	30 1-3/day		
Ketoprofen	1,5-2,5 h	50 1-4/day or 100 1-2/day	phototoxic and allergic reactions	
Phenylbutazon	70 h	200 1-2/day	SLE, pyrazol-allergy, thyroid gland dysfunction is a contraindication	
Meloxicam	20 h	OA 7,5-15/day RA/SpA 15/day	high COX-2-selectivity	
Ibuprofen	2-3 h	max. 800-1200/day	no combination with ASS	

ASS-acetylsalicyl acid, COX-cyclooxygenase, crea-clear.-creatinine-clearance, GI-gastrointestinal, OA-osteoarthritis, RA-rheumatoid arthritis, SLE-systemic lupus erythematodes, SpA-ankylosing spondylitis

Table 1. Characteristics of typical NSAIDs and coxibs (Unger & Baerwald, 2010)

4.2.2 Opioid therapy

If NSAIDs are insufficient or contraindications and interfering side effects, respectively, exist opioids can be considered for effective pain control (Pierer et al., 2010). However, side effects and potential addiction have previously restricted their use in pain therapy. Therefore opioid therapy should only be prescribed within a multimodal pain control concept in advanced inflammatory or degenerative disease if other analgesics are ineffective (Pierer et al., 2010; Siegel et al., 2008). Long term, controlled and randomized studies concerning opioid use in rheumatic diseases are lacking. In clinical practice a positive effect on sleep and musculoskeletal function especially in neuropathic pain, rheumatoid arthritis, osteoarthritis and low back pain can be observed (Pierer et al., 2010; Siegel et al., 2008). Opioids bind to opioid receptors found in the central and peripheral nervous system (Kimura & Walco, 2007, Lang et al., 2010; Siegel et al., 2008). Studies confirm that opioids show mild anti-inflammatory effects (reviewed in Kimura & Walco 2007). Endogenous opioid peptides are released in inflamed regions and bind to upregulated peripheral opioid receptors thereby controlling intrinsic pain pathways (Lang et al., 2010). Tramadol is a weak opioid beneficial especially in osteoarthritis, low back pain and fibromyalgia (Fitzcharles et al., 2005; Goldenberg et al., 2011; Kroenke et al., 2009). Nausea, vomiting, constipation, dizziness, somnolence, cognitive impairment, urinary retention and respiratory depression are major undesirable adverse effects (American Society of Anesthesiologists, 2010; Lang et al., 2010; Winfield, 2008). Therefore long term therapy is not recommended. In chronic nonmalignant pain only mild pain reduction is observed whereas functional outcome (unemployment, necessity of health care) is declining (Siegel et al., 2008). Pain intensity, vital parameters, musculoskeletal function, possible addiction and side effects have to be controlled regularly (Pierer et al.,

2010; Winfield, 2008). Upon initiation of opioids the dosage has to be titrated within the first two to three weeks (Winfield, 2008). After six weeks a significant pain reduction should be documented (Pierer et al., 2010). If optimal pain relief is not occurring opioid rotation should be considered (Kroenke et al., 2009). Exacerbation of pain should always be evaluated and the causes should be detected prior to increasing the dosage. If effective pain control does not occur after three months opioid therapy should be stopped. To avoid withdrawal symptoms a daily reduction of 10 % is strongly recommended (Pierer et al., 2010). Opioids should not be administered in patients with a history of or current substance use disorders (Kroenke et al., 2009). In older patients or patients with renal or liver function impairment the dose has to be reduced 25 % to 50 % (Kroenke et al., 2009; Winfield, 2008). Opioids should be administered with caution in older patients due to high risk of falls leading to fractures. There are insufficient data about the effect of long term therapy with opioids (Pierer et al., 2010). The WHO Three-Step Model for Pain Management provides an international accepted approach for effective pharmacological pain therapy and is demonstrated in Figure 3. The starting therapy step depends on the severity of pain. If the first treatment is insufficient the following step of the model should be initiated. Adjuvant drugs including antidepressants and anticonvulsants can be combined with the medications of the Three-Step Model.

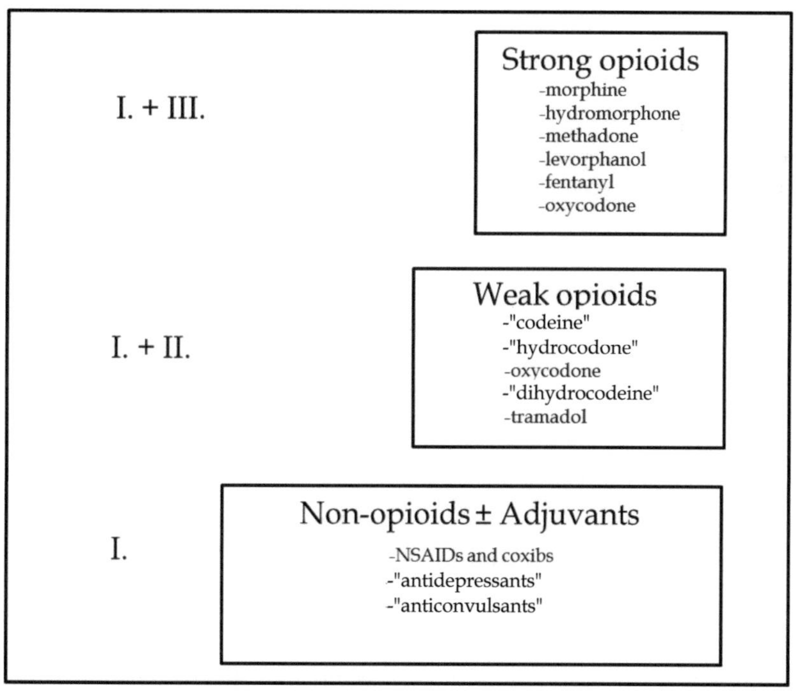

Fig. 3. WHO Three-Step Model of Pain management

4.2.3 Adjuvant drugs

Tricyclic antidepressants like amitriptyline are the most commonly used adjuvant medications to treat patients with rheumatoid arthritis or ankylosing spondylitis (Fitzcharles et al., 2005). Adjuvant drugs play a major role in management of fibromyalgia and seem to be the most effective medications in this condition (Godfrey, 1996). Sleep, mood and fatigue are positively influenced. The anticonvulsants gabapentin and pregabalin provide pain relief especially in neuropathic pain (American Society of Anesthesiologists, 2010; Kimura & Walco, 2007; Kroenke et al., 2009). They have neuromodulatory properties due to binding to calcium-channels in the central nervous system and inhibiting the release of neurotransmitters (American Society of Anesthesiologists, 2010; Kroenke et al., 2009). Cardiovascular side effects as well as somnolence or sedation can limit therapeutic application (American Society of Anesthesiologists, 2010; Kroenke et al., 2009). Antidepressants should be used with caution in older patients due to anticholinergic properties and the high risk of falls (Kroenke et al., 2009). Duloxetine and milnacipran interact with the serotonin and norepinephrine systems. Positive effects on pain und function could be demonstrated especially in fibromyalgia (Goldenberg et al., 2011). Figure 4 shows a stepwise summary of pharmacological and non-pharmacological pain control in rheumatic diseases.

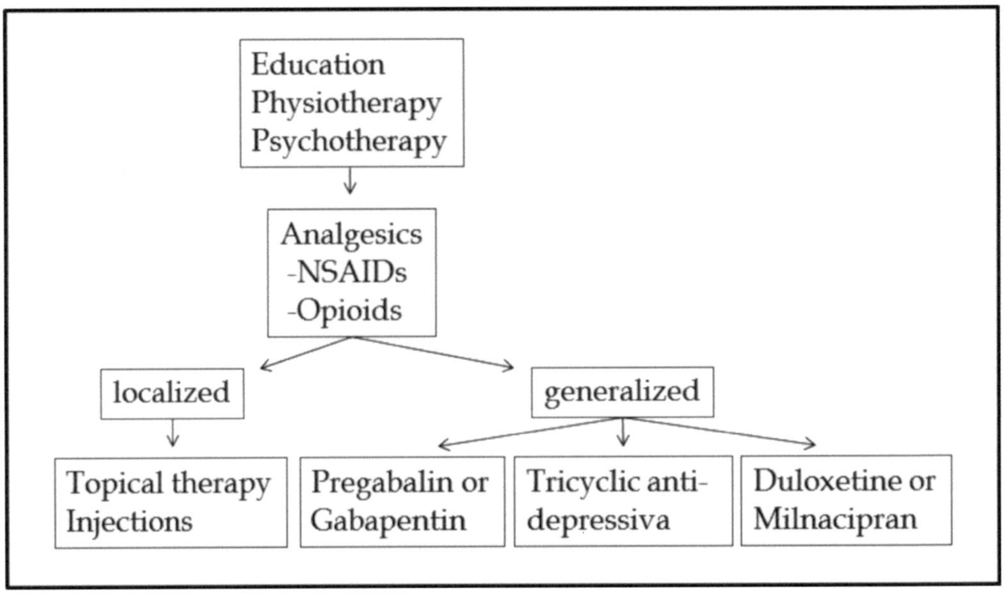

Fig. 4. Pain therapy in rheumatic diseases (Winfield, 2008)

4.2.4 Development of new medication

Pharmacological pain management is restricted due to significant side effects or contraindications of NSAIDs and opioids. Development of new medication is in the focus of current research. Tapentadol hydrochloride is a μ-opioid-receptor agonist and norepinephrine reuptake inhibitor for the treatment of moderate and severe pain exhibiting less gastrointestinal side effects compared to traditional opioids and is effective in neuropathic and/or inflammatory pain (Wade & Spruill, 2009). Cardiovascular and gastrointestinal side effects limit pain control with NSAIDs. Naproxcinod is a new developed COX inhibiting nitric oxide donator (CINOD) which shows an improved safety profile due to release of nitric oxide (NO) (Wallace et al., 2009). NO acts in the vasculature inducing positive effects on blood pressure and mucosal integrity in the gastrointestinal tract (Wallace et al., 2009). Further studies are needed to evaluate the role of dopaminergic agents, N-methyl-D-aspartate (NMDA) receptor antagonists, γ-aminobutyric acid (GABA) agonists, and 5-hydroxytryptamine 3 receptor antagonist in complex pain syndromes with central pain components (Goldenberg et al., 2011).

5. Conclusion

Pain is a cardinal symptom in patients with rheumatic disease. It impacts functioning, quality of life and causes disability. The pain is frequently multifactorial in origin and has both central and peripheral components. Disease activity is only marginally related to the extent of pain severity, and pain-related presentation can differ widely between individuals. Cognitions and emotions contribute to different perception of pain. Although remission of rheumatic diseases can be achieved with use of oral DMARDs or biological therapies, treatment of pain can be a challenge in every day practice. Assessment of pain is pivotal for monitoring therapy response and must take into account various factors. Non-pharmacologic interventions, such as exercise and cognitive-behavioral therapy as well as the use of analgesics such as cyclooxygenase inhibitors or opioids should aim to achieve at better quality of life for patients with rheumatic diseases and should help to maintain function.

6. References

American Society of Anesthesiologists Task Force on Chronic Pain Management and the American Society of Regional Anesthesia and Pain Medicine. (2010). Practice Guidelines for Chronic Pain Management. *Anesthesiology*, 112, pp. (810-835)

Bernau, A. & Heeg, P. (2003). Intraarticular punctures and injections: indications-prevention of infection-technique- complications. *Orthopaede*, 32, 6, pp. (548-570)

Bingham, B.; Ajit, S. K.; Blake, D. R. & Samad, T. A. (2009). The molecular basis of pain and its clinical implications in rheumatology. *Nature Clinical Practice Rheumatology*, 5, 1, pp. (28-37)

Buskila, D.; Langevitz, P; Gladman, D. D.; Urowitz, S. & Smyhte, H. A. (1992). Patients with rheumatoid arthritis are more tender than those with psoriatic arthritis. *The Journal of Rheumatology*, 19, pp. (1115-1119)

Dhanani, S.; Quenneville, J.; Perron, M.; Abdolell, M. & Feldmann, B. M. (2002). Minimal differences in pain associated with change in quality of life in children with rheumatic diseases. *Arthritis & Rheumatism*, 47, pp. (501-505)

Dickens, C.; McGowan, L.; Clark-Carter, D. & Creed, F. H. (2002). Depression in rheumatoid arthritis: a systemic review of the literature and meta-analysis. *Psychosomatic Medicine*, 64, pp. (52-60)

Edwards, R. R.; Wasan, A. D.; Bingham, C. O.; Bathon, J.; Haythornthwaite, J. A.; Smith, M. T. & Page, G. G. (2009). Enhanced reactivity to pain in patients with rheumatoid arthritis. *Arthritis Research & Therapy*, 11, R61, pp. (1-9)

Engel, J. M. (2008). *Interdisziplinäre klinische Rheumatologie* (2n edition), Zeidler, H.; Zacher, J.; Hiepe, F. A., ISBN 978-3- 540-34104-8, Berlin, Heidelberg

Fitzcharles, M.-A.; Almahrezi, A. & Shir, Y. (2005). Pain-Understanding and challenges for the rheumatologist. *Arthritis & Rheumatism*, 52, 12, pp. (3685-3692)

Gerecz-Simon, E. M.; Tunks, E. R.; Heale, J. A.; Kean, W. F. & Buchanan, W. W. (1989). Measurement of pain threshold in patients with rheumatoid arthritis, osteoarthritis, ankylosing spondylitis, and healthy controls. *Clinical Rheumatology*, 8, pp. (467-474)

Godfrey, R. G. (1996). A guide to the understanding and use of tricyclic antidepressants in the overall management of fibromyalgia and other chronic pain syndromes. *Archives of Internal Medicine*, 156, pp. (1047-1052)

Goldenberg, D. L. (2010). The interface of pain and mood disturbances in rheumatic diseases. *Seminars in Arthritis and Rheumatism*, 40, pp. (15-31)

Goldenberg, D. L.; Clauw, D. J. & Fitzcharles, M. A. (2011). New Concepts in Pain Research and Pain Management of Rheumatic Diseases. *Seminars in Arthritis and Rheumatism*, article in press

Grassi, F.; Mileo, A. M.; Monaco, L.; Punturieri, A.; Santoni, A. & Eusebi, F. (1994). TNFα increases the frequency of spontaneous miniature synaptic currents in cultured rat hippocampal neurons. *Brain Research*, 659, pp. (226- 230)

Hochman, J. R.; French, M. R.; Bermingham, S. L. & Hawker G. A. (2010). The nerve of osteoarthritis pain. *Arthritis Care & Research*, 62, pp. (1019-1023)

Iwasaki, A.; Inoue, K. & Hukada, S. (1995). Distribution of neuropeptide-containing nerve fibers in the synovium and adjacent bone of the rat knee joint. *Clinical and Experimental Rheumatology*, 13, pp. (173-178)

Jensen, M. P.; Miller, L. & Fisher, L. D. (1998). Assessment of pain during medical procedures: a comparison of three scales. *The Clinical Journal of Pain*, 14, pp. (343-349)

Kidd, B. L. & Urban, L. A. (2001). Mechanisms of inflammatory pain. *British Journal of Anaesthesia*, 87, pp. (3-11)

Kimura, Y. & Walco, G. A. (2007). Treatment of chronic pain in pediatric rheumatic disease. *Nature Clinical Practice Rheumatology*, 3, 4, pp. (210-218)

Kojima, M.; Kojima, T.; Suzuki, S.; Oguchi, T.; Oba, M.; Tsuchiya, H.; Sugiura, F.; Kanayama, Y.; Furukawa, T. A.; Tokudome, S. & Ishiguro N. (2009). Depression, Inflammation, and pain in patients with rheumatoid arthritis. *Arthritis & Rheumatism*, 61, 8, pp. (1018-1024)

Kroenke, K.; Krebs, E. E. & Bair, M. J. (2009). Pharmacotherapy of chronic pain: a synthesis of recommendations from systematic reviews. *General Hospital Psychiatry*, 31, pp. (206-219)

Lang, L. J.; Pierer, M.; Stein, C. & Baerwald, C. (2010). Opioids in rheumatic diseases. *Annals of the New York Academy of Science*, 1193, pp. (11-116)

Luttosch, F. & Baerwald, C. (2011). Treatment of pain in rheumatic diseases. *Deutsche Medizinische Wochenschrift*, 136, pp. (1598-1600)

Martinez, J. E.; Ferraz, M. B.; Sato, E. I. & Atra, E. (1995). Fibromyalgia versus rheumatoid arthritis: a longitudinal comparison of the quality of life. *The Journal of Rheumatology*, 22, pp. 270-274

Mason, L.; Moore, R. A.; Edwards, J. E., Derry, S. & McQuay, H. J. (2004). Topical NSAIDs for chronic musculoskeletal pain: systematic review and meta-analysis. *BMC Musculoskeletal Disorders*, 19, pp. (5-28)

Merskey, H.; Lindblom, U. & Mumford, J.M. (1986). Pain terms: a current list with definitions and notes on usage. *Pain*, Suppl 3, pp. (215-221)

Mogil, J. S. (1999). The genetic mediation of individual differences in sensitivity to pain and its inhibition. *Proceedings of the National Academy of Scienes USA*, 96, pp. (7744-7751)

Nissalo, S.; Hukkanen, M.; Imai, S.; Tornwall, J. & Konttinen, Y. T. (2002). Neuropeptides in experimental and degenerative arthritis. *Annals of the New York Academy of Sciences*, 966, pp. (384-399)

Pierer, M.; Malysheva, O.; Wagner, U. & Baerwald, C. (2010). Opioids for musculoskeletal pain. *Aktuelle Rheumatologie*, 35, pp. (184-188)

Roddy, E.; Zhang, W.; Doherty, M.; Arden, N. K.; Barlow, J. & Birrell, F. (2005). Evidence-based recommendations for the role of exercise in the management of osteoarthritis of the hip or knee: the MOVE consensus. *Rheumatology (Oxford)*, 44, pp. (67-73)

Schaible, H.-G.; Schmelz, M. & Tegeder, I. (2006). Pathophysiology and treatment of pain in joint disease. *Advanced Drug Delivery Reviews*, 58, pp. (323-342)

Siegel, L.; Pierer, M.; Stein, C. & Baerwald, C. (2008). Opioids in musculoskeletal pain. *Zeitschrift für Rheumatologie*, 67, pp. (646-652)

Skevington, S. M. (1998). Investigating the relationship between pain and discomfort and quality of life, using the WHOQOL. *Pain*, 76, pp. (395-406)

Sokka, T. (2003). Assessment of pain in patients with rheumatic diseases. *Best Practice & Research Clinical Rheumatology*, 17, 3, pp. (427-449)

Tonussi, C. R. & Ferreira, S. H. (1999). Tumor necrosis factor-α mediates carrageenin-induced knee-joint incapacitation and also triggers overt nociception in previously inflamed rat knee-joints. *Pain*, 82, pp. (81-87)

Unger, S. I. & Baerwald, C. (2010). Pain Therapy with selective and non-selective cyclooxygenase inhibitors in rheumatology. *Aktuelle Rheumtologie*, 35, pp. (178-183)

Wade, W. E. & Spruill, W. J. (2009). Tapentadol Hydrochloride: A Centrally Acting Oral Analgesic. *Clinical Therapeutics*, 31, 12, pp. (2804-2818)

Wallace, J. L.; Viappiani, S. & Bolla, M. (2009). Cyclooxygenase-inhibiting nitric oxide donators for osteoarthritis. *Trends in Pharmacological Sciences*, 30, 3, pp. (112-117)

Wendler, J. (2010). Assessment of pain in rheumatology. *Aktuelle Rheumatologie*, 35, pp. (172-177)

Wendler, J.; Hummel, T.; Reissinger, M.; Manger, B; Pauli, E.; Kalden, J. R. & Kobal, G. (2001). Patients with rheumatoid arthritis adapt differently to repetitive painful stimuli compared to healthy controls. *Journal of Clinical Neuroscience*, 8, pp. (272-277)

Winfield, J. B. (2008). *Primer on the Rheumatic Diseases* (13th edition), Klippel, J. H.; Stone, J. H.; Crofford, L. J.; White, P. H., ISBN 978-0-387-35664-8, New York

14

Transition of Care in Rheumatology: Managing the Rheumatic Patient from Childhood to Adulthood

Philomine van Pelt[1,2] and Nico Wulffraat[2]
[1]*Department of Rheumatic Diseases, EMC Rotterdam and Department of Pediatric Rheumatology, EMC Rotterdam*
[2]*Department of Pediatric Immunology, UMC Utrecht*
Netherlands

1. Introduction

1.1 Transition of care

Chronic rheumatic diseases in childhood are an important group of chronic conditions with often severe morbidity and carrying a major impact on growth and development for the affected individual. It is estimated that 30-70% of the patients have continuing disease activity or persisting limitations in functional ability or psychosocial function in their adult life (1-4).

In most countries infants and children with rheumatic diseases are treated by specialist pediatric rheumatologists, nurses and physiotherapists. When such children with chronic diseases reach adulthood (usually between the age of 16 -24), transition to adult health care is needed. This transitional face coincides with the period in which adolescence, or puberty, takes place. Blum and colleagues coined a very useful definition for transition (5). They described transition as 'the purposeful, planned movement of adolescents and young adults with chronic physical and medical conditions from child-centered to adult-oriented health care systems'

The transfer to adult health service requires specific skills and knowledge from the health care providers. When ignored this may result in poor health indicators and loss to follow-up for adolescents with a chronic disease. Basically one needs to recognize that children with severe chronic diseases transgress into a two faced transition to become an adolescent with a chronic rheumatic condition that receives care from a team expert in both pediatric and adult rheumatology. Nowadays, it is generally believed that a multidimensional transition of care is needed (6;7).

In the US a general statement was made by pediatricians and primary health care that transition leading to the transfer of care is one of six primary goals for youth with special healthcare needs {25}

Apart from these issues, other questions to be discussed in this chapter are:

- What is the right time for this transfer of care and who plays a role in this process?
- Which aspects of adolescence play a role in the transfer and transition of care?
- What special preparations are needed for this transfer?
- What does an ideal transition of care system look like?

Most published descriptions of the organization of transition of care for rheumatic diseases refer specifically to Juvenile Idiopathic Arthritis (JIA). Therefore this chapter will also focus on JIA. For the other rheumatic diseases the JIA centered transition programme may serve usefull. However in such cases (for instance SLE, juvenile dermatomyositis, autoinflammatory syndromes) the team also needs to include renal and dermatological expertise.

2. Factors influencing the transfer from pediatric to adult care

2.1 Differences in culture of medical treatment and care in pediatrics and adult medicine

In pediatric medicine, health care should not be limited to the patient's disease. Other aspects of physical development should be taken into account such as growth and puberty. Education and social behavior in the presence of a chronic disease are equally important issues, not only for social development, but also for future opportunities in finding employment. Sport and exercise are important for maintaining social contacts as well as mental and physical health. Furthermore, parents and siblings are also involved in the disease process of the diseased child. Limitations caused by the disease may have an effect on the social life of the whole family.

In adult medicine much attention is given to the rheumatic disease itself, the disease activity and side effects of medications. The impact of the disease on work, family and social life is less important and is hardly discussed by the medical doctor. When supporting staff like nurse practitioners, social workers or physiotherapists are available, these factors are taken into account, which certainly play an important part on issues such as staying in employment, self efficacy, compliance etc. The care for the patient is often structured in a supply-oriented fashion and can be divided into the available separate disciplines. (8;9). If transition programmes are fully patient-oriented they will offer a merge of paediatric and adult care.

Pediatric care	Adult Care
Family-focused (parents strongly involved)	Patient-focused
Generalist, interdisciplinary	Multidisciplinairy
Socially orientated	Disease orientated
Informal atmosphere, relaxed	Formal atmosphere, to the point
Attention for development, school and social functioning	Accent on treatment, self-management and compliance

Table 1. Differences in pediatric and adult care (8;9)

2.2 Who is involved in the transition process?

First and foremost of course, is the adolescent suffering from the chronic (rheumatic) disease, the patient who is transferred to adult care.

Secondly, the paediatric specialist, the person who is responsible for handing over a complete medical file of the patient. The paediatric specialist is usually assisted by allied health professionals such as specialised physical therapists, psychologists and social workers. In addition, the paediatric services together with the adult services are involved in preparing the patient and the parents for the new situation at adult health care.

The adult specialist needs to be prepared for looking after a young patient in adolescent age with a long medical history. Often the disease has already caused irreversible damage and influences growth and development, as well as functional and social performance. One needs to realise that the pattern of joint erosions are often different from adults with RA and that the uveitis so commonly seen in JIA is rare in RA. For young patients visiting the adult department with a relative short disease duration, without such effects of longstanding disease this is of course different. Also, the adult specialist needs to deal with a patient in the adolescence phase. Often the disease has had influence on growth and development, and functional and social outcome. This, however, is different for young patients attending the adult department who had a relatively short disease duration, and who haven't displayed the effects of a longstanding disease.

Finally, the parents and extended family who have been involved in the disease process for a long time as they have had to take care of the medication and appointments at the hospital and sometimes needed to give extra support in nursing their child. When growing up, the child needs less support. The parent is required to release the responsibilities and hand them over to their child. At the adult department all responsibilities must be taken on by the patient themselves. This requires a self confident, considerate and often independent person that is capable to self-manage all aspects of the disease.

3. Aspects of transition

3.1 The concept of self-management

This is described as the transition of the patient from a dependant (childhood) state into a self caring adult person.

As the young child grows up into adulthood via adolescence it will develop a set of tools to cope with this new situation. Such a transition into adulthood (defined by Hardoff (10)) is a period of biological, social and emotional change, in which the adolescent has 4 major tasks:

- to consolidate their identity;
- to achieve independence from their parents;
- to establish adult relationships outside the family;
- to find a vocation.

The adolescent with a chronic disease, however, has additional tasks:

- they have to cope with the disease;
- the treatment and its functional limitations;

- they have to learn to do that independently from the support team which was available to them in their childhood, e.g. the parents and pediatric health services.

Hence, it is not surprising that the value of self-management interventions that train patients to utilize relevant skills is the subject of increased attention (11), see ref White articles [5]. Self-management may be one means of bridging the gap between patients' needs and the capacity of health and social care services to meet those needs.

Self-management is generally held as one of the key elements in a transition program.

But other skills are also important like communication, decision making and assertiveness (12-14). Patients in the adolescent ages were interviewed by Stinson et al (13) about their strategies of gaining control over managing their illness on their own. The two strategies that assisted the process of transition were:

- gaining knowledge and skills to manage the disease and;
- experiencing understanding through social support.

The authors concluded that web-based interventions could be a promising tool in supporting the acquisition of knowledge (13).

Table 2 summarizes the knowledge and skills needed for transition of the adolescent. These items can be prepared by the pediatric and adult health department workers including the specialist, but also parents and peers (healthy as well as those with a chronic disease) are important (12;15).

I: Knowledge for transition
Condition including effects on body, medical history and prognosis
Therapy regimen including names, doses, side effects, rationale, risk of non-adherence
Purposes of tests and procedures
Relevant medical terminology
Specific issues, e.g., antibiotic prophylaxis, immunizations
Role of health care providers, what they do, and how to access their services
Meaning of transition
Differences between pediatric and adult health care
Healthy lifestyles in terms of exercise, nutrition, sun exposure etc
Impact of drugs and alcohol on condition and therapy
Impact of condition and therapy on sexual and reproductive health
Impact of condition and therapy on education and vocation
II: Skills for transition
Health: Feeling confident to see health professional independent of parents Accessing health care independently, including booking appointments, seeking advice and refilling prescriptions Self management of their condition Adherence to therapy and appointments Pain and fatigue management skills

Psychosocial: Independent living skills, self care, meal preparation, hobbies Peer support including independent social life and social competencies
Educational/ vocational: Communication skills Vocational education, work experiences, (part-time) jobs

Table 2. Knowledge and skills needed for transition (12, 15):

Recently several internet based programs for increasing self-management have been developed (16;17).

Interestingly, in a recent survey in our outpatient population of 142 adolescents (age 10-27 years) with JIA , internet is widely used (97.9% of the patients had access to internet) and 77% were daily on the internet. However, only 26% surfed for information about their disease.

The time to start the self-efficacy process with gaining knowledge about disease and related issues should be as young as possible. This will help them to cope with their disease later on in life, its limitations and the opportunities that arise, for instance in finding suitable employment, social activities they can partake in, the importance of taking their medication and monitoring their own health including making own appointments and independently visiting the clinic (15). Data from a UK study supported an early start to transition, whereby 11-14 year-old patients with JIA showing maximum improvement in disease knowledge after 12 months of participation in a transitional care program, which was significantly higher than that of a 17-year-old patient at baseline (18).

3.2 Documentation of disease activity of JIA patients

Despite its name juvenile, JIA is not a disease in childhood only, it may persist into adulthood. In retrospective and cross sectional studies which have been published, complete remission after at least 10 years of disease duration is described in 33-67% of the patients, depending on JIA subtype, and patient population (2;4;19-22). The prognosis is better in the oligoarticular persistent subtype and worse in the systemic group.

Due to higher rates of remission, it is expected that patients with the oligoarticular persistent subtype are lost to follow up. A selection bias of patients after longer disease duration is therefore to be expected. Results of the disease activity of patients with very long disease duration should therefore be analyzed with care as most of the long-term outcome studies of patients with JIA are retrospective and cross-sectional.

Further in this chapter we will highlight the aspect of the tools used to measure disease activity.

3.3 Medication history

Prognosis in RA has improved enormously these last years since intensive combination treatment regimes have been introduced (23). Complete remission is now noted, low DAS scores or other activity scores are commonly used to control disease activity (24;25). Only very recently remission criteria for RA are defined, but studies using these criteria are not published yet (26).

Similar to adults, treatment for JIA has improved dramatically in the past 20 years. Outcome of older patients is therefore hard to compare with younger patients. Patients are treated differently over time and between centers. Before the introduction of MTX and SASP in the 1990's patients were treated with aspirin and corticosteroids.

From the 1990's on the pyramid was dismantled (27). The introduction of DMARDs like MTX and SASP changed prognosis (28;29) (30;31)

Another true revolution was the use of "biologicals" in JIA. Instead of controlling the disease nowadays physicians aim at curing the disease. Especially the follow up of the group of JIA patients in remission without medication, as defined by Wallace (32) will show us in due time whether this is indeed possible.

Following the initial description of the effects of etanercept in adult patients with RA, the first study in children treated with etanercept was described in 2000 by Lovell et al (33). Other biological therapies for children were described in later years. Biological treatment like adalimumab and abatacept, first used successfully in adults with RA are now prescribed to younger patients with JIA. Other biologic agents were not studied in a way that enabled FDA or EMA registration and such drugs are thus still used off label in children.

3.4 Compliance

Compliance is generally defined as a patient's adherence to a recommended course of treatment. Other words used are agreement, conformity, cooperation, respect, submission. Agreement, conformity are difficult terms for adolescents, as they are searching for methods to become independent from the usual carers (parents, but indeed sometimes also the doctor). It is not surprising that compliance in this patient group on their way to independence can be low.

Corticosteroids with known side-effects as a moonface and disfiguring striae have low compliance rates. The combination of alcohol and MTX is not advised, which in turn, can cause delay in therapy. Compliance can be a huge problem in severe, probably life threatening systemic diseases like SLE or systemic JIA.

In the long term, compliance may have an influence on the outcome of JIA patients. As adolescents have a low compliance rate in visiting their doctor, their patient data are lost in the follow-up phase. Changing schools or finding a job sometimes also causes a migration, similarly, when disease activity is quite low, the patients don't make new appointments.

Exact figures are therefore not known.

Kroll described the factors that comprise treatment adherence. In his view, the facilitating strategies are child-centered information, therapy management, behavior modification and parental monitoring (34). Modern techniques can be helpful in improving compliance like internet-based self management programs with telephone support (17) or electronically monitored adherence to medication(35).

Increasing compliance can be supported by parents and other (health) carers. Notwithstanding the above , the main advice for the parent is to "let the patient go".

3.5 Education

Several studies have been done to evaluate educational and occupational outcome of young adults with JIA. Results are conflicting in different countries.

In the USA (36) educational and occupational outcome after a median disease duration of 12.6 years, were similar to adult peers. In Canada, educational level was lower for female patients and unemployment rates were higher(20).

In the UK, Foster et al and Packham et al evaluated in different studies educational attainment and employment status. They concluded excellent educational attainment but a high rate of unemployment among the patients (37;38).

In Germany, also educational achievements of patients were higher but rate of unemployment was lower compared with the age-matched population (4).

The long-term outcome studies evaluated all JIA subtypes, although median disease duration was longer in the UK studies (12.6 years versus 21 and 28 years). Whether lower functional outcome plays a role in unemployment ratio is not known as this is not investigated in all studies.

In some countries more support is given to persons with disabilities. It may be that JIA patients receive sickness or disability benefit and are therefore not included in unemployment figures.

3.6 Psychological aspects

Psychological and social aspects as well as coping strategies are well documented in younger children with JIA (39;40).

Only a few long term outcome studies in adolescents and adults with juvenile arthritis have been published. Significantly impaired physical health but no psychosocial health differences were found compared to the general (Norwegian) population(41). Patients with significant disabilities (Steinbrocker class III or IV) (42) or longstanding disease activity (43), show psychological distress in about one-third of the cases.

Despite reported psychological problems only few patients show social adjustment problems (4;19)). Overall, the literature on psychological outcome has shown contradictory conclusions. This may be due to variations of the measures used, time since onset of disease, inclusion or omissions of controls, the study design, and disease severity or degree of disability. The age seems particularly important because psychosocial adjustment may change as patients pass through life's developmental stages(44).

3.7 Long term outcome of JIA

In longterm follow up studies approximately half of the patients have active disease and/or changes in body structures to a variable extent. Approximately one-third of the patients rated themselves as being functionally limited (3). Little is known about long-term effects of medication, especially the more recently introduced DMARD's and biologicals.

Complete remission in JIA is achieved in 33-67% of the patients, depending on the subtype.

In JIA remission criteria are defined by Wallace et al (32). One of the main differences with adult health care is that complete remission in JIA is defined as "no disease activity", no active joints and low sedimentation rate and or CRP with low physician's global assessment. In adult health care remission used to be defined by low DAS scores but some disease activity may persist.

Remission per subtype JIA

- Systemic	47-76%
- Oligo persistent/extended	35-57%
- Polyarticular RF+	0-15%
- Polyarticular RF –	30-46%
- Enthesitis related	18%
- Psoriatic	33%

(2;4;19;20).

In the past few years, the prognosis for RA has improved enormously since the introduction of intensive combination treatment regimes (23). Complete remission has not been noted, low DAS scores or other activity scores are commonly used to judge disease activity (24;25). However, for instance for patients with JIA the aim of the pediatrician is to reach complete remission of the disease. This is in sharp contrast to the generally accepted disease activity within adult rheumatology. Until very recently, in adult RA new remission criteria have been defined, although new studies using these criteria have not been published yet (26).

The long term complications of JIA and RA are different. Adequate control of inflammation has made Felty syndrome and amyloidosis nowadays very rare complications in JIA, whereas it occurs in 1.4% of adults with RA. In RA, residing functional disability is higher (HAQ >0: is seen in 36% - 72% of patients), as are erosions and other radiological changes like growth deformities, fusion, osteopenia (seen in 25%- 68%).(2;3;19;21;45).

3.8 Developmental aspects

Research has been carried out on the impact of JIA later on in the life of its patients, and important differences between healthy adolescents and young adults suffering from JIA have been found.

For instance in studies done in Europe one of the aspects is the growth difference in JIA patients. In Germany, girls final height is 2 cm shorter than their peers, for boys this is 1 cm (46). In Great Britain, the final height differential is much larger, 4 cm in girls and 4 cm in boys, compared to their peers (47). In the Netherlands, a study is ongoing on the developmental aspects of adolescents with JIA. We found 2 cm decrease in the final height of girls, and only 0,5 cm for boys. Research on growth differences in the United States or South America hasn't been carried out yet.

Growth and final height depends on several aspects.

Malnutrition is common among patients with a chronic disease. Further influence on final height are the age at which the puberty starts, and the clinical progression of puberty and growth spurt (48;49). Possibly abnormalities in the growth hormone axis plays a role (49-51).

A number of (retrospective) studies have been carried out amongst adult women with JIA and the potential influence of JIA on sexuality and fertility and indirectly, on their number of children. No randomized controlled trials are known, all data were retrospectively collected. Conclusions of the authors were that the number of successful pregnancies is comparable to healthy controls, although in our observation this conclusion may be too hasty. The number of miscarriages was not mentioned in any (retrospective) studies, and also fecundity (time to conceive) was not taken into account. More research needs to be done in adult patients (1;52;53).

3.9 Transfer of a complicated medical history

Failure to coordinate care between providers of the pediatric and adult health system adversely affects both quality and efficiency of care. Planning, information and warnings to the next care provider are very important. Documentation of relevant information is important in view of the multidisciplinary nature of transitional care. One can imagine the results of prescribing wrong dosage of for example MTX or TNF blockers on internal organs. Also when medication history is insufficient (eg not mentioning cyclofosfamide) severe physical problems are to be expected.

In a study carried out in the UK it was shown that detailed and extensive documentation significantly improved following participation in a transitional care research program (15).

Nowadays with the support of electronic patient files these problems should be of the past, but these modern techniques are not widely available yet. A summary of medical history and used medication on the past and current medical problems can overcome this problem. Social and psychological issues must also be explained and transferred to social workers within the adult department.

3.10 Transfer of knowledge from pediatrician to adult physician

In 2002, a consensus document on transition of care was approved by the American Academy of Pediatrics, The American Academy of Family Physicians, and the American College of Physicians-American Society of Internal Medicine (54). This consensus statement states that all young people with special health care needs such as rheumatic diseases should have the following: a professional with the appropriate transition care knowledge and skills who attends to the unique challenges of health care transition; a written health care transition plan by the age of 14 including a constantly updated medical summary that is portable and accessible to the youth and family; care guided by the primary and preventive care guidelines for al adolescence and young adults; and affordable, continuous health coverage.

Unfortunately, in 2005, a survey done in Pennsylvania, USA, to evaluate the consensus statement in practice, revealed that 57% of the practices had not started any of the transition guidelines (55).

Also outside the US, the availability of appropriately trained staff and in-service training to maintain staff members' skills and knowledge in adolescence is considered important. In a

Delphi study done in the UK, availability of professionals who were knowledgeable in transitional care was reported to be best practice (56).

However, well trained staff in knowledge of adolescence is rare.

McDonagh described the unmet skills and training needs in health professionals dealing in adolescence. In the below many subjects are mentioned.

	Perceived skill/comfort level (Very low/low) *n* (%)	Perceived knowledge of available information/resources (Very low/low) *n* (%)	Perceived importance of issue being addressed in a rheumatology clinic (moderate/high/very high) N (%)
Suicide risk	15 (68)	13 (59)	19 (86)
STDs/HIV/hepatitis	12 (54)	7 (33)	17 (77)
Gay/lesbian sexuality*	11 (52)	16 (76)	13 (59)
Drug use	10 (45)	13 (59)	20 (91)
Eating disorders	9 (41)	11 (52)	20 (91)
Physical/sexual abuse	9 (41)	6 (27)	20 (91)
Dating/vulnerability	9 (41)	17 (77)	17 (77)
Vocation/employment	7 (32)	9 (41)	20 (91)
Contraception/safe sex	6 (27)	8 (36)	19 (86)
Parental conflict	5 (23)	12 (55)	18 (82)
Driving	5 (23)	9 (41)	18 (82)
Alcohol use	4 (18)	9 (41)	21 (95)
Smoking	4 (18)	7 (32)	20 (91)
Body image*	3 (14)	15 (68)	21 (95)
Peer relations	3 (14)	12 (55)	19 (86)
Nutrition	3 (14)	3 (14)	21 (95)
Depression/anxiety	2 (9)	8 (36)	21 (95)
Psychosomatic complaint	2 (9)	4 (18)	20 (91)
Education*	2 (9)	5 (23)	19 (86)
Exercise	0 (0)	0 (0)	20 (91)

Table 3. (57) Respondents' perceived skill/comfort level in dealing with adolescent issues, their perceived knowledge of resources and their importance in a rheumatology clinic ($n = 22$)

4. Adaptations from pediatric to adult health care

JIA is a heterogeneous group of 7 diseases, comprising from systemic JIA, oligo-articular and poly-articular JIA, enthesitis related JIA (also called juvenile spondylarthropathy), psoriatic arthritis and undifferentiated JIA (58). Only the extended oligo-articular JIA and poly-articular JIA can fit in the diagnosis RA with regards to disease symptoms.

The definition of Rheumatoid Arthritis used to be strict, (ACR criteria 1987), but recently this definition is considered to be imprecise, since also early arthritis with relative short disease duration is treated as RA. However, the term is generally used to describe a symmetrical, persistent, and destructive poly-arthritis often associated with a rheumatoid factor or with positive results in tests for anti-cyclic citrullinated peptide (anti-CCP) antibodies (59).

4.1 Different scoring methods

Most studies describing long term outcome of JIA patients use adult outcome parameters to show for example disease activity, functional outcome or psychosocial outcome ((1;3;20).

But are those the right tools to compare the disease activity in each individual patient from the start of their disease into their adult life? Or even, can we use these parameters to compare RA patients with JIA?

Pediatric multicenter trials have developed a uniformly accepted way of measuring disease activity (60). The initial ACR scores for children (Ped-ACR 30-50-70-90) were adapted from the adult scores (ACR 30-50-70 and 90%). It should be noted however that these ACR/Printo scores were specifically designed for measuring change induced by medication. More recent tools such as JADAS include a single point total score similar to the adult DAS instead of measuring the percentage of change to baseline values. Most used variations in adults with RA are DAS 28 and DAS 44 (61;62). In pediatric rheumatology in 2009 the Juvenile DAS is introduced, variations are the JADAS 10, 27 and 71. The Correlations between the 3 JADAS versions was comparable, but better than the DAS 28 and the CDAI (Clinical Disease Activity Index).

Functional outcome at pediatric age is measured by the Childhood Health Assessment Questionnaire, a derivative from the Health Assessment Questionnaire, which is used for adults. We have compared both questionnaires and used the same adolescents and young adults with JIA. Despite strong correlations in consistency, and independent of age, we found a lack of agreement for the outcome of CHAQ and HAQ (63). This implies that the functional outcome as measured by the CHAQ is not directly comparable to the HAQ when measured at the same time. Direct matching is therefore not possible. Further research in follow-up data is ongoing. When following the patient at an adult age for a longer period, as will be done in transition phase, outcome parameters will have to be comparable to those measured at pediatric age.

A multidimensional assessment questionnaire was proposed including physical, psychosocial and compliance aspects (JAMAR) (64). The JAMAR includes 15 parent or patient-centered measurements or items that assess well-being, pain, functional status, health-related quality of life, morning stiffness, disease activity, disease status and course, joint disease, extra-articular symptoms, side effects of medications, therapeutic compliance, and satisfaction with illness outcome. The JAMAR is proposed for use as both a proxy-report and a patient self-assessment report, with the suggested age range of 7-18 years for use as a self-assessment report. However even this multidimensional score does not measure in detail the consequence of certain limitations for participation in daily life activities. The full impact of certain limitations can only be learned from our patients.

4.2 Models for transition of care

Transition of care for the adolescent with a chronic disease is complex. Many people are involved, the patient, his or her parents, the pediatrician and the adult specialist. Often also other co-workers like social workers or physiotherapists are involved. Therefore a number of health service models have been proposed, including the patient-focussed model, a disease-focussed model, hospital-based model, a team-based outside the health service, a named person, a voluntary organisation and a primary care model (65).

For patients with rheumatic diseases 3 units have described their programs in literature (66-68), all disease focussed models.

While et al developed the disease focussed model of transition further and described 4 models (table)

Models of transition for evaluation
Direct transition (communication and information sharing only)
Sequential transition (includes the development of new services like adolescent clinics)
Developmental transition (includes skill training and support system development)
Professional transition (transfer of expertise only)

Table 4. (11)

When summarizing the most important needs for transition the following key components for the organisation of care can be noted (12):

- Future focused, patient-centered
- Inclusive for parents/ caregivers
- Early start (11-14 years)
- Multidisciplinary, paediatric and adult services, social workers, education
- Dynamic and flexible process in a resilience framework (ITP, Individual Transitional Plan)
    - Coordinated, uninterrupted health care
    - Age and developmentally appropriated
    - Skills training for the young person in communication, decision making, assertiveness, self-management

5. Complications in transition of care

5.1 Complications for the patient

Complications of transition have been well described(6). During transition a whole list of topics needs to be discussed with the adolescent and this is usually the cause of such complications. Some of these topics are for example self care and communication skills: medication is not prescribed because the patient doesn't ask for a recipe; the patient gets pregnant while taking MTX because contraceptives haven't been discussed.

McDonagh suggested a list of topics to be discussed during transition of care are(6):

- decision making

- independent visits
- phoning with own queries
- communication skills
- self care including compliance
- level of parental concern

It is suggested that quality of medical care for young people with chronic disease deteriorates after transfer to adult services has taken place (69).

Potential explanations of deteriorating quality of medical care could be due to:

- reduced therapy goals (low disease activity instead of remission)
- reduced compliance of the adolescent
- insufficient transfer of care by the pediatric and adult health services

A complication in insufficient transfer of medical care of the adolescent with a rheumatic disease can be that the patient is lost in the medical system and not returning to a medical clinic for rheumatic diseases (either returning back to the pediatrician or visiting a different adult department).

It is not clear how many patients are lost in their follow up after their transition to adult health care. Even in large outcome studies of adult patients with JIA exact numbers can not be determined (2-4).

There are numerous reasons why these patients are missing from the medical system after their transfer to adult health care:

- Their disease may be in remission
- They may have moved or even migrated abroad
- There is insufficient availability of (adequate) rheumatologists
- There is insufficient preparation for adult health care (failure of transition of care process)
- Non compliance of the patient:
  Too busy with study, new home, new friends or new job to visit a rheumatologist
  Loss of confidence in adult care
  No interest in own health
  Incapacity to deal with independent self-care

Apart from the risk of no-shows, there are potential problems that the patient finds it difficult to cope with such as:

- their persistent disease activity to which insufficient attention is given
- their reduced functional ability whereby no additional help is offered
- the side effects of their medication
- psychological symptoms like depression
- insufficient self care, ongoing dependency on parents or partner

In pediatric health care, the medical approach is from a multi-disciplinary perspective whereby the patient's whole well-being is taking into account.

5.2 Complications for the carers

Most adult rheumatologists are not trained in adolescent medicine and the subjects associated with adolescence and their subsequent handling of the rheumatic disease. Also some professionals may simply not like looking after adolescents and find their non-compliance and uncommunicative behaviors an irritation in an adult clinic (6).

The adolescent patient (as any other healthy person of this age range) requires special attention as he or she is in a period of transition from a dependant to an independent state. At adolescence the child's focus shifts away from family to peers. This important move should be no different for chronically ill adolescents. Adolescents begin to adopt a multitude of new social and emotional roles and learn to cope with altered bodily functions.

Adolescents with a chronic disease are constantly struggling with independence. At the same time, their illness often keeps them tied physically, emotionally and financially to their families.

Moreover, a chronic disease like JIA or its treatment may interfere with the normal growth process like muscle strength and sexual maturity (70).

Factors which play a role during normal adolescence are

- Independence and assertiveness
- Peer relationships
- School at work
- Physical appearance
- Sexuality
- Death and dying

Besides culture differences, adult rheumatology services are frequently different from pediatric rheumatology services in the following aspects(6):

- Time available for consultation
- Continuity of care in terms of the same doctor at consecutive visits
- Format of referrals to allied professionals, usually by short paper referrals rather than detailed in person overview during a meeting of the rheumatology team.

When these issues are not taken into account during the transition phase transfer, problems are expected.

6. Future developments

6.1 Optimal organization of transition of care

Papers and textbooks dealing with transition of care often provide interesting descriptions, theories and hypothesis rather than solid empirical data. The importance of a transition program for adolescents with JIA is widely recognized but the lack of solid data from studies to base the policy on is remarkable. Just very few studies have been published with data to support current programs (14). Most published studies evaluating transitional care have been for patients with diabetes mellitus, with programs targeted at improving patient education, staff continuity or delivery of service.

This existing evidence supports the use of educational programs, joint pediatric and adult clinics and specific young adult clinics. Evidence for patients with rheumatic disease however have not been published yet, most likely because outcome markers for these chronic diseases are rather complex, while in diabetes disease specific biochemical indicators like HbA1c are used.

When summarizing the most important needs for transition in rheumatology, the following key components can be distinguished(7;12;71):

- Medical care in the transition phase should be focused on the future of the adolescent patient, and centred around the young adult
- Health care should include parents as well as support health staff
- Start of the transitional process should be addressed at the start of the adolescence (11 - 14 years)
- The medical approach should be from a multidisciplinary perspective, and include both paediatric and adult services, as well as social workers and educational experts
- It should be a dynamic and flexible process in a resilient framework (ITP, Individual Transitional Plan)
  - Coordinated, uninterrupted health care
  - Appropriate for age and developmental stage
  - Include skills training for the young person in communication, decision making, assertiveness, self-management(72)
  - Make plans for the future (peer support including independent social life and social competencies, education, housing)
- Policy regarding contact after transfer to adult services
- Evaluation process: audit; regular review of policy; participation of young people and parent in evaluation and future development of the service
- Where possible, linking families to share information and experiences

Regarding the medical documentation and administrative transfer an electronic patient file will be very helpful. Important information is then always available for every health care provider. Wherever possible, during the visits, the patient can also ask for the recall of the summary of the appointments as well as their blood test results, therefore creating an excellent knowledge of disease.

Individualized transition plans (ITP) are important for a successful transfer to adult health care. Such plans need to incorporate items on the basic domain on organs and their function (pain, swelling, LOM), then activities of daily life (walking, sitting, standing, self hygiene) and participation in the society (walking to school, work, computer use, cooking, house-cleaning, relations); (adapted from the international classification of functioning (73)). The young person has to be trained in knowledge and skills during transition. The skills and knowledge can be prepared by the pediatric and adult health department workers including the specialist, but may also include and important support from parents and peers (healthy as well with a chronic disease) (15).

During the transition phase the ITP should be reviewed regularly by the transition coordinator. Omissions are easily identified and additional attention can be given to the patient.

And last but not least we need to include the patient's opinion and learn to listen to them. This is not as obvious as it seems, as illustrated by the experience of describing disease activity of psoriasis. Where doctors measure numbers of plaques and percentage of affected skin area, our (adolescent) patients only care about skin lesions in their faces. From their viewpoint it can be stated that only if facial lesions regress, there is significant disease improvement.

In order to create a substantial foundation based on factual data that results in a successful transfer in rheumatic diseases we need to define:

What is the best parameter to measure a successful transfer:

Would this be disease activity results, functional outcome or psychosocial parameters?

Furthermore, we need to determine which test (pediatric or adult version) will be used to measure the parameter in adolescent age.

When successful transfer is defined, research can be done to consider the right timing, for the individual patient, in a transition phase guided by both pediatric and adult carers with the inclusion of parents and peer support.

7. Acknowledgements

The authors received un unconditional grant from the Dutch Arthritis Association; Pfizer (formerly Wyeth) and Roche.

8. References

[1] Packham JC, Hall MA. Long-term follow-up of 246 adults with juvenile idiopathic arthritis: social function, relationships and sexual activity. Rheumatology (Oxford) 2002; 41(12):1440-1443.
[2] Packham JC, Hall MA. Long-term follow-up of 246 adults with juvenile idiopathic arthritis: functional outcome. Rheumatology (Oxford) 2002; 41(12):1428-1435.
[3] Minden K. Adult outcomes of patients with juvenile idiopathic arthritis. Horm Res 2009; 72 Suppl 1:20-25.
[4] Minden K, Niewerth M, Listing J, Biedermann T, Bollow M, Schontube M et al. Long-term outcome in patients with juvenile idiopathic arthritis. Arthritis Rheum 2002; 46(9):2392-2401.
[5] Blum RW. Introduction. Improving transition for adolescents with special health care needs from pediatric to adult-centered health care. Pediatrics 2002; 110(6 Pt 2):1301-1303.
[6] McDonagh JE, Southwood TR, Ryder CA. Bridging the gap in rheumatology. Ann Rheum Dis 2000; 59(2):86-93.
[7] White PH. Transition: a future promise for children and adolescents with special health care needs and disabilities. Rheum Dis Clin North Am 2002; 28(3):687-703, viii.
[8] Fleming E, Carter B, Gillibrand W. The transition of adolescents with diabetes from the children's health care service into the adult health care service: a review of the literature. J Clin Nurs 2002; 11(5):560-567.

[9] Schidlow DV, Fiel SB. Life beyond pediatrics. Transition of chronically ill adolescents from pediatric to adult health care systems. Med Clin North Am 1990; 74(5):1113-1120.
[10] Hardoff D, Chigier E. Developing community-based services for youth with disabilities. Pediatrician 1991; 18(2):157-162.
[11] While A, Forbes A, Ullman R, Lewis S, Mathes L, Griffiths P. Good practices that address continuity during transition from child to adult care: synthesis of the evidence. Child Care Health Dev 2004; 30(5):439-452.
[12] McDonagh JE. Young people first, juvenile idiopathic arthritis second: transitional care in rheumatology. Arthritis Rheum 2008; 59(8):1162-1170.
[13] Stinson JN, Toomey PC, Stevens BJ, Kagan S, Duffy CM, Huber A et al. Asking the experts: exploring the self-management needs of adolescents with arthritis. Arthritis Rheum 2008; 59(1):65-72.
[14] Crowley R, Wolfe I, Lock K, McKee M. Improving the transition between paediatric and adult healthcare: a systematic review. Arch Dis Child 2011; 96(6):548-553.
[15] Robertson LP, McDonagh JE, Southwood TR, Shaw KL. Growing up and moving on. A multicentre UK audit of the transfer of adolescents with juvenile idiopathic arthritis from paediatric to adult centred care. Ann Rheum Dis 2006; 65(1):74-80.
[16] Stinson J, McGrath P, Hodnett E, Feldman B, Duffy C, Huber A et al. Usability testing of an online self-management program for adolescents with juvenile idiopathic arthritis. J Med Internet Res 2010; 12(3):e30.
[17] Stinson JN, McGrath PJ, Hodnett ED, Feldman BM, Duffy CM, Huber AM et al. An internet-based self-management program with telephone support for adolescents with arthritis: a pilot randomized controlled trial. J Rheumatol 2010; 37(9):1944-1952.
[18] McDonagh JE. Transition of care from paediatric to adult rheumatology. Arch Dis Child 2007; 92(9):802-807.
[19] Flato B, Aasland A, Vinje O, Forre O. Outcome and predictive factors in juvenile rheumatoid arthritis and juvenile spondyloarthropathy. J Rheumatol 1998; 25(2):366-375.
[20] Oen K, Malleson PN, Cabral DA, Rosenberg AM, Petty RE, Cheang M. Disease course and outcome of juvenile rheumatoid arthritis in a multicenter cohort. J Rheumatol 2002; 29(9):1989-1999.
[21] Manners PJ, Bower C. Worldwide prevalence of juvenile arthritis why does it vary so much? J Rheumatol 2002; 29(7):1520-1530.
[22] Nordal E, Zak M, Aalto K, Berntson L, Fasth A, Herlin T et al. Juvenile idiopathic arthritis; Ongoing disease activity and changing categories in a long-term Nordic cohort study. Arthritis Rheum 2011.
[23] van der Kooij SM, Goekoop-Ruiterman YP, Vries-Bouwstra JK, Guler-Yuksel M, Zwinderman AH, Kerstens PJ et al. Drug-free remission, functioning and radiographic damage after 4 years of response-driven treatment in patients with recent-onset rheumatoid arthritis. Ann Rheum Dis 2009; 68(6):914-921.
[24] Soubrier M, Lukas C, Sibilia J, Fautrel B, Roux F, Gossec L et al. Disease activity score-driven therapy versus routine care in patients with recent-onset active rheumatoid arthritis: data from the GUEPARD trial and ESPOIR cohort. Ann Rheum Dis 2011; 70(4):611-615.

[25] Bakker MF, Jacobs JW, Welsing PM, Vreugdenhil SA, Booma-Frankfort C, Linn-Rasker SP et al. Early clinical response to treatment predicts 5-year outcome in RA patients: follow-up results from the CAMERA study. Ann Rheum Dis 2011; 70(6):1099-1103.

[26] Felson DT, Smolen JS, Wells G, Zhang B, van Tuyl LH, Funovits J et al. American College of Rheumatology/European League Against Rheumatism provisional definition of remission in rheumatoid arthritis for clinical trials. Arthritis Rheum 2011; 63(3):573-586.

[27] Levinson JE, Wallace CA. Dismantling the pyramid. J Rheumatol Suppl 1992; 33:6-10.

[28] Reiff A, Shaham B, Wood BP, Bernstein BH, Stanley P, Szer IS. High dose methotrexate in the treatment of refractory juvenile rheumatoid arthritis. Clin Exp Rheumatol 1995; 13(1):113-118.

[29] Ravelli A, Viola S, Ramenghi B, Di Fuccia G, Ruperto N, Zonta L et al. Evaluation of response to methotrexate by a functional index in juvenile chronic arthritis. Clin Rheumatol 1995; 14(3):322-326.

[30] Gedalia A, Barash J, Press J, Buskila D. Sulphasalazine in the treatment of pauciarticular-onset juvenile chronic arthritis. Clin Rheumatol 1993; 12(4):511-514.

[31] van Rossum MA, Fiselier TJ, Franssen MJ, Zwinderman AH, ten Cate R, Suijlekom-Smit LW et al. Sulfasalazine in the treatment of juvenile chronic arthritis: a randomized, double-blind, placebo-controlled, multicenter study. Dutch Juvenile Chronic Arthritis Study Group. Arthritis Rheum 1998; 41(5):808-816.

[32] Wallace CA, Ruperto N, Giannini E. Preliminary criteria for clinical remission for select categories of juvenile idiopathic arthritis. J Rheumatol 2004; 31(11):2290-2294.

[33] Lovell DJ, Giannini EH, Reiff A, Cawkwell GD, Silverman ED, Nocton JJ et al. Etanercept in children with polyarticular juvenile rheumatoid arthritis. Pediatric Rheumatology Collaborative Study Group. N Engl J Med 2000; 342(11):763-769.

[34] Kroll T, Barlow JH, Shaw K. Treatment adherence in juvenile rheumatoid arthritis--a review. Scand J Rheumatol 1999; 28(1):10-18.

[35] Rapoff MA, Belmont JM, Lindsley CB, Olson NY. Electronically monitored adherence to medications by newly diagnosed patients with juvenile rheumatoid arthritis. Arthritis Rheum 2005; 53(6):905-910.

[36] Gerhardt CA, McGoron KD, Vannatta K, McNamara KA, Taylor J, Passo M et al. Educational and occupational outcomes among young adults with juvenile idiopathic arthritis. Arthritis Rheum 2008; 59(10):1385-1391.

[37] Foster HE, Marshall N, Myers A, Dunkley P, Griffiths ID. Outcome in adults with juvenile idiopathic arthritis: a quality of life study. Arthritis Rheum 2003; 48(3):767-775.

[38] Packham JC, Hall MA. Long-term follow-up of 246 adults with juvenile idiopathic arthritis: education and employment. Rheumatology (Oxford) 2002; 41(12):1436-1439.

[39] LeBovidge JS, Lavigne JV, Donenberg GR, Miller ML. Psychological adjustment of children and adolescents with chronic arthritis: a meta-analytic review. J Pediatr Psychol 2003; 28(1):29-39.

[40] Huygen AC, Kuis W, Sinnema G. Psychological, behavioural, and social adjustment in children and adolescents with juvenile chronic arthritis. Ann Rheum Dis 2000; 59(4):276-282.

[41] Ostile IL, Johansson I, Aasland A, Flato B, Moller A. Self-rated physical and psychosocial health in a cohort of young adults with juvenile idiopathic arthritis. Scand J Rheumatol 2010; 39(4):318-325.

[42] David J, Cooper C, Hickey L, Lloyd J, Dore C, McCullough C et al. The functional and psychological outcomes of juvenile chronic arthritis in young adulthood. Br J Rheumatol 1994; 33(9):876-881.

[43] Packham JC, Hall MA, Pimm TJ. Long-term follow-up of 246 adults with juvenile idiopathic arthritis: predictive factors for mood and pain. Rheumatology (Oxford) 2002; 41(12):1444-1449.

[44] Oen K. Long-term outcomes and predictors of outcomes for patients with juvenile idiopathic arthritis. Best Pract Res Clin Rheumatol 2002; 16(3):347-360.

[45] Bloom BJ, Smith P, Alario AJ. Felty syndrome complicating juvenile rheumatoid arthritis. J Pediatr Hematol Oncol 1998; 20(5):511-513.

[46] Minden K. Adult outcomes of patients with juvenile idiopathic arthritis. Horm Res 2009; 72 Suppl 1:20-25.

[47] Packham JC, Hall MA. Long-term follow-up of 246 adults with juvenile idiopathic arthritis: functional outcome. Rheumatology (Oxford) 2002; 41(12):1428-1435.

[48] Souza LS, Machado SH, Brenol CV, Brenol JC, Xavier RM. Growth velocity and interleukin 6 concentrations in juvenile idiopathic arthritis. J Rheumatol 2008; 35(11):2265-2271.

[49] Simon D. Puberty in chronically diseased patients. Horm Res 2002; 57 Suppl 2:53-56.

[50] Souza L, Machado SH, Bredemeier M, Brenol JC, Xavier RM. Effect of inflammatory activity and glucocorticoid [corrected] use on nutritional variables in patients with juvenile idiopathic arthritis. J Rheumatol 2006; 33(3):601-608.

[51] De Benedetti F, Meazza C, Martini A. Role of interleukin-6 in growth failure: an animal model. Horm Res 2002; 58 Suppl 1:24-27.

[52] Peterson LS, Mason T, Nelson AM, O'Fallon WM, Gabriel SE. Psychosocial outcomes and health status of adults who have had juvenile rheumatoid arthritis: a controlled, population-based study. Arthritis Rheum 1997; 40(12):2235-2240.

[53] Ostensen M. Pregnancy in patients with a history of juvenile rheumatoid arthritis. Arthritis Rheum 1991; 34(7):881-887.

[54] Rosen DS, Blum RW, Britto M, Sawyer SM, Siegel DM. Transition to adult health care for adolescents and young adults with chronic conditions: position paper of the Society for Adolescent Medicine. J Adolesc Health 2003; 33(4):309-311.

[55] White PH. On the road to adulthood for youth with rheumatic diseases: what health care professionals can do. Arthritis Rheum 2008; 59(8):1054-1057.

[56] Shaw KL, Southwood TR, McDonagh JE. User perspectives of transitional care for adolescents with juvenile idiopathic arthritis. Rheumatology (Oxford) 2004; 43(6):770-778.

[57] McDonagh JE, Southwood TR, Shaw KL. Unmet education and training needs of rheumatology health professionals in adolescent health and transitional care. Rheumatology (Oxford) 2004; 43(6):737-743.

[58] Petty RE, Southwood TR, Manners P, Baum J, Glass DN, Goldenberg J et al. International League of Associations for Rheumatology classification of juvenile idiopathic arthritis: second revision, Edmonton, 2001. J Rheumatol 2004; 31(2):390-392.

[59] Combe B, Landewe R, Lukas C, Bolosiu HD, Breedveld F, Dougados M et al. EULAR recommendations for the management of early arthritis: report of a task force of the European Standing Committee for International Clinical Studies Including Therapeutics (ESCISIT). Ann Rheum Dis 2007; 66(1):34-45.

[60] Giannini EH, Ruperto N, Ravelli A, Lovell DJ, Felson DT, Martini A. Preliminary definition of improvement in juvenile arthritis. Arthritis Rheum 1997; 40(7):1202-1209.

[61] Prevoo ML, 't Hof MA, Kuper HH, van Leeuwen MA, van de Putte LB, van Riel PL. Modified disease activity scores that include twenty-eight-joint counts. Development and validation in a prospective longitudinal study of patients with rheumatoid arthritis. Arthritis Rheum 1995; 38(1):44-48.

[62] van der Heijde DM, 't Hof MA, van Riel PL, Theunisse LA, Lubberts EW, van Leeuwen MA et al. Judging disease activity in clinical practice in rheumatoid arthritis: first step in the development of a disease activity score. Ann Rheum Dis 1990; 49(11):916-920.

[63] van Pelt PA, Kruize AA, Goren SS, van der NJ, Uiterwaal CS, Kuis W et al. Transition of rheumatologic care, from teenager to adult: which health assessment questionnaire can be best used? Clin Exp Rheumatol 2010; 28(2):281-286.

[64] Filocamo G, Consolaro A, Schiappapietra B, Dalpra S, Lattanzi B, Magni-Manzoni S et al. A new approach to clinical care of juvenile idiopathic arthritis: the Juvenile Arthritis Multidimensional Assessment Report. J Rheumatol 2011; 38(5):938-953.

[65] Chamberlain MA, Kent RM. The needs of young people with disabilities in transition from paediatric to adult services. Eura Medicophys 2005; 41(2):111-123.

[66] McDonagh JE, Shaw KL, Southwood TR. Growing up and moving on in rheumatology: development and preliminary evaluation of a transitional care programme for a multicentre cohort of adolescents with juvenile idiopathic arthritis. J Child Health Care 2006; 10(1):22-42.

[67] Rettig P, Athreya BH. Adolescents with chronic disease. Transition to adult health care. Arthritis Care Res 1991; 4(4):174-180.

[68] Tucker LB, Cabral DA. Transition of the adolescent patient with rheumatic disease: issues to consider. Pediatr Clin North Am 2005; 52(2):641-52, viii.

[69] Beresford B. On the road to nowhere? Young disabled people and transition. Child Care Health Dev 2004; 30(6):581-587.

[70] KyngAs HA, Kroll T, Duffy ME. Compliance in adolescents with chronic diseases: a review. J Adolesc Health 2000; 26(6):379-388.

[71] Scal P, Evans T, Blozis S, Okinow N, Blum R. Trends in transition from pediatric to adult health care services for young adults with chronic conditions. J Adolesc Health 1999; 24(4):259-264.

[72] Olsen DG, Swigonski NL. Transition to adulthood: the important role of the pediatrician. Pediatrics 2004; 113(3 Pt 1):e159-e162.

[73] World Health Organization. International classification of functioning, disability and health: ICF. Geneva: World Health Organization; 2001. Ref Type: Generic